ANATOMY OF MASOCHISM

THE PLENUM SERIES IN SOCIAL/CLINICAL PSYCHOLOGY

Series Editor: C. R. Snyder
University of Kansas
Lawrence, Kansas

Current Volumes in the Series:

ADVANCED PERSONALITY
Edited by David F. Barone, Michel Hersen, and Vincent B. Van Hasselt

ANATOMY OF MASOCHISM
June Rathbone

AVERSIVE INTERPERSONAL BEHAVIORS
Edited by Robin M. Kowalski

CULTURES, COMMUNITIES, COMPETENCE, AND CHANGE
Forrest B. Tyler

HANDBOOK OF SOCIAL COMPARISON
Theory and Research
Edited by Jerry Suls and Ladd Wheeler

HUMOR
The Psychology of Living Buoyantly
Herbert M. Lefcourt

PERSONAL CONTROL IN ACTION
Cognitive and Motivational Mechanisms
Edited by Miroslaw Kofta, Gifford Weary, and Grzegorz Sedek

PHYSICAL ILLNESS AND DEPRESSION IN OLDER ADULTS
A Handbook of Theory, Research, and Practice
Edited by Gail M. Williamson, David R. Shaffer, and Patricia A. Parmelee

THE REVISED NEO PERSONALITY INVENTORY
Clinical and Research Applications
Ralph L. Piedmont

SOCIAL COGNITIVE PSYCHOLOGY
History and Current Domains
David F. Barone, James E. Maddux, and C. R. Snyder

SOURCEBOOK OF SOCIAL SUPPORT AND PERSONALITY
Edited by Gregory R. Pierce, Brian Lakey, Irwin G. Sarason, and Barbara R. Sarason

---

A Continuation Order plan is available for this series. A continuation order will bring delivery of each new volume immediately upon publication. Volumes are billed only upon actual shipment. For further information please contact the publisher.

ANATOMY OF MASOCHISM

JUNE RATHBONE
University College London
London, England

Kluwer Academic/Plenum Publishers
New York, Boston, Dordrecht, London, Moscow

Library of Congress Cataloging-in-Publication Data

Rathbone, June
Anatomy of masochism/June Rathbone.
p. cm — (The Plenum series in social/clinical psychology)
Includes bibliographical references and index.
ISBN 0-306-46593-0
1. Sadomasochism. 2. Interpersonal relations. 3. Masochism.
I. Title II. Series.
HQ79.R28 2001
306.77'5—dc21 2001029649

ISBN: 0-306-46593-0

233 Spring Street, New York, N.Y. 10013

http://www.wkap.nl/

A C.I.P. record for this book is available from the Library of Congress

10 9 8 7 6 5 4 3 2 1

Printed in the Unites States of America

PREFACE

When a 'love'-relationship is not loving, it is usually sadomasochistic. This has been my experience. In the third edition of *Sexual Deviation* (1996, edited by Ismond Rosen) Mervin Glasser reiterated: "… it can be seen that there is always an element of deception in masochism, always an arrogant contempt and assertion of control hidden behind the humiliation and submission … one is led to recognize that there is always an element of deception in any perversion since … sado-masochism is so ubiquitous a feature in the perversions" (ch.12, p. 292).

Is dominance/submission inevitable? Personally, I am not prepared to accept that there is no alternative for human beings to a relationship of dominance and submission. In 1807 Georg Wilhelm Friedrich Hegel published his *Phenomenology of Mind* and was engaged in revising it shortly before he died in 1831. It influenced the development of Karl Marx, as can be seen from *The Economic and Philosophical Manuscripts of 1844*. Possibly its best known section is 'Lordship and Bondage'. Here, as Marx puts it, "Hegel conceives the self-creation of man as a process" and his analysis of the Master-Slave opposition becomes the motive principle of the historical process, of the history of our human civilization: Man was born and history began with the first fight for prestige, for Recognition—a fight to the death unless one capitulated. It ended in the appearance of a Master and a Slave. Thus, Man at his origin is always either Master or Slave. The history of the interaction between men and of their interaction with Nature is the history of the interaction of warlike Masters and working Slaves.

Anton Chekhov believed he had to squeeze 'the lackey' out of himself. In his 1899 short story, *The Lady with the Little Dog*, Anna Sergeyevna tells Gurov of her Councillor husband, Von Dideritz: "What he does at that job of his I don't know—I only know that he's a lackey." But of course, with time, Gurov's fleeting, exploitative affair with her takes a mysterious turn and they realize that, loving each other, they have a long way to travel and the most complicated and difficult part is only just beginning.

Alfred Hitchcock obtained satisfaction from manipulating his actors and his audience and there have been dictators whose obsession for manipulating has been far less benign. However, is there not a cryptic adversarial element in everyday human relations? Do families not spread themselves at the expense of single residents in a shared dwelling? Is there not a one-upmanship amongst friends: "You've read her latest novel, I expect, haven't you?" Most of us will have encountered the blinkered competition and cruel bureaucracy to which hierarchical systems give rise.

What is the difference between domination and leadership? Norman Dixon offers some telling comments on leadership in his book *On the Psychology of Military Incompetence* (1976): "Good leadership is synonymous with inspiring confidence in those who follow, and confidence is born of results" (p. 212); "... leadership is no more than exercising such an influence upon others that they tend to act in concert towards achieving a goal which they might not have achieved so readily had they been left to their own devices" (p. 214); "... leadership depends upon a proper understanding of the needs and opinions of those one hopes to lead, and the context in which the leadership occurs. It also depends on good timing" (p. 215). None of these observations could apply to domination, rather their opposites. Domination destroys confidence and pleasure in achievement. It has no interest in cooperation. It has no empathy and is more likely to be brutal than sensitive with respect to timing.

There are those who use other people as if they were addictive substances. They present a similar psychic economy to those who do not deal with the problems, the overwhelming emotions, the mental pain facing them on a psychological level, but instead become aware of an overpowering need for medication, food, tobacco, alcohol, opiates or sex. These 'others', if they are sexual partners, play almost no role in the subjects' inner world; they are more objects of need than of desire, mainly perhaps a sleeping pill. But they are not necessarily sexual partners. Those who constantly engage in dispersing strong emotions, including pleasurable ones, in action, are often alexithymic, unable to distinguish one affect from another, only impelled to evacuate unbearable affective arousal. They frequently complain that they feel empty, misunderstood, out of touch with the people who are important to them but who neglect them. These 'others' are narcissistic objects (Kohut, 1971), almost transitional objects (Winnicott, 1953), teddy bears to soothe, to be mastered, to be bitten and torn, punished as often as loved. But these 'others' can only assuage the addictive need for a short time. As Joyce McDougall writes in *Theatres of the Body* (1989): " ... what they offer is rarely enough for the desperate, raging infant hidden within these unhappy adults ... the 'others' who allow themselves, unconsciously, to be manipulated into living out another individual's unacknowledged psychological crises have also found a characterological way of solving the same problem" (p. 96).

The five BBC Reith Lectures of 1999 were delivered by Anthony Giddens, the Director of the London School of Economics, on the theme of Globalization. In his fourth lecture, he expounds his concept of a democracy of the emotions in sexual relations, parent-child relations and in friendship. He points out that in the traditional family, both women and children lacked rights; sexuality was dominated by reproduction and regulated by the concept of womanly virtue. A double standard with respect to the sexes, far from being the quintessential creation of the Victorian period, as is often alleged, was in fact central to almost all non-modern societies in one version or another. It involved a dualistic view of female sexuality: the virtuous woman on the one hand and the libertine on the other. (Estela Welldon explores this concept in the context of motherhood. Her disturbing book *Mother, Madonna, Whore: The Idealization and Denigration of Motherhood* (1988) is drawn from her clinical experience as a consultant psychotherapist specializing in sexual deviance. Several of the male sadomasochists I interviewed clearly carried this dualistic representation of womanhood, which is so prominent in the writing of Leopold von Sacher-Masoch, himself. At its most basic it is the infant's incapacity to tolerate good and bad in the same person.) Giddens continues his lecture by delineating what he sees as the alternative to the traditional family: a couple, a unit based on emotional communication or intimacy, communication being the means of establishing the tie in the first place and the chief rationale for its continuation "I want," he says, "to use the idea of what I call the 'pure relationship' ... based upon emotional communication, where the rewards derived from such communication are the main basis for the relationship to continue." This pure relationship—and he emphasizes that it is an ideal for the future—has different dynamics from more traditional social ties. It depends upon active trust, upon opening oneself up to the other, self-disclosure being the basic condition of intimacy. This pure relationship is also implicitly democratic, for a good relationship is one of equals, where each party has equal rights and obligations, each person has respect for the other and wants the best for the other. Since it is based on communication, an understanding of the other person's point of view is essential. Relationships function best if people don't hide too much from each other, if there is mutual trust, but trust cannot be taken for granted—it has to be worked at. Finally, a good relationship is free from arbitrary power, coercion or violence. A democracy of the emotions is as important for the quality of our lives as public democracy. It does not imply lack of discipline, according to Giddens, or absence of authority but it puts them on a different footing. Sexual equality is not only a core principle of democracy, it is also relevant to happiness and fulfilment." Giddens ends with a moving picture of his great aunt: "She married young, and was with her husband for over 60 years. She once confided to me that she had been deeply unhappy with him the whole of that time. In her day there was no escape." A sadomasochistic relationship with a vengeance, one might surmise.

This book might almost be dedicated to Giddens' great aunt. A survey of the previous literature on masochism is undertaken in Part I. Papers taking a purely psychological approach are reviewed first, then empirical studies. But first of all Freud's writings on masochism, or more accurately, sadomasochism, are given special consideration, together with the critical response they have evoked over time

Part II reports on the interviews conducted with 48 self-declared sadomasochists (43 male, 5 female) and with 35 controls (26 male, 9 female). These interviews probed early family relationships and revealed that, in terms of attachment theory, the index group as a whole suffered greater insecurity of emotional attachment than the control group. Coherence was significantly diminished in the index group and this was irrespective of depression, which was measured in both groups. The overlap between sadomasochism and depression is discussed. A computer-driven variant of the classic Stroop color-naming task provided evidence for a sadomasochistic mind-set, which was confirmed by free recall of words composing the presentation. Details concerning chronicity, practice and motivation of sadomasochism were obtained by questionnaires, direct discussion and correspondence. What emerged as a major feature, distinguishing index subjects from controls, was an early background which afforded little opportunity for the development of a theory of mind, and which resulted in a lack of empathy and a preoccupation with the physical. In many cases, as anticipated, there was evidence for a physiological addiction which began with prolonged pain or stress in childhood. This would most likely be mediated by the endogenous opioids, neuronal hormones which are actually produced by protracted pain or stress and which have been shown to be strongly addictive (Olson *et al.*, 1980–87).

Sadomasochists, whether openly practising or not, are people who are sensitized to dominant or submissive behavior, who may be regarded as experts on the subject of control. Helplessness in childhood makes control a key issue for the sadomasochist. This is discussed in Part III, together with the differences in attitude, in mental processing and in behavior which are likely to separate those who acknowledge their sadomasochism from those who do not. Finally, the wider effects of this form of sexuality are considered.

June Rathbone
University College London

ACKNOWLEDGMENTS

Completion of this book brings an opportunity to express my gratitude to the many people who have generously helped me to reach this point.

I would like to thank my PhD Supervisor in the Department of Psychology, University College London, Professor Peter Fonagy, FBA, for his sound advice, encouragement, patience and good humour. Discussions with Mr Richard E. Rawles and Dr A. R. Jonckheere, also in the Department of Psychology, UCL, were helpful, thought-provoking and lively. Professor Cedric Smith of the Galton Laboratory and Professor David Wilkie of the Department of Biology, UCL, both took a kindly interest in my research, providing explanations of statistical procedures and of physiological processes, respectively. Mr Simon Zielinski, MSc, of the Department of Psychology, UCL, gave me invaluable practical help by programming the computer-driven task which constituted a strand of the research, and subsequently solving several software problems for me. Equally invaluable was the unflagging assistance of Dr Gillian Truslove, now retired from the Galton Laboratory, UCL, who urged me on and helped me to enter data into the computer and to find typographical errors in the text.

I am grateful to Professor Mary Main and Dr Erik Hesse of the Department of Psychology, University of California at Berkeley, for their instruction in the Adult Attachment Interview and for permission to indicate its method of classification in Appendix 2, to Professor Ian Gotlib of the Department of Psychology, Northwestern University, Evanston, Illinois, for sending me his validated word-list to incorporate in my own word-presentation, to Professor Glenn Wilson and Dr Chris Gosselin of the Institute of Psychiatry, London, for permitting me to adapt two of their well-tested questionnaires for my own use, to the American Psychiatric Association for permitting me to quote material from the Diagnostic and Statistical Manual of Mental Disorders in Appendix 1.

I would like to express my gratitude to Eliot Werner, Executive Editor, and Dr Rick Snyder, Series Editor, for their assistance, open-mindedness and encouragement in the preparation of this book for publication in the Social/Clinical Psychology series of Plenum Press.

Finally I wish to thank all the people who came for interview, spared me their time and spoke so frankly of personal matters.

CONTENTS

Chapter 6

Chapter 7

Chapter 8

Part I

AN EXAMINATION OF MASOCHISM

CHAPTER 1

FREUD'S WRITINGS ON MASOCHISM EXAMINED IN DETAIL

SUMMARY

Finding an explanation of masochism was a problem which occupied Freud throughout his career. It led him to radical revision of basic psychoanalytic theory. His writings on masochism, or more accurately, sadomasochism, are therefore considered in detail chronologically and their accuracy is examined in the light of direct personal observation over more than twenty years. Tracing the evolution of his views has also entailed consideration of what he meant by the term 'instinct'. Freud's exposition of sadomasochism has evoked much critical response over time. Only a selection of comment is undertaken here: those commentaries dealing (a) with masochism in women, (b) with the validity of his proposed etiology of beating fantasies, and (c) with the development of his conceptualization of masochism and its practical repercussions. The value of such critique and development of theory is recognized, but the accuracy of Freud's portrait of masochism is upheld.

INTRODUCTION

Part of Freud's impact on psychology was by turning things on their heads. Consider, for instance, these two fundamentally opposed formulations: "The function of a nervous system is to keep its possessor informed about the world" (Nathan, 1988, p. 1). "The nervous system is an apparatus which has the function of getting rid of the stimuli that reach it" (Freud, 1915*a*, p. 120). Both true, neither original (Freud always attributed the principle of constancy to Fechner, 1873), but which is likely to lead to new perspectives? And bear in mind that the less obvious antedates the obvious by more than seventy years. Freud made few claims to originality—he, if anyone, knew that almost everything has been said and done before—but where daring is coupled with right judgment, the outcome can come close to originality. Add to this the fact that, in the psychological literature, whereas most empirical studies address the question 'what?' and most theoretical papers the question 'how?', Freud stands virtually alone in having the courage to ask the more daunting question 'why?'—thus impacting on subsequent generations, obloquy and opprobrium notwithstanding (after Ian Suttie (1935) we have Jeffrey Masson (1984) and Morton Schatzman (1992)). That a hypothesis cannot be proved does not render it invalid. That an observation is not acceptable does not make it untrue—for the ultimate grudge against Freud is for his pessimism—even the intolerable may be true. He is accused of weaving a web of conjecture on the basis of a few spoilt Viennese neurotics—my own view is that many, if not most, of his insights sprang from observation of those nearest to him and, above all, of himself.

In fact, trying to explain masochism without Freud would be like trying to explain gravity without Newton. The all-pervasive and fundamental quality of masochism, together with its patent infantilism, points to a genesis in early childhood; however modified in its adult manifestation, masochism has its roots in sexuality, specifically where this has taken a deviant path. Who, then, could be more qualified to throw light upon its etiology than Freud, who steadfastly attributed prime importance to the relationships and events of early childhood and to sexuality in the development of the human individual?

Since there is a lot of ground to cover, the style of this section will be blunt, not polished, and certainly not academic. Freud's concepts will be discussed to some extent from the basis of direct personal observation. An immediate *caveat* must enter at this point. Personal observation must be treated with caution: it can be distorted by subjective reactions; it cannot be assumed to be objective or generally valid. There is a tendency to overstate what has become a conviction as a result of direct personal observation. Such evidence may thus be termed—as one wishes—'anecdotal' or 'empirical' in a radically different sense of the word than the usual academic one. In defence of this more general definition, it might be pointed out that numerical data with accompanying statistical analysis can be and have been falsified, whereas the accuracy of the personal observations which follow can readily be verified (or challenged) by anyone who cares to look for himself. The convention of supporting assertions by citing other authors, who have in turn supported their assertions by citing yet other authors, undoubtedly has a validatory value but possibly a modest one. At worst, it may be a paper credential which comes rather cheaply. Unless otherwise indicated, the observations which follow have been made repeatedly, that is to say, the same observation has been made hundreds, rather than tens, of times. There is, of course, the danger of misinterpretation but with each recurrence the chance of this must surely diminish since each time the situation presents itself there is a possibility of some feature in it being so salient as to correct any previous misconstruction. In most cases, interpretation does not enter, since the observations relate to plain, concrete facts.

Over the decades, Freud's ideas have been borrowed, often without acknowledgement, his formulations paraphrased, usually without improvement, and his theories potted, invariably with impoverishment. There has been much misrepresentation. Here, wherever possible, they will therefore be presented simply in the form of quotation, chiefly from the Stracheys' translation. This will inevitably result in a naive impression and stylistic monotony but these seem a small price for accuracy, which is the overriding goal.

THE EVOLUTION OF FREUD'S VIEWS TRACED CHRONOLOGICALLY FROM THE ORIGINAL

Freud's first approach to masochism is summarized in a paragraph added in 1909 to *The Interpretation of Dreams* (1900): "There is a masochistic component in the sexual constitution of many people, which arises from the reversal of an aggressive, sadistic component into its opposite" (p. 159). What are here called 'mental' ('*ideelle*') masochists will later be termed, in an expanded concept (Freud, 1924*a*), 'moral' ('*moralische*') masochists. In *Three Essays on the Theory of Sexuality* (1905), sadism and masochism are described as "the most common and the most significant of all the perversions" (p. 157). Krafft-Ebing's (1886) emphasis on humiliation or subjection, Schrenck-Notzing's (1899) on pleasure in pain (algolagnia) are noted. The roots of sadism can be seen in normal sexual aggressiveness on the part of the male: "the biological significance of it seems to lie in the need for overcoming the resistance of the sexual object". This aggressive component of the sexual instinct has, however, "become independent and ... usurped the leading position." Masochism represents a passive sexual attitude, "the extreme instance of which appears to be that in which satisfaction is conditional upon suffering physical or mental pain at the hands of the sexual object". Masochism is still regarded at this time only as a transformation of sadism, though a footnote added in 1924 gives the gist of Freud's later view that there may be a primary masochism. The castration complex and a sense of guilt are among the factors which may combine "to exaggerate and fixate the original passive sexual attitude" (p. 158). Several other key observations on masochism are made in the *Three Essays*, either in the original (1905) text or in later additions to it. To mention them in the order in which they occur: "every pain contains in itself the possibility of a feeling of pleasure"; "active and passive forms are habitually found to occur together in the same individual ... although the active or the passive aspect of the perversion may be the more strongly developed" (p. 159); "the organ which, more than any other, represents the passive sexual aim is the erotogenic mucous membrane of the anus" (p. 198).

This is perhaps the moment to interrupt exposition in order to take stock of Freud's propositions so far. Two, just touched upon, are crucial. Freud himself considered the following of sufficient importance to quote it in 1924 as the basis of erotogenic masochism: "in the case of a great number of internal processes sexual excitation arises as a concomitant effect, as soon as the intensity of those processes passes beyond certain quantitative limits ... it may well be that nothing of considerable importance can occur in the organism without contributing some component to the excitation of the sexual instinct" (1905, pp. 204–205). He took the trouble to underline his adherence to this view with a footnote added in 1924 to the proposition, just preceding: "If we assume that a similar erotogenic effect attaches even to intensely painful feelings, especially when the pain is toned down or kept at a distance by some accompanying condition, we should here have one of the main roots of the masochistic-sadistic instinct" (1905, p. 204). The question 'why?' is being addressed on a basic, physical level. This is why von Sacher-Masoch described himself as a 'supersensualist' and de Sade preferred "this shock of pain, infinitely keener and more vigorous" than simple pleasure. This is why amyl nitrite is inhaled at sadomasochistic rituals "to prolong masochistic activity and endure more pain" (Litman & Swearingen, 1972, p. 83). In fact, before Freud's observation could be dismissed, another answer would have to be found to the straightforward question: why should some masochists insist on physical pain when the easier option of humiliation is also available? The delineation of erotogenic zones of the body and the pregenital sexual organization is equally important. The masochist is living proof of a sadistic-anal phase of sexuality to which he has regressed (and the coupling of the two epithets, after all so strangely assorted, one of Freud's most brilliant insights). It is a specific requirement of some masochists to be defecated upon in order to obtain satisfaction; the event of an involuntary bowel motion is tantamount to sexual satisfaction for others; one of my interviewees described how his 'dominatrix' compelled him to retain a painful object in his rectum throughout their dinner together; soiled linen and bespattered lavatory-pans are incessant masochistic provocations. The reaction-formations of cleanliness and orderliness, characteristic of obsessional neurosis, find their counterpart in the extreme messiness and slovenliness liable to be achieved habitually by the masochist—both attesting to a sadistic-anal derivation. The anal component is also apparent in the behavior of both with respect to money. The obsessive is typically parsimonious whilst the masochist can be relied upon to get into fresh financial difficulties almost as soon as he is extricated from the last quagmire. Incidentally, remarkable support for the 'sadistic-anal' concept is to be found in the book *Culture, Health and Illness* by Cecil Helman (1990), an anthropologist working in primary health care. One patient in his Massachusetts study (Helman, 1985) of psychosomatic disorders expressed himself thus: "I tend to hold lots of things inside ... anger, tension, hostility, any kind of fear—I think of them as being crammed into my colon" (Helman, 1990, p. 233).

In *Instincts and Their Vicissitudes* (1915*a*), we find Freud still maintaining that masochism can only be derived from sadism (though again a footnote added in 1924 points to his subsequent revision of this view). Here he puts forward a model for this transformation, not of *content* but of *aim*, whereby the change of object results in a change from activity to passivity: "In the case of the pair of opposites sadism-masochism, the process may be represented as follows:

(a) Sadism consists in the exercise of violence or power upon some other person as object.
(b) This object is given up and replaced by the subject's self. With the turning round upon the self the change from an active to a passive instinctual aim is also effected.
(c) An extraneous person is once more sought as object; this person, in consequence of the alteration which has taken place in the instinctual aim, has to take over the role of the subject.

Case (c) is what is commonly termed masochism. Here, too, satisfaction follows along the path of the original sadism, the passive ego placing itself back in phantasy in its first role, which has now in fact been taken over by the extraneous subject" (pp. 127–128). 'Extraneous' here is a good rendering of Freud's '*fremd*' (strange, alien). The masochist's partner is in fact peripheral, expendable. Worth mentioning also is that Freud points explicitly to a parallel, at stage (b), with obsessional neurosis: "the desire to torture has turned into self-torture and self-punishment, not into masochism" (p. 128). The explanation of what he would later (Freud, 1924*a*) designate as erotogenic masochism is reiterated and developed in his obvious and ongoing concern to penetrate the dynamic relations of sadism and masochism. Sadism aims originally at mastering rather than inflicting pain, "but when once the transformation into masochism has taken place, the pains are very well fitted to provide a passive masochistic aim; for we have every reason to believe that sensations of pain, like other unpleasurable sensations, trench upon sexual excitation and produce a pleasurable condition, for the sake of which the subject will even willingly experience the unpleasure of pain. When once feeling pains has become a masochistic aim, the sadistic aim of *causing* pains can arise also, retrogressively; for while these pains are being inflicted on other people, they are enjoyed masochistically by the subject through his identification of himself with the suffering object" (1915*a*, pp. 128–129). Having enunciated the concept which later analysts would take to their bosoms as projective identification, Freud adds that "feelings of pity cannot be described as a result of a transformation of instinct occurring in sadism, but necessitate the notion of a *reaction-formation* against that instinct" (p. 129). A point of some weight, applying equally to masochism which pursues its aims with equal ruthlessness. The other major contribution at this time is the explicit linking of masochism and narcissism: "the instinctual vicissitudes which consist in the instinct's being turned round upon the subject's own ego and undergoing reversal from activity to passivity are dependent on the narcissistic organization of the ego and bear the stamp of that phase" (p. 132).

The twentieth in the series of *Introductory Lectures on Psycho-Analysis* (Freud, 1916–1917), on 'The sexual life of human beings', contains a comprehensive list of perversions which might have been compiled yesterday and a caution of special relevance to masochism: "we must learn that each of these groups is to be found in two forms: alongside of those who seek their sexual satisfaction in reality are those who are content merely to imagine that satisfaction, who need no real object at all, but can replace it by their phantasies" (*S.E.* 16, p. 306).

The case history of the 'Wolf Man' (who, despite casting aspersions before his relatively recent death on 'the Professor's' methods and interpretations, nevertheless allegedly used to answer the telephone: "Wolf Man speaking"!) was completed in November 1914 but only published four years later (Freud, 1918). It forms therefore, both in time and in a specific portion of its content (p. 26), a bridge with '*A Child is Being Beaten*' (Freud, 1919). It also marks a radical change of approach to the paired components of the sexual instinct, sadism and masochism, in that it introduces the Oedipal situation into their etiology. The three-and-a-half-year-old child gave up masturbating very soon after his Nanya's rebuke. "*His sexual life, therefore, which was beginning to come under the sway of the genital zone, gave way before an external obstacle, and was thrown back by its influence into an earlier pregenital organization.* As a result of the suppression of his masturbation, the boy's sexual life took on a sadistic-anal character" (pp. 25–26). Besides becoming a tormentor, he began to have masochistic beating phantasies: "the content of these was of boys being chastised and beaten ... the heir to the throne being shut up in a narrow room and beaten". The figure carrying out the beating was his 'all-powerful' father: "he was in this way able to renew his first and most primitive object-choice, which, in conformity with a small child's narcissism, had taken place along the path of identification ... in conformity with his higher stage of development, identification was replaced by object-choice" (p. 27). When his father returned home (significantly for attachment theory (Bowlby 1969, 1973, 1980), after prolonged absence) the boy tried to provoke punishment with repeated tantrums. "In accordance, moreover, with the motives which underlie masochism, this beating would also have satisfied his sense of guilt" (p. 28).

Sadomasochism is becoming more complex, 'overdetermined', and is seen as serving more than one function. Several later writers have levelled this as a criticism. For instance, Maleson (1984) and Grossman (1986) both trace the evolution of Freud's concept, pointing out how and where he shifts his ground. Their critical commentaries are given in some detail later. Many of their objections are theoretically irrefutable, others can be tackled, but from a practical point of view one is tempted to say 'so what?'! How could such a complex phenomenon as masochism be anything other than heterogeneous? Most behavior shows individual differences and is overdetermined, so how could it be otherwise than that masochists behave diversely and are formed in different ways? The point is that in his pioneering work over the years, by a process of continuing scrutiny sometimes requiring the revision of previous views, Freud shed light on most of these ways. Without him, we wouldn't have got out of the harbour, so let us proceed!

'*A Child is Being Beaten*', Freud (1919) relates, was a recurrent phantasy of early childhood which first came to his notice through the reluctant confessions of patients suffering from hysteria or obsessional neurosis but which was probaby of more general incidence. It "was invariably cathected with a high degree of pleasure and had its issue in an act of pleasurable auto-erotic satisfaction" (p. 180). He delves into its history first for females: "The little girl's beating-phantasy passes through three phases, of which the first and third are consciously remembered, the middle one remaining unconscious. The two conscious phases appear to be sadistic, whereas the middle and unconscious one is undoubtedly of a masochistic nature; its content consists in the child's being beaten by her father, and it carries with it the libidinal charge and the sense of guilt ... had primarily a genital significance and developed by means of repression and regression out of an incestuous wish to be loved by the father" (pp. 195–196). Before delineating the history of the phantasy for males, Freud mentions what he sees as a confounding factor: "My male cases ... included a fairly large number of persons who would have to be described as true masochists in the sense of being sexual perverts. They were either people who obtained their sexual satisfaction exclusively from masturbation accompanied by masochistic phantasies; or they were people who had succeeded in combining masochism with their genital activity in such a way that, along with masochistic performances and under similar conditions, they were able to bring about erection and emission or to carry out normal intercourse. In addition to this there was the rarer case in which a masochist is interfered with in his perverse activities by the appearance of obsessional ideas of unbearable intensity" (pp. 196–197). Some important general observations on adult masochism follow: it may be "deeply embedded since infancy"; in both phantasies and performances the masochistic attitude "coincides with a *feminine* one" of which the individual is often himself aware; "on the other hand the persons who administer chastisement are always women" (p. 197). Returning to the childhood phantasy: "the original form of the unconscious male phantasy was not the provisional one ... 'I am being beaten by my father', but rather: *'I am loved by my father'*. The phantasy has been transformed by the processes with which we are familiar into the conscious phantasy: *'I am being beaten by my mother'*. The boy's beating-phantasy is therefore passive from the very beginning, and is derived from a feminine attitude towards his father. It corresponds with the Oedipus complex just as the female one (that of the girl) does; only the parallel relation which we expected to find between the two must be given up in favour of a common character of another kind. *In both cases the beating-phantasy has its origin in an incestuous attachment to the father*" (p. 198). The crucial difference between the sexes is underlined: "in the case of the girl the unconscious masochistic phantasy starts from the normal Oedipus attitude; in that of the boy it starts from the inverted attitude, in which the father is taken as the object of love" (pp. 198–199). A further elucidation: "the boy evades his homosexuality by repressing and remodelling his unconscious phantasy: and the remarkable thing about his later conscious phantasy is that it has for its content a feminine attitude without a homosexual object-choice" (p. 199). This goes straight to the root of something, vague yet pervasive, of which one becomes aware in contact with an adult male masochist who is not overtly homosexual. It is difficult to define more precisely than 'a vein of homosexuality'. (This personal observation antedates an empirical study carried out in 1994 (Rathbone, 1999) by over twenty years, but it was confirmed in the case of many sadomasochistic subjects participating in that study. It was also confirmed in a recent British television feature entitled *Kinsey's Paedophiles.* In this TV profile (9pm, Monday 10 August 1998, Channel 4, in the *Secret History* series) Alfred Kinsey's associates attested that in his later years the famous researcher increasingly sought personal satisfaction in homosexual relations—his masochism is also well attested (Jones, 1997) and is discussed in Part III.) After broadening the enquiry to seek the motive for repression in general, Freud returns to the Oedipus complex, "the nuclear complex of neuroses. I hope that in this paper I have raised an expectation that the sexual aberrations of childhood, as well as those of mature life, are ramifications of the same complex" (p. 204).

In introducing the death instinct in *Beyond the Pleasure Principle* (1920*a*) Freud raised, and is still raising, hoots of incredulity on all sides, particularly among later psychoanalysts, though physicians have long given it implicit credence when they have counted a 'will to live' as an important influence on whether or not a patient who is seriously ill will recover. What is often overlooked is Freud's own initial tentativeness. At the end of his argument he casts himself as "*an advocatus diaboli,* who is not on that account himself sold to the devil" (p. 59). He envisages future discoveries in biology which "may be of a kind which will blow away the whole of our artificial structure of hypotheses". He stands by it to this extent: "I cannot deny that some of the analogies, correlations and connections which it contains seemed to me to deserve consideration" (p. 60).

There is no doubt that this period was a turning point in Freud's perception of masochism—"there *might* be such a thing as primary masochism" (p. 55). Tentativeness dropped away as the change of approach was consolidated in the publications which followed (Freud, 1923*b*, 1924*a*), but their material can hardly receive the consideration it merits without a considerable digression.

Definitions of Instinct

First then, and long overdue, what did Freud mean by an 'instinct' ('*Trieb*', drive)? It soon becomes clear that he meant a force, a tendency, operating on several different levels. In his *Three Essays on the Theory of Sexuality,* he writes: "By an 'instinct' is provisionally to be understood the psychical representative of an endosomatic, continuously flowing source of stimulation, as contrasted with a 'stimulus' which is set up by *single* excitations coming from *without*. The concept of instinct is thus one of those lying on the frontier between the mental and the physical" (Freud, 1905, p. 168). In *Instincts and Their Vicissitudes*: "If now we apply ourselves to considering mental life from a *biological* point of view, an 'instinct' appears to us as a concept on the frontier between the mental and the somatic, as the psychical representative of the stimuli originating from within the organism and reaching the mind, as a measure of the demand made upon the mind for work in consequence of its connection with the body" (Freud, 1915*a*, pp. 121–122). In *The Unconscious*: "An instinct can never become an object of consciousness—only the idea that represents the instinct can. Even in the unconscious, moreover, an instinct cannot be represented other than by an idea. If the instinct did not attach itself to an idea or manifest itself as an affective state, we could know nothing about it" (Freud, 1915b, p. 177). *In Beyond the Pleasure Principle*: "the organism's 'instincts'—the representatives of all the forces originating in the interior of the body and transmitted to the mental apparatus" (Freud, 1920*a*, p. 34). The nature of instinct is conservative: *"an instinct is an urge inherent in organic life to restore an earlier state of things"* (p. 36). With the introduction of the death instinct and after the recognition that libido could also be directed to the ego in the form of narcissism, the dualism between the sexual instincts and the instincts of self-preservation, the ego-instincts, became a dualism between the sexual or life instincts and the death instinct. About the life instincts, Freud is extremely clear: "the essence of the processes to which sexual life is directed is the coalescence of two cell-bodies" (Freud, 1920*a*, p. 56).

"And even though it is certain that sexuality and the distinction between the sexes did not exist when life began, the possibility remains that the instincts which were later to be described as sexual may have been in operation from the very first, and it may not be true that it was only at a later time that they started upon their work of opposing the activities of the 'ego-instincts'" (Freud, 1920*a*, p. 41). Support for this suggestion comes from David Wilkie of the Biology Department, University College London. In yeast, the hybrid diploid cell is achieved by the fusion of two haploid yeast cells, each possessing a 'mating-type' gene, which controls this 'sexual' process. This is exactly analogous to the fusion of male and female gametes in human beings, producing as it does a hybrid diploid cell. Another analogous feature of the yeast hybrid cell is its capability of proceeding through meiotic division to generate a tetrad of haploid progeny, the equivalent of gametes (Wilkie, 1992, and personal communication).

It seems probable, however, that in the sentence just quoted and even more at other points in his argument, Freud was not only thinking at the biological but at an even more fundamental level. At the back of his mind, there seems to be the notion of instincts as primordial physical forces, manifesting biologically with the advent of life on earth, eventually reaching the mental life and behavior of human beings. It is surely this conception which causes him to describe Eros as a unifying, constructive force, in continuous opposition to the death instinct whose work is disintegration and destruction.

Freud insisted that the death instinct worked silently, unperceived (1923*a*, p. 258; 1930, p. 119). *In Beyond the Pleasure Principle,* he examined at some length the truth of the assumption that "all living substance is bound to die from internal causes" (Freud, 1920*a*, p. 44). His examination is chiefly at a biological, indeed a cellular, level. On this biological level, considerable evidence for a death instinct exists. There are several clinical disorders, such as Werner's syndrome, associated with premature senility. There is the Hayflick limit for cells in culture. The tissue-culturist, Leonard Hayflick (1965), found that, in standard culture conditions where the medium was regularly renewed, diploid human cells had a limited life span. Skin fibroblasts taken from a youngish adult would produce 50–60 cell divisions, from an 80-year-old perhaps only 20 divisions, before the cells stopped dividing and a 'crisis period' set in. After about 9 months, the whole culture would be dead. *In vivo* there is the phenomenon of apoptotic cell death.

"It is generally considered that the union of a number of cells into a vital association—the multicellular character of organisms—has become a means of prolonging their life. One cell helps to preserve the life of another, and the community of cells can survive even if individual cells have to die. We have already heard that conjugation, too, the temporary coalescence of two unicellular organisms, has a life-preserving and rejuvenating effect on both of them. Accordingly, we might attempt to apply the libido theory which has been arrived at in psycho-analysis to the mutual relationships of cells. We might suppose that the life instincts or sexual instincts which are active in each cell take the other cells as their object, that they partly neutralize the death instincts (that is, the processes set up by them) in those cells and thus preserve their life; while the other cells do the same for *them,* and still others sacrifice themselves in the performance of this libidinal function" (Freud, 1920*a*, p. 50).

A hypothesis which must have raised many an eyebrow, yet in his review article in *Nature,* April 1992, 'Social controls on cell survival and cell death', Martin Raff of the Department of Biology, University College London, sets forth precisely the same hypothesis: "... in all of these cases, cells deprived of survival signals die by typical programmed cell death.

Thus, the idea that cells require signals from other cells to avoid killing themselves is not new. What is novel is the suggestion that these cases are only examples of a general mechanism that may operate in most cells, at least in higher animals" (Raff, 1992, p. 398).

And even if, at the other extreme, the death instinct could only be accorded validity on a conceptual level, it is worth reflecting that the sciences would not exist—particularly psychology, aspiring to be a science—without metaphor (Hoffman *et al.* 1990). Cognitive processes *require* language, symbolism and metaphor—the human brain cannot function creatively, probably cannot function at all on any human level, without them (Hermans *et al.* 1992, particularly p. 26).

Despite the taboo on teleological thinking, it is worth considering the proposition that mortality is a stern argument in support of determinism, and determinism necessitates a death instinct—not a circularity since no doubt attaches to the reality of death. If individuals are determined, there can be no change, let alone progress, except by replacing the individuals. When they have, to a greater or lesser extent, actualized their limited potential, the broom must descend and sweep them out of the way. The 'teleological' stigma actually rests entirely on equating 'cause' with 'purpose', in other words on the definition of 'cause'. When it is really the effect we are concerned with, this can be something of a semantic quibble. When death incontrovertibly exists and all living organisms are (arguably) internally determined, whether the constant replacement of individuals is the effect of a *random* cause or the result of an inscrutable purpose is of limited importance. Most of us would have less difficulty in accepting that the behavior and the life span of an amoeba are determined. Freud, however, drew no special line of demarcation between man and other animals. Certainly, in the case of the masochist, we are dealing with behavior which is rigidly determined indeed, and persistently self-destructive. Taking also into account his preoccupation with the macabre—in the pornographic literature the macabre is quite as much in evidence as, for instance, beating or bondage—is it really so fanciful to see a death instinct at work in him?

The Final Picture Begins to Take Shape

After this lengthy détour, let us return to the track—the evolution of Freud's views on masochism—which has now reached *The Ego and the Id* (1923*b*). Several concepts discussed in this work reappear as important parts of the final picture. One of these is still concerned with the two new classes of instincts, Eros and the death instinct, which are given further support by the physiological processes of anabolism and catabolism (p. 41). Now the proposition, foreshadowed in the clause, "wherever the original sadism has undergone no mitigation or intermixture..."

(Freud, 1920*a*, p. 54), is explicitly examined, namely that of their fusion (*'Mischung'*) and *'de*-fusion' (*'Ent*mischung') (1923*b*, pp. 41–42). Another concept moving into prominence in its definitive form is the superego (*'das Über-Ich'*, partly the former *'Ich-Ideal'*), derived from a transformation, by a process of identification and introjection, from the earliest object-cathexes, and thus "the heir to the Oedipus complex" (p. 48). This leads to the postulate which assumes utmost importance in Freud's final depiction of masochism—that of an unconscious sense of guilt: "In the end we come to see that we are dealing with what may be called a 'moral' factor, a sense of guilt, which ... refuses to give up the punishment of suffering" (p. 49). A footnote gives an interesting hint of Freud's view of the possibility of 'curing' masochism: "One has a special opportunity for influencing it when this *Ucs.* sense of guilt is a 'borrowed' one—when it is the product of an identification with some other person who was once the object of an erotic cathexis" (p. 50).

In 1924 many threads come together in what is almost certainly Freud's most comprehensive statement. He opens *The Economic Problem of Masochism*: "The existence of a masochistic trend in the instinctual life of human beings may justly be described as mysterious from the economic point of view. For if mental processes are governed by the pleasure principle in such a way that their first aim is the avoidance of unpleasure and the obtaining of pleasure, masochism is incomprehensible. If pain and unpleasure can be not simply warnings but actually aims, the pleasure principle is paralysed—it is as though the watchman over our mental life were put out of action by a drug.

Thus masochism appears to us in the light of a great danger, which is in no way true of its counterpart, sadism. We are tempted to call the pleasure principle the watchman over our life rather than merely over our mental life" (Freud, 1924*a*, p. 159). At last, an adequate statement about the phenomenon of masochism. Not that it is a perversion, a sexual deviation amongst other curious deviations, but that it is grossly and fundamentally abnormal. It is *contra naturam*, because it opposes the pleasure-unpleasure principle. There would surely be few psychologists who would wish to dispute the primacy of this principle. The whole edifice of behaviorism is built upon it. The fact that masochism is sometimes literally a danger to life itself is attested by the deaths ensuing on rituals such as 'bondage' and hypoxyphilia (sexual arousal by oxygen deprivation)—about 50 a year in the United States according to coroners' records of thirty years back (Litman & Swearingen, 1972) and almost certainly more numerous today.

It is significantly in *The Economic Problem of Masochism* that Freud undertook, as a preliminary, an important rexamination of the pleasure principle and sought to clarify its relation to the death instincts and the erotic life instincts. It could not be correct that the Nirvana principle, Fechner's (1873) principle of constancy, and the pleasure principle, supposedly allied to it, are entirely in the service of the death instincts "whose aim is to conduct the restlessness of life into the stability of the inorganic state", warning against the disturbances of the libido, the life instincts. In our perception of stimuli, "there are pleasurable tensions and unpleasurable relaxations of tension", notably in the case of sexual arousal. Pleasure and unpleasure must depend on some qualitative factor: "Perhaps it is the rhythm, the temporal sequence of changes, rises and falls in the quantity of stimulus". Freud had considered this possibility in *Beyond the Pleasure Principle*: "the factor that determines the feeling is probably the amount of increase or diminution in the quantity of excitation *in a given period of time*" (Freud, 1920*a*, p. 8); "is the feeling of tension to be related to the absolute magnitude, or perhaps to the level, of the cathexis, while the pleasure and unpleasure series indicates a change in the magnitude of the cathexis *within a given unit of time*?" (p. 63). In living organisms the Nirvana principle, belonging to the death instinct, has been modified by a fusion with libido to become the pleasure principle: "The *Nirvana* principle expresses the trend of the death instinct; the *pleasure* principle represents the demands of the libido; and the modification of the latter principle, the *reality* principle [Freud, 1911, p. 219], represents the influence of the external world. None of these three principles is actually put out of action by another. As a rule they are able to tolerate one another, although conflicts are bound to arise occasionally from the fact of the differing aims that are set for each—in one case a quantitative reduction of the load of the stimulus, in another a qualitative characteristic of the stimulus, and, lastly [in the third case], a postponement of the discharge of the stimulus and a temporary acquiescence in the unpleasure due to tension" (Freud, 1924*a*, pp. 160–161).

As mentioned in the next chapter, a very different postponement of discharge and acquiescence in unpleasure is described with precision by Theodor Reik (1939, pp. 43–45), not in connection with the reality principle but in the context of masochism. In considering what he rightly sees as a quintessential characteristic of masochism, the suspense factor, he traces how an anxious pleasure progressively becomes a pleasurable anxiety and ends in impotence.

Much of what follows upon Freud's (1924*a*) opening statement about masochism, quoted above, and the unravelling of the three principles was either set out or foreshadowed in the earlier writings already considered—its history is that which has been cursorily examined in a chronological manner up to this point. The remaining material is new and substantial.

Let us return with Freud to the theme of the paper: "Masochism comes under our observation in three forms: as a condition imposed on sexual excitation, as an expression of the feminine nature, and as a norm of behavior. We may, accordingly, distinguish an *erotogenic*, a *feminine* and a *moral* masochism" (p. 161). This lucid premiss has led to an astonishing amount of confusion, mostly through careless reading and relaying. Feminists have fallen on it like furies (Mitchell, 1974; Mitchell & Rose, 1982; Cixous, 1976; Dinnerstein, 1977; Chodorow, 1978; Gallop, 1982; for thoughtful overviews of feminist attitudes and reactions, see Young-Bruehl, 1990, and Frosh, 1987, pp. 52–58, 174–207; see also the following section of this chapter discussing 'Developments and critical commentaries on Freud'). Freud's transgression was, of course, to equate femininity with passivity. He did so reluctantly, and with subsequent reservations ("we far too readily identify activity with maleness and passivity with femaleness, a view which is by no means universally confirmed in the animal kingdom" (Freud, 1930, p. 106); "even in the sphere of human sexual life you soon see how inadequate it is to make masculine behavior coincide with activity and feminine with passivity" (Freud, 1933, p. 115)). At no time did he assert that *all* women are masochists, though it must be admitted that he sometimes came near to implying it (1933, p. 116). If it is accepted that the female's sexual role is, by comparison with the male's, an essentially passive one—animal behavior, at least in most of the higher species, would seem to suggest it—then Freud's designation constitutes an extremely accurate observation. Sexual masochism could justly be described as 'feminine' (a) because the masochist adopts an overtly passive role in the rituals he devises, (b) because he usually, according to my own observation, has latent homosexual tendencies and is indeed, as documented in the empirical studies which are reviewed in Chapter 3 (e.g., Gosselin & Wilson, 1980), not infrequently a transvestite, sometimes also a practising, self-declared homosexual, (c) because his strongest libidinal (inverted Oedipal) attachment has often been to his father, not his mother.

Having made the important statement: "the first, the erotogenic, masochism—pleasure in pain—lies at the bottom of the other two forms as well" (Freud, 1924*a*, p. 161), Freud starts by considering 'feminine' masochism, the perversion (this term has become 'politically incorrect', as have the milder descriptors, 'sexual deviance' or 'sexual aberration', but '*Perverse*' is Freud's word for those practising the 'variance' and 'perversion' is the term adopted by his commentators, so it will also be employed where appropriate in this historical survey): "masochistic—and therefore often impotent—subjects whose phantasies either terminate in an act of masturbation or represent a sexual satisfaction in themselves. The real-life performances of masochistic perverts tally completely with these phantasies, whether the performances are carried out as an end in themseves or serve to induce potency and to lead to the sexual act" (pp. 161–162). It is worth noting in the last sentence that with phantasies and performances (*'Veranstaltungen'*) Freud points to two out of the three factors seen as quintessential to masochism by Theodor Reik (1939), phantasy and the demonstrative factor, the other, already mentioned, being the suspense factor. Freud goes on to give a fair listing of what are still, over seventy years on, the commonest masochistic phantasies and practices: "being gagged, bound, painfully beaten, whipped, in some way maltreated, forced into unconditional obediance, dirtied and debased" (p. 162). This leopard, at any rate, is evidently not one to change his spots very much—a point which might reflect upon the value of the 'empirical' findings, reviewed in Chapter 3 and by Rathbone (1999), when weighed against the expenditure of time, effort and money involved in obtaining them! Freud concludes his description by noting that the masochist imposes strict limitations on what is done to him, and embarks on precisely what is missing in the empirical studies: "The obvious interpretation, and one easily arrived at, is that the masochist wants to be treated like a small and helpless child, but, particularly, like a naughty child" (p. 162). He observes, with equal accuracy, that "the material is very uniform ... But if one has an opportunity of studying cases in which the masochistic phantasies have been especially richly elaborated, one quickly discovers that they place the subject in a characteristically female situation" (p. 162). "This superimposed stratification of the infantile and the feminine" is a very accurate portrayal indeed. A male masochist (and in this, his most important discussion of the subject, Freud clearly recognizes that the perversion is to be found overwhelmingly in males), struggling to achieve 'normal' heterosexual coitus, is constantly impeded by the irruption of infantile and feminine impulses. What he really wants is to suck, to be cuddled, to wet the bed, to have a bowel motion; he wants, as Freud puts it, to be copulated with (*'Koitiertwerden'*).

"Being castrated—or being blinded, which stands for it—often leaves a negative trace of itself in phantasies, in the condition that no injury is to occur precisely to the genitals or the eyes," Freud continues (p. 162). A personal observation I have made, and therefore not necessarily generally applicable, is that, in practice, when denied the punishing rituals he craves, the frustrated masochist will often nonetheless seek to damage his genitals or his eyes in a minor, nondefinitive way. He will, for instance, wear painfully tight trousers, rub soap into his eyes, read small print hour after hour by inadequate light. As Freud notes, "being castrated" is one of his aims.

"A sense of guilt, too, finds expression in the manifest content of masochistic phantasies; the subject assumes that he has committed some crime (the nature of which is left indefinite) which is to be expiated by all these painful and tormenting procedures. This looks like a superficial rationalization of the masochistic subject-matter, but behind it there lies a connection with infantile masturbation. On the other hand, this factor of guilt provides a transition to the third, moral, form of masochism" (p. 162). The observation of the displacement of guilt is an important one, with far-reaching applications. In life, the masochist is noticeably *not* guilty about behavior to which guilt might be expected, with some justification, to adhere, but he blames himself for events over which he had no control.

The masochistic perversion "is entirely based on the primary, erotogenic masochism, on pleasure in pain", and Freud now turns his attention to this. It arises by the mechanism first proposed in the *Three Essays* (1905, pp. 204–205). After quoting his original formulation, he gives the proposition further definition and extends it: "the occurrence of such a libidinal sympathetic excitation when there is tension due to pain and unpleasure would be an infantile physiological mechanism which ceases to operate later on. It would attain a varying degree of development in different sexual constitutions; but in any case it would provide the physiological foundation on which the psychical structure of erotogenic masochism would afterwards be erected" (1924*a*, p. 163).

How did Freud know that pain and stress trench upon sexuality? In all probability, the example (1905, p. 203) of the schoolchild, becoming sexually excited and even experiencing something akin to orgasm under the stress of an examination, was an experience he had had, possibly on more than one occasion, himself. It will be seen that in extending the concept he has, in fact, also modified it, making a distinction not only between child and adult but also between physiological and psychological mechanism. This is undoubtedly because he is about to shift his ground or, more accurately, his angle or his level, in order to account for "the regular and close connections of masochism with its counterpart in instinctual life, sadism."

And this is precisely what Maleson (1984), Grossman (1986) and many other critics object to. What they are really saying, beneath their critiques, is: "Tell us please—is London a metropolis or is it in England? Is Paris in France or is it in Europe? No, no, just tell us! Is it—yes or no?" I submit that the creative mind does not function in terms of 'either-or' but in terms of 'and-and', that the nearest approximation to truth is sometimes, indeed, a paradox. Freud tells us in his obituary of Charcot: "He used to look again and again at the things he did not understand, to deepen his impression of them day by day, till suddenly an understanding of them dawned on him" (Freud, 1893, p. 12). In 1914, *On the History of the Psycho-analytic Movement*, he tells us that he learnt "to follow the unforgotten advice of my master, Charcot: to look at the same things again and again until they themselves begin to speak" (p. 22). In the letter he contributed to *Le Disque Vert*, only a month after completing *The Economic Problem of Masochism*, he tells us yet again the two lessons learnt from Charcot: "that one should never tire of considering the same phenomena again and again (or of submitting to their effects), and that one should not mind meeting with contradiction on every side provided one has worked sincerely" (1924*b*, p. 290). He saw it as a fact that masochism had a physiological basis and equally as a fact that masochism and sadism were present together in the same individual. His explanation of the first fact was inadequate, inappropriate, as an explanation of the second. *"La théorie, c'est bon, mais ça n'empêche pas d'exister,"* as Charcot once observed (Freud, 1893, p. 13). What threw most light on the second fact was, almost certainly, a third fact for Freud, namely the destructiveness of both sadism and masochism. He thus turned to the two classes of instincts in order to explain their coexistence.

"... We arrive at another derivation of masochism, which, however, is not in contradiction with the former one ... The libido has the task of making the destroying instinct innocuous, and it fulfils the task by diverting that instinct to a great extent outwards—soon with the help of a special organic system, the muscular apparatus—towards objects in the external world. The instinct is then called the destructive instinct, the instinct for mastery, or the will to power. A portion of the instinct is placed directly in the service of the sexual function, where it has an important part to play. This is sadism proper. Another portion does not share in this transposition outwards; it remains inside the organism and, with the help of the accompanying sexual excitation described above, becomes libidinally bound there. It is in this portion that we have to recognize the original, erotogenic masochism" (1924*a*, pp. 163–164). The concept, recently introduced (1923*b*, pp. 41–42), of fusion and *de*fusion is invoked in the next step of the argument: "a very extensive fusion and amalgamation, in varying proportions, of the two classes of instincts takes place, so that we never have to deal with pure life instincts or pure death instincts but only with mixtures of them in different amounts. Corresponding to a fusion of instincts of this kind, there may, as a result of certain influences, be a *de*fusion of them. How large the portions of the death instincts are which refuse to be tamed in this way by being bound to admixtures of libido we cannot at present guess." The final step of the argument is that primal sadism "which has been directed outwards, projected, can be once more introjected, turned inwards, and in this way regress to its earlier situation. If this happens, a secondary masochism is produced, which is added to the original masochism" (p. 164). Erotogenic masochism derives 'its changing psychical coatings' (*'seine wechselnden psychischen Umkleidungen'*) from the succeeding phases of sexual development: the fear of being swallowed up (the oral stage), the wish to be beaten (sadistic-anal), phantasies of castration (phallic), and finally (from the genital stage) "the situations of being copulated with and of giving birth, which are characteristic of femaleness". At each stage the father is the agent. However much detractors might wish to dismiss all this as 'spinning a yarn', it is not so easy to dismiss, since it encompasses what is, in fact, the predominant content of masochistic phantasies. And as a parting fact, though not a new one since it was delivered already in the *Three Essays* (1905, p. 193), the frequent masochistic preoccupation (as a result of regression) with the buttocks: "The nates are the part of the body which is given erotogenic preference in the sadistic-anal phase, like the breast in the oral phase and the penis in the genital phase" (1924*a*, p. 165).

Moral masochism, the third form (the designation which present-day psychologists and psychiatrists demolish as a loose blanket-term, applied to a multitude of diverse character traits and behavior, and therefore of no meaning), "is chiefly remarkable for having loosened its connection with what we recognize as sexuality ... The suffering itself is what matters" (p. 165). Whether it is caused by a love-object, by someone indifferent, by impersonal powers or circumstances, is of no importance, provided it satisfies an unconscious sense of guilt. All that matters is to "maintain a certain amount of suffering" (p. 166). The 'need for punishment' arises from a tension between the ego and the superego. *'Gewissensangst'* ('conscience anxiety') is the ego's response to the perception that it has not come up to its ideal. It fears the displeasure of the superego because the latter came into being through the introjection of the two parents and retained, probably in exaggerated form, "their strength, their severity, their inclination to supervise and to punish ... Kant's Categorical Imperative is thus the direct heir of the Oedipus complex" (p. 167). Behind the parents lay all the influences of tradition and to their imagos are later linked "the influences of teachers and authorities, self-chosen models and publicly recognized heroes ... the dark power of Destiny which only the fewest of us are able to look upon as impersonal" (p. 168)—least of all the masochist who "always turns his cheek whenever he has a chance of receiving a blow" (p. 165).

Freud makes a distinction between ultramorality and moral masochism: "In the former, the accent falls on the heightened sadism of the super-ego to which the ego submits; in the latter, it falls on the ego's own masochism which seeks punishment, whether from the super-ego or from the parental powers outside ... the sadism of the super-ego becomes for the most part glaringly conscious, whereas the masochistic trend of the ego remains as a rule concealed from the subject". The next statement is low-key, but its practical significance is momentous: "Conscience and morality has arisen through the overcoming, the desexualization, of the Oedipus complex; but through moral masochism morality becomes sexualized once more, the Oedipus complex is revived and the way is opened for a regression from morality to the Oedipus complex. This is to the advantage neither of morality nor of the person concerned. An individual may, it is true, have preserved the whole or some measure of ethical sense alongside of his masochism; but, alternatively, a large part of his conscience may have vanished into his masochism" (p. 169). Day-to-day contact with a masochist eventually brings the realization that there is no conscience in operation; there is only a vicious circle of guilt, demanding punishment, punishment giving erotic satisfaction, thus creating more guilt, requiring further punishment. The mechanism is ruthless—it will stop at nothing.

We have surely all met with the behavior of the 'moral' masochist at some time or other—their name is legion, and we are all to some extent among them: "the masochist must do what is inexpedient, must act against his own interests, must ruin the prospects which open out to him in the real world and must, perhaps, destroy his own real existence" (pp. 169–170). In *The Ego and the Id* (1923*b*, p. 54) Freud, characteristically, turned an accepted view around—that the suppression of aggressiveness resulted from moral standards. In fact, the more aggression is controlled, the harsher do these standards become. This idea, which reappears on several subsequent occasions, is restated and developed here in the context of moral masochism: "The situation is usually presented as though ethical requirements were the primary thing and the renunciation of instinct followed from them. This leaves the origin of the ethical sense unexplained. Actually, it seems to be the other way about. The first instinctual renunciation is enforced by external powers, and it is only this which creates the ethical sense, which expresses itself in conscience and demands a further renunciation of instinct." In standing conventional wisdom on its head, Freud is, in a sense, pleading clemency for the moral masochist: his lot would have been easier had he, in the course of time, grown less scrupulous in turning his aggression away from others. Is this a contradiction of what has been said previously about conscience vanishing into masochism? In that it reflects the complexity of reality, it is more paradox than contradiction, for, on the one hand, there have been heroes and martyrs to whom one would have to attribute nobility as well as masochism; on the other, there is usually an element of self-deception attached to masochistic scruple. Maybe an important determining factor for conscience is the degree of regression. The nature of the relationship between conscience and renunciation of instinct continues to occupy Freud as a general problem. He tackles it again and takes his argument into much greater detail, relating it to ambivalence, in *Civilization and its Discontents* (1930, pp. 123–133). Here, however, he pursues it no further but simply brings the paper to its cheerless conclusion: "Thus moral masochism becomes a classical piece of evidence for the existence of fusion of instinct. Its danger lies in the fact that it originates from the death instinct and corresponds to the part of that instinct which has escaped being turned outwards as an instinct of destruction. But since, on the other hand, it has the significance of an erotic component, even the subject's destruction of himself cannot take place without libidinal satisfaction" (p. 170).

The Economic Problem of Masochism was apparently the culmination of Freud's exposition of masochism. Subsequent papers contain no new ideas of major importance, but his consideration of specific aspects is well worth mentioning. In choosing to write at all about *Dostoevsky and Parricide* (1928), he points to the fact that masochism occasionally goes hand in hand with artistic, particularly literary, ability. All masochists are phantasts; it seems that a few possess gifts adequate to breaking out of the prison of stereotypy, harnessing the primary processes for actual artistic achievement, though masochism remains evident in their works. With Dostoevsky's own life and *The Brothers Karamazov* there came a golden opportunity to explore the central importance of the father, of an ambivalent attitude towards him and also towards castration, in the etiology of masochism. After outlining the normal course of the Oedipus complex, Freud points out: "A further complication arises when the constitutional factor we call bisexuality is comparatively strongly developed in a child ... Of the two factors which repress hatred of the father, the first, the direct fear of punishment and castration, may be called the normal one; its pathogenic intensification seems to come only with the addition of the second factor, the fear of the feminine attitude" (pp. 183–184). As is amply evidenced in his phantasies and behavior, a masochist both fears and desires castration. He invariably reacts to father figures ambivalently.

In *Civilization and its Discontents* (1930) Freud looks particularly at the destructive instinct directed outwards in the form of aggression. As to sadomasochism and its derivation in terms of the two classes of instincts, he simply reaffirms his previous convictions, but there is a disarming candour about his own attitude to the controversial theory: "In sadism, long since known to us as a component instinct of sexuality, we should have before us a particularly strong alloy of this kind between trends of love and the destructive instinct; whilst its counterpart, masochism, would be a union between destructiveness directed inwards and sexuality—a union which makes what is otherwise an imperceptible trend into a conspicuous and tangible one ... To begin with it was only tentatively that I put forward the views I have developed here, but in the course of time they have gained such a hold upon me that I can no longer think in any other way. To my mind, they are far more serviceable from a theoretical standpoint than any other possible ones; they provide that simplification, without either ignoring or doing violence to the facts, for which we strive in scientific work. I know that in sadism and masochism we have always seen before us manifestations of the destructive instinct (directed outwards and inwards), strongly alloyed with erotism; but I can no longer understand how we can have overlooked the ubiquity of non-erotic aggressivity and destructiveness and can have failed to give it its due place in our interpretation of life" (Freud, 1930, pp. 119–120).

The *New Introductory Lectures on Psycho-Analysis* (1933) bring, in 'Anxiety and Instinctual Life' (Lecture XXXII), further confirmation that it was precisely the phenomenon of sadomasochism which caused Freud to revise his theory of the two opposing classes of instincts: "we have argued in favour of a special aggressive and destructive instinct in men not on account of the teachings of history or of our experience in life but on the basis of general considerations to which we were led by examining the phenomena of sadism and masochism ... Both phenomena, sadism and masochism alike, but masochism quite especially, present a truly puzzling problem to the libido theory; and it is only proper if what was a stumbling-block for the one theory should become the corner-stone of the theory replacing it" (p. 104). Finding an explanation of masochism was thus a crucial and long-standing goal of Freud's thinking. For this reason, if for no other, it behooves us to listen to what he has to say about it. As to its treatment, he makes his opinion clear in *Analysis Terminable and Interminable* (1937): "Even to exert a psychical influence on simple masochism is a severe tax upon our powers" (p. 243).

A Few Further Remarks

Many other allusions to masochism in Freud's works have, of necessity, gone unmentioned in this survey. There are also many ideas which have extreme relevance to masochism. Since space is limited, it might be wise to mention one of the less obvious: "But I have had good reason for asserting that everyone possesses in his own unconscious an instrument with which he can interpret the utterances of the unconscious in other people" (Freud, 1913, p. 320). "It is a very remarkable thing that the *Ucs.* of one human being can react upon that of another, without passing through the *Cs.*" (Freud, 1915*b*, p. 194). The masochist has not only a remarkable ingenuity in his methods of provocation—he has an uncanny and malevolent intuition. However great the pains taken to conceal the spot at which provocation is most successful, he will unerringly divine it. This acute but highly specialized receptivity—for in most respects his narcissism makes him grossly insensitive to others (Lewinsky, 1944)—may well be because of the unusually large input of the primary processes in his mental life.

The evidence of functioning on the level of the primary processes is abundant and is linked to regression: "Unconscious processes only become cognizable by us under the conditions of dreaming and of neurosis—that is to say, when processes of the higher, *Pcs.*, system are set back to an earlier stage by being lowered (by regression)" (Freud, 1915*b*, p. 187). Freud repeatedly used the metaphor of the negative and the positive of one and the same picture to convey the relation of a neurosis to a perversion: "*neuroses are, so to say, the negative of perversions*" (1905, p. 165). How do these "older, primary processes, the residues of a phase of development in which they were the only kind of mental process" (Freud, 1911, p. 219) become evident? In suspensions of logic, puzzling ellipses, glaring yet unperceived contradictions, bizarre associations which are meaningful only in the unconscious of the masochist (Lenzer, 1975). There is a belief in 'the omnipotence of thoughts' and an assumption that trivial details of personal background are not only of intrinsic interest but are common knowledge, requiring no explanation. Newly encountered people are liked, disliked, have characteristics attributed to them simply because they bear a name significant in the past. There are strange formulations: for instance (a personal observation), age is stated again and again, despite repeated correction, as "when I was half-past-three" or "when I was about half-past-eight", because a clock face is being visualized, specifically a large round clock at the dock gates, essential for calculating the tides, of huge significance since seagoing was the charismatic occupation of an idealized father. Similarly (another personal observation), a fervent aspiration, voiced whenever opportunity allows, that somehow the arts and the sciences should be brought together, derives from two childhood incidents: a painter once explained what he was trying to capture in his landscape, and father once explained the workings of the ship's engine-room, the intensity of both experiences lying in the respect the child received from a god-like father. Above all, there is the proclivity to phantasize, a predilection for ghost stories, for science fiction, for make-belief, for dressing up.

In concluding this examination of Freud's writings on masochism I would like to make two points. The first is that, in direct personal observation over twenty years, I have found that they are extremely accurate. The second point is a much broader one. Scientific classification has proceeded in the direction of the smaller and more specific for so many generations that the practitioner of today finds his teeth chattering if he even dares to turn and glance back in the other direction where the old encompassing classifications loom out of the mist to unnerve him. But the 'families'and 'genera' not only had once, but retain still, their value for a scientific understanding. Does 'acid' or 'alkaline' become meaningless directly a complex molecular structure has been determined?

DEVELOPMENTS AND CRITICAL COMMENTARIES ON FREUD

It would hardly be an exaggeration to say that all subsequent psychoanalytic writers on masochism comment on Freud. How could it be otherwise since they all come out of Freud? Necessarily they allude to his concepts, either developing, modifying or challenging them (for a general review of the psychological literature on masochism see the next chapter and Rathbone (1999)). The present discussion, attempting to represent the views of later commentators on Freud, is extremely selective: those dealing with masochism in women, those examining the validity of his observations on beating fantasies and those specifically looking at the development of his conceptualization of masochism and its practical repercussions.

Feminist Issues

Helene Deutsch (1925) sees the masculinity complex in women, arising from the universal bisexuality in which they share, as flaring up 'with elemental force' in the female reproductive functions. Deutsch (1930) defines her aim: "to examine the genesis of 'femininity', by which I mean the feminine, passive-masochistic disposition in the mental life of women" (p. 48). She takes Freud's observations on the consequences of the anatomical differences between the sexes a stage further. "The most difficult factor in the 'anatomical destiny' of the woman is," she writes, "the fact that at a time when the libido is still unstable, immature and incapable of sublimation, it seems condemned to abandon a pleasure-zone (the clitoris as a phallic organ) without discovering the possibility of a new cathexis" (p. 51). The wishful phantasy of a child (from her father) is 'a very unreal and uncertain substitute'. "The hitherto active-sadistic libido ... is deflected in a regressive direction towards masochism. In place of the active urge of the phallic tendencies, there arises the masochistic phantasy: 'I want to be castrated', and this forms the erotogenic masochistic basis of the feminine libido" (p. 52). Deutsch opines that the Oedipus complex in girls is, in fact, inaugurated by the castration complex (cf. Freud, 1925, p. 256; 1931, p. 230; 1933, p. 194), which persists because it contains not only the masculinity complex but also "the whole infantile set towards femininity" (p. 53). Subsequently the woman's attitude towards reproduction and towards her child is "permeated by pleasure-tendencies of a masochistic nature" (p. 53).

In '*A Child is Being Beaten*' Freud wrote of the repression of an erotic *phantasy* but Deutsch speaks in more than one connection of the repression of masochistic instinctual tendencies and the danger attending this repression. Since these tendencies are, even by Deutsch's scenario, the result of suppressed sadism, there is something intrinsically implausible about this concept. What is supposed to happen to sadism when its passive successor is repressed? She simply does not say, but goes on to talk of narcissism and object choice "of an affectionate and passive type" (p. 55). Even if one can swallow her "masochistic triad: castration, rape and parturition" (p. 57), the ultimate improbability is reached with her extraordinary generalization: "In the deepest experience of the relation of mother to child it is masochism in its strongest form which finds gratification in the bliss of motherhood" (p. 58). With that she has, of course, clearly parted company with Freud.

In challenging the premisses of Helene Deutsch, with great good sense it must be said, Karen Horney (1935) directs her arguments simultaneously against those of Sandor Rado (1933): "Rado affirms that he is concerned only with pathologic phenomena, but from his deduction as to the origin of feminine masochism, one cannot but conclude that the sex life of the vast majority of women is pathologic. The difference between his views and those presented by Deutsch, who affirms that to be feminine is to be masochistic, is thus seen to be theoretical rather than factual" (Horney, 1935, p. 242).

Women *may* derive masochistic satisfaction from masturbation, menstruation, intercourse and childbirth—this Horney grants—but what is the genesis and frequency of occurrence? Where are the data to support these assertions? Penis envy is a working hypothesis, not a fact. "How a libido-cathexis of an organ [the clitoris] can be sadistic and then turn inward, seems mysterious" (p. 244). Rado's assumption that the narcissistic shock sustained by the little girl on discovering her inferior genitalia spoilt all sexual pleasure for her would be more accurately named the greediness principle than the pleasure principle. Why should she be sexually excited by the pain of her discovery, adopt the pain as a substitute gratification and thence develop an enduring, lifelong masochistic attitude? Reactions such as this, assumed by Rado, certainly exist but they are an expression of masochistic tendencies, not their root.

Freud's hypothesis that pathological phenomena are merely the magnification of 'normal' processes, for all its force, must have limitations, even with respect to the Oedipus complex, under differing cultural conditions. The ubiquity of feminine masochism is the impression which results when cultures with other customs are excluded from the picture. The self-assertive Soviet woman would hardly take beating as a token of affection, as her peasant predecessor might have done under tsarist patriarchy. Omission of the factor of social conditioning leads to overvaluation of the causative role of anatomical differences. Civilized people may engage in painful or uncomfortable activities for realistic, not masochistic motives; in primitive societies, suffering may be a magical defense against danger.

Is masochism a collective term for very complex phenomena? "The suffering may concern the physical or the mental sphere. There is some gratification or relief of tension connected with it, and that is why it is striven for" (p. 252). After enumerating the overlapping economic and emotional factors bearing down upon the women of her day and militating against their autonomy, Horney expostulates: "it is hard to see how any woman may escape becoming masochistic to some degree, from the effects of the culture alone, without any appeal to contributory factors in the anatomical-physiological characteristics of woman, and their psychic effects" (p. 256).

It should be remembered, amidst the feminist resentment which is here being set in motion (the clinical sociologist, Melvyn L. Fein, has recently undertaken a detailed comparison of radical feminism with Marxism (Fein, 1999, pp. 91–122)), that Freud himself was *not* without sympathy for the social subjection of women. Elisabeth Young-Bruehl (1990) acknowledges this basic fact (p. 25). She anthologizes all his writings concerning women, providing an introduction which is highly informative with respect to the feminist debate, and an excellent running commentary. As she points out, Freud fully anticipated the controversy his views would evoke (Freud, 1931, p. 230). The root of the controversy lay in Freud's relatively late perception of the importance of the female infant's preoedipal attachment to her mother and its developmental implications. Amongst her introductory remarks to *The Psychogenesis of a Case of Homosexuality in a Woman* (Freud, 1920*b*), Young-Bruehl notes that "in the essays he wrote on female psychology in the next decade, Freud again and again challenged his female trainees and colleagues to follow in the direction of this case, that is, to investigate the female's mother-bond" (pp. 241–242). That they did and are still doing, relevantly to the present study, in connection with beating fantasies.

BEATING FANTASIES

Ruth Lax (1992) reports clinical material on five female patients for whom "mother was perceived as the judge, prosecutor, and punisher" (p. 466), "aggressor/castrator" (p. 472). Their beating fantasies had two aspects: "the girl, 'at a price', is unconsciously gratified since her father, in regressed form, via the beating, commits the incestuous act. The second aspect relates to mother, who, as the unconscious meaning also indicates, is the real punisher administering the 'actual' beating" (pp. 466–467). Identification with her forms 'the oedipal law' (the prohibition of oedipal wishes) but later "identification with mother's successful womanliness may merge with the idealized mother image of early childhood and become incorporated in the feminine ego ideal aspects of the superego" (p. 470). "These internalized identifications form the core of the female superego. Such a resolution is optimal though perhaps infrequent" (p. 472), Lax concludes.

Twenty years previously Novick & Novick (1972) looked, not like Lax at adults, but at 111 children, both boys and girls, attending Anna Freud's Hampstead (North London) Clinic. Beating wishes in the anal phase and beating games in the phallic phase appeared universally but fantasies only in a few and with the onset of the latency period. In the case of the girls, they found, like Lax, that "the beaten victim of the fantasy consciously personified the child herself" (p. 239). Freud had stated that the second, 'unmistakably masochistic' stage of the girl's fantasy always remained repressed. They distinguished between a 'transitory' fantasy and one which was 'fixed', which did not follow Freud's pattern. There was more to it, "and this remainder contained the main libidinal and narcissistic pleasure of the fantasy—hence the reluctance of the children to disclose it. It stood for an early masochistic tie to the mother. In this extension, someone important, often a woman, felt very sorry for the beaten child, and in many versions, the child was then regarded as a very important and special person" (pp. 240–241). One child fantasized that his mother applied soothing lotion to his buttocks (the culmination so favoured in the adult pornographic formula and thereby supporting the Novicks' finding). Thus although "the beating fantasy is not formed until the phallic-oedipal stage is reached, the primary determinants of the beating wish which is discharged in the fantasy are pre-oedipal" (p. 241). The 'transitory' fantasy was more often found in girls and spontaneously modified to a passive-feminine sexuality. The 'fixed' fantasy arising at puberty in a group of disturbed boys became the permanent focus of their sexuality. It was rooted in an early sadomasochistic relationship with their mothers but multiply determined and serving multiple functions. In line with Freud's (1919) remarks on his male subjects, the Novicks concluded that "a beating fantasy in a boy was indicative of severe disturbance in ego and drive development" (p. 241).

Novick and Novick (1987) reiterate these findings but extend their material to adults and the scope of their study to a penetrating delineation of other factors in masochistic development. The mother is central in all these factors. In the beating fantasies, it may be the father who carries out the punishment, but this is "a displacement of aggression from the more frightening, but more important, primary object to the father" (p. 366). The actual father was often an ineffectual or absent figure.

Wayne Myers (1980/81), reporting his work over fifteen years with a woman (an analysis interminable if ever there was one!), finally also unearthed an unconscious fantasy of being beaten by her mother. Her lifelong masturbatory fantasy of being beaten by her father was a screen.

Thus, it may be that Freud's account was tinged by a Victorian patriarchal attitude. My own view is that he nevertheless put his finger on something extremely important when he pointed to an inverted oedipal attachment in the incipient male masochist. He also had a great deal more to say about masochism than his 1919 account of beating fantasies, and it is to critiques of his persevering attempts at conceptualization that we now turn.

Developing Conceptualization

Franklin Maleson (1984) makes many of the same observations as William Grossman (1986), whose paper is considered below. *Descriptively*, writes Maleson, the term masochism is applied to sexual perversion, to manifestly nonsexual character pathology, to many actions, attitudes or thoughts having only an element of suffering or renunciation in common. *Dynamically*, the term may suggest a harsh superego, conflicts over aggression, sadistic-anal regression or fixation, object-holding needs stemming from deprivation, feminine traits, rape or beating wishes, either conscious or unconscious. *Theoretically*, and potentially dangerously for clinical interpretation, a death instinct, sadistic and masochistic component sexual drives, erotogenic masochism or innate feminine proclivities toward pain may be implied.

Maleson then traces the evolution of Freud's use of the term 'masochism', finding two major threads: (1) an oscillation between masochism as instinctual drive and as forms of behavior; (2) a progressive broadening of the descriptive application from the sexual to the nonsexual (moral masochism). In Freud's (1905) exploration of infantile sexuality, masochism signified sexual excitement associated with pain, a normal developmental capacity which might endure and become extreme as an ultimate perversion. (Maleson's use (p. 327) of the word 'capacity' is actually, if one wants to quibble, a subtle distortion—Freud simply pointed to the occurrence of the phenomenon.) In 1919, Freud broadened its application to characterological behavior derived from an oedipal beating fantasy, with hypersensitivity towards father figures. He changed his position in 1924 when he created a conceptual unity of primary or erotogenic masochism, feminine masochism and moral masochism. Erotogenic masochism resulted from a fusion of the death instinct with libido which 'tamed' it. That portion of the death instinct which was directed outward, constituting 'sadism proper', might be redirected against the self through guilt as 'secondary masochism' or taken up by the superego. Masochistic perversions and fantasies were thus related to oedipal guilt, to erotogenic masochism and, above all, to feminine masochism in that they placed the subject in situations of being castrated, copulated with, or giving birth. Even in moral masochism, the detachment from libido was illusory. The superego was an introjection of the child's first objects as part of the resolution of the Oedipus complex, becoming desexualized by instinctual defusion but resexualized in three stages: (1) unconscious guilt is translated into need for (parental) punishment; (2) beating by the father stands for a passive sexual relation to him; (3) regression takes place from morality to the revived Oedipus complex. Metapsychologically, all masochism is ultimately based on erotogenic masochism. The sexual and nonsexual are linked via the beating fantasy. However, the centrality of the beating fantasy in cases of moral masochism has since been questioned with observations that sexual and moral masochism are generally not manifest in the same individual. (Personally, I would not wish to contradict this general observation, but it should be noted that Berliner (1958, p. 40) wrote: "There is no sexual masochist who is not also a severe moral masochist".) More recent views, desexualizing the term except for the perversion, have stemmed from ego and superego analysis, object relations theory and studies of narcissism and aggression. Dynamic formulations explain masochism as revenge through martyred induction of guilt, the need for punishment of forbidden wishes, the active anticipation of passively feared dangers, the control of others through provoking punishment, attempted merger to prevent loss of an unloving object, the expression of dependent, passive strivings, and the repair of narcissistic mortification. Characterological masochism has come to be considered an overdetermined composite, sometimes used for ineffective, self-damaging behavior, sometimes for failure to progress therapeutically. Turbulent relationships may be called sadomasochistic when what is meant is violent. This is misleading since a 'sadomasochistic view of sexuality' implies that violence is an integral part of sexual pleasure whereas the narrower 'violent' view may promote fear and withdrawal from sexual relations. (Certainly there are masochists, such as T.E. Lawrence, who repudiate 'normal' sexual relations (Turner, 1991). Whether this is because they fear them as violent, whether they abstain from other forms of sexual activity, possibly more violent—these are other questions.) Freud's equating of masochistic with passive/feminine and sadistic with active/masculine has been largely questioned by later analysts. Use of the term masochistic may be based on value judgments and conceptions of the normal which differ from person to person.

Maleson proceeds to contrast metapsychological and clinical concepts of masochism. For Freud in the *Three Essays* (1905) a perversion was a lingering over an intermediate sexual aim, a component instinct which broke through repression. His comment: "Clinical analysis of extreme cases of masochistic perversion shows that a great number of factors (such as the castration complex and the sense of guilt) have combined to exaggerate and fixate the original passive sexual attitude" (p. 158), anticipated the later concept of perversions within the framework of the structural theory, not component drives but overdetermined compromises serving several functions. In *Instincts and Their Vicissitudes* (1915*a*) sadism was primary, masochism its redirected form, but the instinctual aim in both cases was satisfaction through pain as a source of sexual pleasure, especially convenient for the sadist enjoying masochistic suffering vicariously. Yet still Freud suggested that, as perversions encountered clinically, they are overdetermined and involve multiple identifications, defense and the apparent erotogenic potential of pain. These clinical complexities were explored further in '*A Child is Being Beaten*' (1919) where beating fantasies were seen to develop in phases of which the most crucial, being beaten by the father, arose from incestuous oedipal love, a genital wish transformed through guilt, repression and regression. Males had a feminine attitude toward the father. Finally, in *The Economic Problem of Masochism* (1924*a*), masochism became primary but, within Freud's new structural model, sadism and masochism were no longer considered as component sexual instincts pushing through repression but as products of instinctual fusion attaching ultimately to different mental agencies in manifest behavior. They were thus no longer pure drives nor yet behavior of the whole person. Why was masochism assigned to the ego rather than the id? The concepts of primary masochism and the death instinct have been widely challenged, as has that of an underlying erotogenic masochism which changes its psychical coating with the oral, sadistic-anal, phallic and genital phases of sexual delopment (Brenner, 1959). The more current concepts of 'erotization' or 'libidinization of pain' might be applicable to various associations of pain and gratification but they fail to convey a clinically useful mechanism. (It is difficult to pinpoint any substantial difference between the 'current' designations and Freud's, beyond a *penchant* for jargon. If the difference is taken to lie in a distinction between pain as an accompaniment and pain as a cause, Freud's is, on a physiological level, probably the more correct, and would appear to convey 'a clinically useful mechanism', were it only appreciated.)

Freud's concept of feminine masochism, based on erotogenic masochism, supported by the feminine fantasies of male perverts, was elaborated by Deutsch (1925, 1930) as the result of woman's anatomical destiny. It has since been criticized and reformulated, as has the idea of masochism as a component sexual instinct. Freud's starting points for the latter were clinical description of sadomasochistic perversions and universal bisexuality to account for these paired opposites regularly occurring in the same individual. The hypothesized component instincts were then said to cause the clinically manifested perversions, thus endowing sadism and masochism with double meanings, as both instincts and behaviors. "The potential for inaccurate interpretation is obvious," Maleson concludes, "... vastly overdetermined phenomena should not be reductionistically viewed as simple biological forces or id wishes" (p. 350). (This being the main thrust of the critique, and a valid one, it can only be reiterated that Freud made diverse approaches to masochism precisely because he realized that it was overdetermined. Since he was blazing a trail through entirely uncharted territory, he could hardly take account of all aspects of this overdetermination at one and the same time.)

William Grossman (1986) explains in a footnote that his paper was already completed when Maleson's appeared, that the two papers generally agreed but comparison would be too tedious to undertake. Grossman outlines the development of the concept of masochism from the sexology of Krafft-Ebing and Havelock Ellis to the present. He points out that, in applying his new method, Freud reformulated the problem of masochism, which had never been precisely defined. The relation of partners in the perversion became the model for the relation between intrapsychic agencies. Masochism became a fundamental theoretical concept of drives and structure. The evolution of psychoanalytic theory and technique was, in its turn, influenced by the effort to use such an ill-defined idea as masochism as a theoretical concept. It is now clear that it is an imprecise term, of descriptive or evocative value, best used to refer to fantasies where "the association of pleasure and unpleasure is motivated and obligatory" (p. 381) and to the perversion which is their enactment. (He appears to be unaware of the sticky wicket created by 'unpleasure' at one end of his better definition!) The seeking for pain may be a significant factor in many complex clinical situations, as recognized also by Maleson (1984).

'Masochistic' behavior is to be found both in normal people and in a variety of pathological syndromes. In practice it may be difficult to decide whether pain is covertly sought, whether self-injury is deliberate. Much depends on whether this is conscious or unconscious, whether character, perversion, neurosis or psychosis is under consideration, whether emphasis is placed on aggression or on sexual satisfaction. 'Masochistic' behavior has different consequences when it is found in different character types, and some of these never come to analysis or are not analysable when they do.

Masochistic fantasy, preoccupied with combining the pleasurable with the unpleasurable, points to a set of relations betweeen affects and between people, the roles of subject and object being characteristically interchangeable. The solitary enactment of such a fantasy may unconsciously contain another person as participant or spectator.

Unpleasure inevitably involves vicissitudes of aggression. The emphasis may be on punishment, propitiation or pain. The need may be to extract pleasure from adversity, to deflect aggression from an object which is both needed and feared, or to obtain satisfaction in a passive mode. Unpleasure may be sought for excitement, for relief of tension, to avoid some other pain, for another kind of satisfaction, or to escape 'real' pain and passivity. If masochism is dissected conceptually it dissolves into component issues of pleasure and unpleasure, aggression, activity and passivity relating to authority, important identifications, impulse control and reality testing.

Freud's (1896) idea that hysteria was the negative of an unconscious perversion was so strikingly original that one tends to forget how many of his ideas about sexuality and the perversions were taken over from Krafft-Ebing and other contemporaries. The importance Krafft-Ebing (1886) ascribed to masochism probably contributed to the diffusion of the concept to cover what might better be regarded as vicissitudes of aggression. In striving to establish sadism and masochism as fundamental instinctual components of the libido and to relate them to the oral, anal and genital zones which had both sexual and self-preservative aspects, Freud had to find both sexual and self-preservative components for sadism and masochism. He also had to explain why they were directed from the start at objects. As a pair, he thought one of them had to be primary. Finally, in relating them to bisexuality, he had to explain how they led to normal masculinity and femininity, on the one hand, or to sadistic and masochistic perversions, on the other. Krafft-Ebing believed masochism arose out of erotogenic pain, sexual bondage and sexual activity in which pain and emotional bondage could play varying roles. The psychopathic disposition to 'sexual ecstasy' might be awakened, as in Jean-Jacques Rousseau's case, by childhood beating, but such events were only subsidiary factors in the etiology of masochism.

Grossman now traces, with more than a hint of criticism, the evolution of Freud's views on masochism. In the *Three Essays on the Theory of Sexuality* (1905) Freud noted Krafft-Ebing's emphasis on pleasure in humiliation or subjection and Schrenck-Notzing's on pleasure in pain or cruelty, and, Grossman says, sought thereafter some way of integrating these two views, the one emphasizing interpersonal, the other erotogenic, factors. By 1924, in *The Economic Problem of Masochism,* the triad of "erotogenic pain, subjugation to a sexual object, and sexual activity in which the other factors played a part had acquired a developmental and structural significance" (p. 394) as erotogenic, moral and feminine masochism. (Having confused us with this misordering, Grossman goes on to point out how Freud confused us with his original definitions and brought down on his head the subsequent wrath of the feminists.) When Freud equated erotogenic masochism with a primary masochism (the critique proceeds) "derived from libidinally bound destructive instinct", he found the "elegant, if unsatisfactory" solution to two problems: the analogy with narcissism and the unitary origin of masochism and sadism. The clinical observation that masochism was sadism turned against the self could be retained as secondary masochism. Between 1905 and 1924, there had been *Instincts and Their Vicissitudes* (1915*a*) and *'A Child is Being Beaten'* (1919) where Freud considered masochism in terms of object relationship, more specifically, the Oedipus complex. The fantasy represented a sexual relation between father and child, in which the child's role was a feminine one, and to which attached, most importantly, a sense of guilt, opening the way to the later concept of moral masochism. With this concept, "Krafft-Ebing's requirement of a *conscious* link with sexuality was discarded, as was a requirement that suffering should come from a love object. In moral masochism, the important thing was that unconscious guilt required punishment" (pp. 397–398).

Grossman continues by examining the manner in which the prototypes for psychoanalytic concepts changed. In 1905, the perversions were prototypes for the mental life of childhood. In *Beyond the Pleasure Principle* (1920*a*), the child throwing away his toy and regaining it became the normal prototype of pathological repetition, "a complex and motivated behavior of infancy expressing aggression" (p. 399). Freud turned his attention from the conversion of activity into passivity to the opposite process in the mastery of trauma, the acquisition of the love object's power, pointing to mechanisms for the patterning of aggression, and beyond that, to the relations between the ego and the external world. In this prototype of children's play, developed and related to masochistic practices by later investigators such as Lewinsky (1944) and Loewenstein (1957), frustration is made to yield pleasure (whereas in moral masochism suffering provides narcissistic satisfaction). However, Grossman insists, a prototype is not a cause, and children's games are a far cry from the physical and emotional anguish investigated by Fraiberg (1982) and Glenn (1984*a,b*), though both may give rise to phenomena that, descriptively, could be called masochism. The theoretician may find in the games a model of parent-child interaction that leads to the establishment of the ego ideal and the superego: the child's self-control of aggression, its affective control of the parent's aggression and even the parent's affect. Ambiguities in using the term masochism also of adults with severe character pathology arise from unresolved problems in superego development. Self-damage may be a function of a sense of guilt, but it may also represent a need to express fantasy in action or a primitive conception of reality, leading to crises in regulating aggression. "The term masochism is used to allude to a variety of developmental end-points for which we have no reason to assume a common developmental pathway" (p. 405). "Some of the trouble we have with Freud," Grossman modestly concludes, "comes from his mixture of the old and the new ways of thinking" (p. 410).

No one would wish to deny the value of these critiques, only to suggest that their value should be assessed in the light of one of Grossman's introductory remarks: "While it is not my intention to offer a theory of masochism ..." (p. 381). Freud, however, did.

CHAPTER 2

SURVEY OF PSYCHOLOGICAL LITERATURE (1926 ONWARDS)

SUMMARY

The aim of this survey has been to look at as many aspects of the complex phenomenon of masochism as possible, rather than to list as many authors as possible with their dates, ranging them into camps and hanging some conceptual tally over their tents. The process of plucking one idea from a paper or book of many pages, encapsulating it in one sentence and thereby disposing of the work of many weeks or years has always seemed to me an unfair and futile one. Inevitably I have done this too, but I have also attempted to convey the contents of many of the papers considered as thoroughly as possible, with occasional assesssments, and have arranged these synopses in chronological order. Freud's writings and subsequent commentaries upon them have already been considered in the previous chapter. Here it will therefore be a case of indicating briefly where an author has used and possibly developed some particular aspect of Freud's views on masochism. It is hoped that the method employed in this survey, though unstandard and unwieldy, may nevertheless achieve its aim of covering most psychological approaches to the problem of masochism published since Freud.

Along well-worn Freudian lines and concentrating on the erotic zones of the body, Isidor Sadger (1926) points to unsatisfactory breast-feeding, weaning, toilet training and dissuasion from masturbation as inevitable creators of ambivalence in the infant. Tolstoy's earliest recollection of being tightly swaddled is quoted as the source of his lifelong passion for freedom and hatred of coercion. (Times do not appear to have changed much, as can be seen from Figure 9.1 in Chapter 9!) "Just as the suckling or the very young infant learns to love all those who stimulate and satisfy its sexuality, so it learns, on the other hand, to hate all those who in any way interfere with its sexual life" (p. 486). Jealous older siblings may add fuel to this smouldering ambivalence. "Whoever hates more than he loves, that is, whoever originally felt more keenly the withdrawal of sexual stimuli than he had felt the positive pleasure these had afforded, will have a tendency to sadism. Sadists are all vigorous haters" (pp. 489–490). An originally strong genital erotism in homosexuals tends towards masochism. Especially where cleansing by the mother or romping with the father has led to painful-pleasurable stimulation, "it is very easy for the excessive craving of the sexual organs, so fraught with feelings of voluptuous pain, to become linked with the primary feeling of being in the power of some stronger being; this again forms the bridge to masochism in the strict sense" (p. 490). A rather simplistic view, more likely to account for universal or sporadic sadomasochistic impulses than extreme cases of masochism, unless the factors Sadger examined are quantitatively exaggerated.

Nine years before Freud's death, in his paper on the erotization of anxiety, René Laforgue (1930) suggests that connections existing between anxiety and forepleasure enable anxiety to be utilized as a substitutive gratification. Many people obviously derive satisfaction from causing others anxiety, from experiencing it themselves through ghost stories or from lingering over reports of horrifying catastrophes. Obtaining submission through causing anxiety is, indeed, an educational method widely employed by parents, teachers and dictators. The power of the army sergeant or the policeman may depend largely on an erotic need in its dual aspect of actively causing anxiety or passively experiencing it. Investigations have linked anxiety with the act of birth, the damming-up of libido and castration, but clinical observations have also shown that anxiety-formation constitutes the main aim and pleasure-gain of some individuals—a surrogate for orgasm.

Laforgue describes several cases in which the anxiety generated relates to a primal scene which is revivified for its pleasure content, orgasm often being construed by the watching child as anxiety, and by the adult as *'la petite mort'*. If the earliest sexual excitement of an infant is felt as anxiety and fixated as such, the link is already forged between sexual satisfaction and the fear of death—a link often encountered in the masochist, though Laforgue points to it only in the hypochondriac. His cases of anxiety-neurosis and phobia, with their regression to oral and anal stages of libidinal development, might in fact be called sadomasochists, as suggested by his definition of anal anxiety: "We know that anal love will torture and even kill the love-object. These sadistic wishes rouse great anxiety; on the one side there is the anxiety of killing the love-object by the omnipotence of thought, and, on the other, the anxiety of being forced to allow oneself to be killed by the love-object and thus belong to it. It is not clear to what extent the awful fulfilment as well of these sado-masochistic tendencies is experienced in this anxiety" (p. 320).

Karl Menninger's (1938) book *Man Against Himself* has a far wider scope than masochism, certainly than the masochistic perversion. The term 'masochism' occurs rarely and the short subsection of the chapter on 'Antisocial Behavior' headed 'Perversions' deals chiefly with homosexuality. Highly anecdotal, 'antediluvian', as one can almost hear a present-day critic charge—Freud himself was still alive—the work has, nevertheless, much light to cast on masochism, particularly in its provocative and vengeful aspects, and also an unusual quality of thoroughness. The fact that he is writing for a general readership, far from resulting in superficiality, has eliminated jargon and sharpened the arguments, since he assumes that he is preaching to the unconverted. His references on the somewhat obscure subject of asceticism are particularly valuable.

Menninger's central theme is "the opposition and interaction of aggressive, self-punitive, and erotic components of the self-destructive tendency". He ranges the manifestations of this tendency from the irreversible, suicide, through 'chronic' suicide (asceticism, martyrdom, invalidism, alcohol addiction, neurotic, criminal and perverse behavior, psychosis), 'focal' suicide (self-mutilation, malingering, repeated surgery, engineered accidents, impotence and frigidity), to organic suicide (high blood pressure and other cardiovascular disease, eye affections, hyperthyroidism, gastrointestinal problems, arthritis, tuberculosis, asthma, skin complaints and headaches). He points out in relation to these ailments that continuous stimulation (introverted rage) leads to continuous symptomatology and ultimately to organic changes. He summarizes the report of a case of hypertension and concludes: "The treatment enabled him to assimilate the original episode [a severe whipping at the hands of his mother] into the totality of his experience so that it could undergo modification in the light of his intelligence and in this way save his vasomotor system from the excessive burden of a constant reaction to a tremendous unconscious and otherwise unexpressed emotion" (p. 381). Without even using the word, he conveys the whole essential mechanism of repression and its release.

Theodor Reik's work on masochism merits consideration in some detail since it was, and arguably is still, the most accurate depiction and the most substantial contribution to an understanding of the phenomenon after Freud's. Its importance lies in the 'nitty-gritty'. Reik (1939) initiates his search for the quintessential characteristics of masochism with three examples. First, the phantasy of a young girl that she enters a butcher's shop, undresses and lies waiting whilst the butcher cuts up some calves. Assistants prod her body and then the butcher himself hauls her about. As he takes the knife he puts his finger into her vagina and she has an orgasm. Second, one of the phantasies by which a 37-year-old father of three achieves potency. A series of young athletes are ritually sacrificed to Moloch. The high priest tests the genitals of each victim for weight, some are rejected but then those found worthy of sacrifice to the god are cut away. Ejaculation occurs when the high priest holds up the knife. Identification is with the next victim in line as he is obliged to watch the preceding execution. Third, the actual ritual required by a middle-aged pervert who is impotent. From time to time he visits a prostitute, enquiring if she gives Russian lectures, which for him connote terrifying pogroms and prison scenes. He instructs her to scold him like a naughty child and threaten a severe beating with a club. He obediently takes down his trousers and often even before he receives a blow on the buttocks he ejaculates.

In none of these three examples, perhaps accidentally, Reik points out, does the perception of pain receive any significance, rather is the pleasure in anxiety or terror. Otherwise, all the accepted characteristics of masochism are present: the passivity, the impotent submission to another person, the terrible, degrading treatment and its concomitant sexual excitement. The three elements which, with varying intensity, constitute the inevitable essence of masochism are, however, as already mentioned in the previous chapter, the peculiar significance of phantasy, the suspense factor and the demonstrative factor. They are intimately associated and only different modes of expression of a deeply hidden essential.

The significance of phantasy is as a preparation for producing sexual tension. It can already be observed in the original scenes which initiated the perversion. The young girl had lived near a slaughterhouse and, together with her slightly older brother, watched their uncle and his fellow-butchers cutting up animals. Afterwards, in their garden, she would lie waiting on a bench until her brother came to cut her up with strokes of the hand. The preliminaries were pleasure-toned. Waiting to be slaughtered, anticipation of being handled produced sexual tension in her even at that time. In the Moloch scene, terrible future possibilities are phantasized, the material coming again from childhood, but its religious elaboration deriving from later reading. As a boy, his elder brother had shown him the results of a phimosis operation and ensuing phantasies involved their stern father who would operate (or cause a doctor to operate) on his own penis in due course. Homosexual stirrings had mixed with the need for punishment springing from masturbation. In the Moloch phantasy, he takes his place before the altar in a series of brothers, experiencing the anxiety of him who is next.

Reik now considers how masochism differs from other perversions in which the preliminaries of a desired situation are phantasized, noting that it is indeed the essence of perversion to linger in phantasy on the preparatory activities rather than progress to genital satisfaction. In sadism and voyeurism, phantasies will produce sexual tension, but satisfaction can also come about opportunistically without such preparation. With masochism, as with that other perversion with a passive goal, exhibitionism, phantasy is an indispensable preliminary in order to attain sexual excitement. Both depend on the reaction of a partner, and if it is not the desired one, then almost no sexual effect is produced. However, phantasy is not quite as important for the exhibitionist as for the masochist, for the former may decide to expose himself as soon as he sees a group of young girls approaching. The mere sight of a dog whip may be sufficient to produce sexual excitement in a masochist, but this is only when there has been a long phantasy preparation since the distant past. The material has been gone over so often that everything is prepared, and the glimpse of a whip can simply precipitate it at any moment, like the first notes of an old familiar melody. The fetishistic mechanism of substituting the detail for the whole is not peculiar to the excitability of any perversion. The erotogenic effect of surrogate details may indeed be seen in the field of normal sexuality. The masochistic perversion is, however, a realization of imagined situations with which the person has long concerned himself, the staging of a drama. The performance which actualizes the dramatist's phantasy conception is exposed to accidents and adaptations to the means at hand. It depends on the cooperation of the actors and usually falls short of the conception. Owing to this theatrical element, it seldom becomes a matter of 'deadly earnest' as with the sadist (cf. Freud, 1924*a*, p. 162). A peculiar feature is the tendency to 'synchronization'. In the Moloch phantasy, the sexual excitement ran a temporal course corresponding to the course of events, ejaculation always occurring at the point at which the high priest held up the knife. Masochistic situations are often conserved for years unchanged or with minor substitutions of people, times or places. Eventually a new situation may appear and be long maintained in its turn, with the old 'worn out' content obtruding now and then. These cycles create the impression that the masochistic phantasy is at length superseded because it has lost its power to excite, but the tenacity of phantasy is characteristic of masochism. Reik notes further that the phantasy is often verbal as well as visual. The masochist will then require to hear just those abusive or humiliating words in a certain order in actuality. It can become a stage story capable of extension to many suffering actors, drawn from later reading, the nucleus persisting through decades. The different scenes are selected according to their capacity for exciting and discarded on a diminution of their sexually stimulating value. Thus, to conservatism is opposed a need for variation, the 'successful' phantasy giving the most satisfactory orgasm. Identification is, of course, with the victim, but also with the active terrifying figure and sometimes with an onlooker who knows the feelings of both. Sometimes details are modified until they show consistency; at other times considerations of reality are ignored, a little like poetic licence. Most phantasies, elaborated from a core of reality, were first accompanied by sexual excitement and then recalled to consciousness when excitement recurs. In the desexualized form of masochism, phantasy construction is less discernible because it has spread over the whole life of the individual. The life configuration of the martyr, for instance, is based on an unconscious phantasy, only rarely on the possibly conscious one of being the victim of a hostile fate. Impersonal forces take the place of the abusing sexual partner, and hinder the attainment of his life purpose, causing him frustration and disgrace (cf. Freud, 1924*a*, pp. 165–170). Since the whole life story is acted out under the blows of destiny, there is no need to elaborate an isolated masochistic phantasy.

Reik next points to two features which distinguish masochistic from normal sexual gratification: the preponderance of the anxiety factor and the tendency to prolong the act. (It might be remarked *en passant* that there is a tendency 'to prolong' in general. For instance, an excruciating dawdling over meals is a typical masochistic provocation.) Sexual tension vacillates between pleasure and anxiety and is maintained instead of pressing towards discharge. It is better designated 'suspense', for tension denotes excitation, tending to reach a climax and subsequent discharge, whereas suspense connotes uncertainty, hesitation, being poised with no definite duration or termination of this state—an 'agony of suspense', or, conversely, the child's expectation of Father Christmas or the thriller-reader's of a solution. Being hung on some contraption is a masochistic practice which presumably gives a functional objectivity to the sensation of suspense. The masochist seeks to prolong the forepleasure or, more importantly, to avoid the end-pleasure, because it involves anxiety. The child's practice of reserving the best piece of food for the end can result in his renouncing it entirely, thus changing from self-control to an ascetic characteristic. This conflict of desire for the end-pleasure yet avoidance of it by the entrenched masochist results in a characteristic vacillation between the pleasurable and the fearful, a pleasurable-displeasure. He strives to 'have his cake and eat it,' but the striving tapers off into discontent, into a pleasureless ejaculation or the dissipation of tension without gratification. Most typically, in this alloy of pleasure-seeking and self-torture, the tension never rises until it flows over into gratifying orgasm but is maintained as suspense. Ultimately the anxiety associated with end-pleasure is displaced, and the increase in tension which could lead to orgasm is avoided also, leading to impotence. Wilhelm Reich's (1932) assertion that the masochist is incapable of increasing the tension is refuted by Reik. It is incorrect that each increase is immediately inhibited and transformed into displeasure so that end-unrest takes the place of end-pleasure. That occurs only as a final stage when fear of end-pleasure has become too great. Originally each increase in tension was desired, so long as it did not lead to orgasm, but of course it increased anxiety since orgasm brought the threat of castration and death. Reik (1939) sees the suspense factor as a double need, between anxiety and pleasure, determined by doubt, whether to step over the forbidden boundary or pull back before the fearful consequences. Not pleasant in the beginning, it becomes so as a substitute for orgasm. "Instead of the pleasure which brings with it an anxiety, there now appears an anxiety which produces a pleasure" (p. 44).

When there has been no punishment, abuse or pain before sexual intercourse, the suspense factor will inhibit gratification. Preliminary punishment or humiliation is an alternative which permits orgasm. Without it, there appears in place of the climax a suspense which leads to a disturbance of potency and finally to impotence. But even in masochistic practices, the suspense factor still operates, as with the middle-aged man visiting the prostitute. The scene falls into two parts: expectation of a blow, to which the abuse and threats have led up, and the masochistic practice itself. The waiting for the blow is more important libidinously than the actual blow and may precipitate ejaculation. It is a pleasing anxiety in face of punishment or humiliation. In the masochistic scene, therefore, the tension vacillating between pleasure and anxiety, is directed towards punishment, whereas in the phantasy it is directed towards the end-pleasure, which is not attained without preliminaries or else is transformed into terminal discontent. The suspense factor in phantasy is the former sexual tension transformed by unconscious anxiety; in the masochistic scene, a later stage, the anxiety has become pleasant. An anxiety-fraught pleasure has become a pleasurable anxiety.

Relating forepleasure with suspense, Reik points out that forepleasure anticipates end-pleasure of which it is a sampling, whereas suspense also anticipates future punishment, sampling a dish which is desired but forbidden. It is thus forepleasure plus foredispleasure and is transformed progressively into the latter, as when the first twinges of toothache cause one to test the tooth with one's tongue, repeat this to confirm the ache and continue touching the tooth lest it ache of its own accord suddenly and overwhelmingly. This is in order to prepare or harden oneself for pain and for the dentist, in order to prevent anxiety becoming too great; it is seeking out the very thing about which one is anxious, out of anxiety, an intentional seeking of foredispleasure to be better prepared for greater discomfort, an active rather than a passive role. The conversion of passive into reflexive (cf. Freud, 1915*a*, p. 128) also spreads tension over a longer time and thereby transforms strong into moderate excitement. The fore-displeasure does not come as a surprise to the masochist but by his instructions. His punishment or humiliation is selected by him, at a chosen time and according to his own rhythms, thus diffusing excitement over a definite period and diminishing anxiety. Instead of suffering anxiety, he has produced the suffering as master of his own destiny. He has anticipated all these terrors—"the masochistic mechanism is in its intentions a flight towards something lying ahead ... the psychic preparedness for discontent" (p. 48).

Passing to the third striking characteristic of masochism, the demonstrative feature, which invariably places suffering and humiliation in a showcase, Reik disagrees with Lampl-de Groot (1937) and Menninger (1938) who emphasize narcissism. The exposure of the body in masochistic practices might be termed exhibitionism but for two considerations: first, the exhibitionist displays what is thought to be beautiful or stimulating; second, the masochist displays in order to be provocative. Occasionally exposure suffices to touch off satisfaction, as with the girl's phantasy of lying naked in the butcher's shop, enjoying the feeling of being degraded and being ignored by the butchers, or the middle-aged man, exposing his buttocks to the prostitute. In cases where conscious pride is taken in the body, the punishment or pain which follows is perceived as more severe, the disgrace deeper. Where the body seems hateful or disgusting, its exposure will contribute to masochistic pleasure and sexual excitement. A shameful display of bodily or psychic awkwardness, the embarrassing situation, being watched while urinating or defaecating, are all enjoyed with the same anxious-pleasant feeling which accompanies corporal punishment.

This demonstrative feature is clearly recognizable in the desexualized forms of masochism, but Reik disagrees with Wilhelm Reich (1932) in calling this inhibited exhibitionism. It is a demonstrative concealment or an exhibition with reversed implications. A girl who would always refer to her lack of attractiveness precisely when she could have taken pride in it, wallowing in her own defects before an obligatory onlooker or listener, is hardly a case of inhibited exhibitionism, rather a divided or ambiguous attitude. If the masochist's suffering goes unnoticed, it loses its enjoyable character, though he may also strike the pose: "I bear no malice even if my heart breaks" (p. 54). The characters of Dostoevsky and Tolstoy expose their weaknesses voluptuously; Rousseau and Baudelaire confess as flamboyantly as the Christian martyrs, and ascetics display before their audience or, in the last resort, before God. In the history of a persecuted people, the association of being loved with being punished reaches the religious plane as the conviction of being chosen for a great mission. Increase in deprivation betokens the proximity of salvation and victory, even as increase in pain indicates the imminence of orgasm for the pervert.

The attention of others must be drawn through clumsiness or bad behavior, extending even to criminal acts, or through self-ridicule. In the clown, Pagliaccio, the laugh should not only conceal suffering but also betray it. Self-flagellation before a mirror is not really solitary since the spectator, himself, must witness the exposure and the beating, and share the pleasure, rather similarly to self-pity where a sympathetic mother is unconsciously present. The attempt to put a phantasized situation into execution by this mirror-beating scene, in which one person has taken over the role of the second, is a step away from phantasy and towards seeking an actual partner.

Most masochists feel that their exposure is shameful. Even if there is an exhibitionism with reversed signs this is not narcissism, which is an attitude of self-love expressing itself in self-satisfaction. Narcissus had no need to draw the attention of others when he fell in love with his mirror image. The narcissism of the masochist is, in Reik's view, deranged at the deepest level. If narcissism were represented by a gourmet, revelling in the solitary reading of food-books, masochism would best be represented by the man bearing emotive placards in front of a hunger demonstration. The demonstrative feature has the primary and essential goal, often unconscious, of evoking definite reactions in the environment. It is provocative, and in this it shows already the intimate relationship between masochism and sadism.

If one might point to one shortcoming of Reik's otherwise most impressive account of masochism, it would be that he fails to mention the 'deeply hidden essential' of which his three characteristics (the importance of phantasy, the suspense factor and the demonstrative factor) are only different modes of expression.

In his book *Masochism in Modern Man* (1941), Reik repeats this material, still without repairing the crucial omission just mentioned. He derives masochism from sadism and emphasizes the defiance, stubbornness and vengeful pride of the masochist, aiming, not at pain, but at pleasure, sooner or later, in his own way, at 'victory through defeat'. It is a pity that Reik points so frequently to the uniqueness and superior wisdom of his own insights over those of other analysts, but this boastfulness may perhaps be overlooked in someone who knows his subject so concretely and in such depth. His findings with respect to masochism will doubtless continue to be expanded and supplemented (for instance, in the physiological sphere, since he deals only with the psychological), may be peripherally modified, but are unlikely to be invalidated since they are deadly accurate. They are also presented with sufficient reiteration to drive them home.

One might take issue with one or two points. In summarizing (p. 30) Freud's conception of the origin of masochism, Reik explains the postulated fusion of the erotic and death instincts but omits Freud's concept of instinctual *de*fusion. Part III on the dynamics of masochism contains a chapter, 'The Impatience of Patience' (p. 110) in which Reik opines that the childhood punishments and humiliations of many masochists were not out of the ordinary but perceived hypersensitively. This disregards many cases of actual trauma in childhood. Even more could one disagree with the statement (Part IV: Ego-Gains, chapter on 'The Anticipated Rehabilitation'): "It has furthermore to be admitted that the damage caused by a masochistic character almost exclusively concerns his own person and hardly, and then only indirectly, others" (p. 261). Although Reik derives masochism from sadism, he does not give due weight to actual sadistic behavior in the entrenched masochist, only to role reversal and mocking. Equally doubtful is the curious assertion (Part VIII: Cultural Aspects, chapter on 'Marginal Problems') that erotogenic masochism, "the mixture of pleasure and pain or anxiety in early childhood", can only be reconstructed, never observed, and "would *only* amount to a physiological factor which makes masochism possible" (p. 374, italics added). But these are isolated criticisms of a major psychological study, demanding the greatest respect even today, or perhaps especially today.

Hilda Lewinsky (1944) summarizes the accepted view of masochism, largely due to Freud, as the turning of sadism upon the self, combined with a residue of primary erotogenic masochism. Besides the division into feminine and moral masochism, other accepted tenets are anal fixation and skin-erotism (cf. Freud, 1905, p. 169), avoidance of castration-anxiety and observance of superego prohibitions regarding genitality and sadism by avoiding responsibility for sexual satisfaction. Lewinsky, however, challenges the view that masochism is simply the passive counterpart of sadism and believes it can be accounted for without recourse to a death instinct. She centralizes narcissistic gains. The anticathexis set up by pain, draining all other psychical systems (Freud, 1920*a*, p. 30), means an increase of narcissistic libido, and the love object is used to induce this increase. Passivity, if ordering a specific form and degree of pain can be called passivity, is often an expression of strength and narcissistic tendencies. But as Eidelberg (1934) shows, the 'masochistic mechanism' by means of which external frustrations are rendered innocuous is an extremely active one, similar to the child's repetitive play. Lewinsky agrees with Ferenczi (1925, 1926) that the masochist only enjoys suffering specified by himself, thus saving his pride, sparing himself surprise and tension, and ensuring the concerned attention of the love object. Mortification or injury which is inflicted impersonally causes strong displeasure.

Education demands that the child should learn to endure tension as part of growing up. The masochist is not really adult—he is playing at toughness and his ego-ideal of invulnerability is supremely narcissistic. The hero of fairy tale and saga, the troubadour and the Romantic also glorify the masochistic attitude, but the cruelties of masochistic phantasy are most closely matched in reality by initiation rites and martyrdom in a religious or political cause, where the ability to endure suffering strengthens narcissism. Suffering becomes ecstatic because it makes the martyr equal to his god and sanctification confers approval posthumously.

The child may indeed see the grown-up as cruel and hard but, Lewinsky points out, the grown-up also smiles, even encourages, when struck with aggressive intent by the child. This is what the masochist acts out: "to be grown up is to find nothing painful, and to be grown up is—according to Freud—the most influential desire of childhood" (Lewinsky, 1944, p. 152). The masochist's capacity for suffering is, however, a myth, as noted by Wilhelm Reich (1932)—he wishes he could endure tension but in reality his threshold of tolerance is inferior, hence the phantasies of martyrdom, hence the staging of endurance and helplessness with the assistance of a partner. (A low pain threshold was, incidentally, attested to by no less a practising masochist than T.E. Lawrence.) Sexual excitation overrides pain, and Lewinsky supposes that the pain could not be borne at all without it, but it is this component, with its great narcissistic gain, which makes masochism so difficult to cure. Jeanne Lampl-de Groot (1937) found masochistic phantasies deriving from the Oedipus complex more easily dissolved than those serving to avoid 'narcissistic mortification', but Lewinsky goes further. Masochism is not just a flight from narcissistic wounds but an attempt to increase narcissistic libido, a search for heightened narcissistic cathexis. (Freud's (1920*a*) description of the anticathexis ensuing upon a breach in our protective shield against stimuli is again invoked as model for such an increased narcissistic cathexis, but the mechanism, as applied by Lewinsky to masochism, remains obscure.)

Does changing "I do not want to be beaten" to "I want to be beaten" correspond to a change of anxiety into libido? Lewinsky cites Freud's (1905, p. 203) observation of the sexually exciting effect an examination may produce on the schoolchild and quotes Laforgue (1930, p. 313) on anxiety being eroticized to the point where it becomes a substitute for normal orgasm. (Both citations might nowadays be related to stress-produced endogenous opioids as probable mediators of such effects.) In sadistic phantasies, to cause anxiety is often more important than to cause pain. It is a sign of power which the child sees as characteristic of the grown-up. To tolerate anxiety is a sign of maturity, and Lewinsky emphasizes that this view is shared by both child and grown-up. Like all perversions, masochism is a defense against castration-anxiety but this accepted finding might be extended to anxiety in general. The fact that anxiety is latent and does not become conscious as painful is an immense gain for the masochist. In this the change from passively suffering to deliberately orchestrating, in accordance with the repetition compulsion, plays an important part.

Changing "I want to be beaten" to "I want to be loved", Lewinsky likens the masochist to a pasha forcing the environment to minister to his desires. The environment, or more specifically the partner, having little feeling, cannot be hurt. This may mask sadistic impulses but, more importantly, it preserves an immense egocentricity. He craves strong feelings probably to reassure himself that his feelings are not dead, even to reassure himself against death itself. The pleasure principle has ostensibly been superseded by the reality principle, but he aims at the wholesale erotization of the reality principle. After punishment for nonfulfilment of tasks, he does not mend his behavior. "He projects his super-ego into the outer world and lives in a protracted, continual masturbation-phantasy" (p. 154). His need for punishment, for the presence of the object at all costs but without giving anything in return, can only mean an unpleasant relationship. Being loved would call for loving in return, for actions as well as feelings he does not want to give or cannot give.

Lewinsky looks briefly at precursors to the masochistic situation: weaning, where the mother is cruel and frustrating but is at least present, ministering to hunger; the smack for running off the pavement, where the degree of anxiety the mother transfers to the child will determine whether he loves her for saving him or hates her for smacking him. In the adult masochistic situation, the object is used to augment narcissistic libido, to permit the subject to receive attention and excitement without concern or reciprocity. This remains Lewinsky's main conclusion and her explanation for the great difficulty in treating masochism. She might well have added a corollary concerning the pathological laziness of her pasha figure.

Otto Fenichel (1945) accepts Freud's theories of masochism, except for the concept of primary masochism. He sees many masochistic phenomena appearing in analysis as "a strengthening of a passive-receptive giving oneself up for the sake of the pleasure of regaining participation in omnipotence" (p. 74). He likens some mechanisms in masochistic behavior to what Freud described as the 'signal' function of anxiety. Fantasies and rituals abound in castration threats, but castration is invoked in order to annul it.

Bertram Lewin's book *The Psychoanalysis of Elation* (1950) is both erudite and extreme. He invests the nursing of the infant at the breast with overriding developmental importance and confines himself almost exclusively to an oral interpretation of human behavior. The oral triad, consisting of the active wish to eat, the passive wish to be devoured and the wish to sleep, is established in the nursing situation, where physiological needs soon become psychological wishes. The sense of being engulfed just before falling asleep reappears, Lewin believes, in 'feminine' masochistic fantasies: "The sinking, falling, yielding, passive giving way that is expressed in the phobias as a fear of death and of being devoured is a replica of the passive erotic relaxation that follows upon nursing ... in its three attitudes at the breast, potentially, the baby would be, in successsion or in overlap, a cannibal, a masochist, and a suicide" (p. 116).

Lewin concludes his investigation of elation with the observation that reality, with its frustrations and deprivations, is viewed by the manic through rose-tinted spectacles, which "like many other paired and pink objects ... stand for the breasts. Reality is seen monochromatically through the rosiness of the mood at the breast" (pp. 181–182). Although far from Lewin's intention, this observation may help to elucidate the curious insistence of the pornographic literature of flagellation that white buttocks quickly become pink.

René de Monchy (1950) considers masochism as a pathological and as a normal phenomenon in the human mind, but considers it only from the instinctual point of view. He envisages a possible sublimation of masochistic impulses in the same way that aggressive drives can be sublimated and made useful to the individual and society. "The widely prevalent masochistic tendency to devotion and sacrifice can hardly be always labelled as pathological ... European culture of today is characterized by unusually strong tensions. The question arises whether one of the causes may not be the pronounced tendency to condemn and eliminate the masochistic impulses" (pp. 96–97). He echoes Freud's (1921) observations on the willing subordination of the individual to the typical organized group, the army or the church. He points to saints, idealists, reformers, artists, scientists as examples of those who deliberately sacrifice themselves and thereby "belong to the great ones of this world" (p. 97).

In 1948, Robert Eisler expanded his lecture to the Psychiatric Section of the Royal Society of Medicine to a book (Eisler, 1951) by the addition of copious notes and references in support of his main thesis that man was originally *le bon sauvage.* As well as wide-ranging erudition, he shares the propensity for wishful thinking and sweeping generalization of his mentor, C.G. Jung. His argument is supported in the main by anthropological, linguistic and mythological studies which dart from epoch to epoch, occasionally jolting down to earth with an allusion to a modern sex-crime. Apparently urban man went down the cul-de-sac of the Hamadryas baboon (to which the modern sadistic murderer could be a throwback), "armed with long powerful canine teeth for the fierce and passionate combats … which allowed only the strongest, tallest and most formidable males to transmit their individual characteristics" (p. 30). "It is obvious," he pronounces, "that the peaceful, food-collecting pygmies, ignorant of war, who inhabit the jungles and virgin forests, must be descended from the non-fighting, howler-monkey type Primates whose sexual behavior pattern survives 'archetypally' and atavistically in the average client of the public brothel … " (pp. 30–31).

"The sadist," he explains initially, "is obviously a person of feeble sympathetic resonance … The masochist, too, is a person of subnormal emotional sensitivity whose need … must therefore be assuaged by a strong dose of pain directly inflicted upon his or her own organism" (p. 26). From this momentous observation, we embark on prehistory, noting the turning point at the end of the pluvial period when the herd of harmless, frugivorous ape-men was driven by hunger to become a hunting pack. The blood-letting religious rites of the Maenads, the Hebrews, the Norsemen, the Berbers (to name but a few) all derive from this day of the wolf, as does the masochist's fascination with his naked 'Venus in Furs'.

Eisler's final hope of avoiding war is that this 'Fall', in the biblical sense, is reversible. If man was originally "a peaceful, frugivorous, non-fighting and not even jealous animal" (p. 51), he might (one suspects through Free Love) throw off "the fatal wolf's mask" (p. 52). The only light on sadomasochism emanates from the Notes—the quotations, bibliographic material and biographical details of de Sade and von Sacher-Masoch, though these are transparently tendentious.

Marie Bonaparte (1951) reviews Freud's two theories of sadomasochism. The first (*Three Essays on the Theory of Sexuality*), that masochism was derived from a primary sadism, was modified after the dualism of life and death instincts had been expounded to accept a primary erotogenic masochism (*The Economic Problem of Masochism*). She then cites passages from the Marquis de Sade (*Histoire de Juliette: Les Prospérités du Vice*, 1792), justifying sadomasochism as a sharper pleasure, and indicates their points of agreement with Freud's theories. She makes a distinction between aggressive and death instincts, tracing the former to the unavoidable penetration of the single living cell in the course of nutrition, reproduction and trauma. In the case of all mammals, there must be not only the penetration of ovum by sperm but the female body by the male penis, leading in the human female to psychical confusion between erotic and wounding penetration. Flight from the male or the acceptance of "some homeopathic dose of masochism" (p. 180) ensues. Turning from a phylogenetic to an ontogenetic consideration of masochism, she observes that coitus is always first viewed by the human child as an aggressive act. As a result, the little girl may either recathect her innate portion of masculinity as a defense or accept her role with "a truly feminine masochism" (p. 182); the little boy may either identify masochistically with his mother or accept his future role as male aggressor. Since pain and distress like other powerful stimuli have a concomitant sexual excitation, often awakened by "the whippings of ill-inspired upbringers", the human imagination permits the adult sadist to identify with his victim and enjoy the pain he inflicts, from his safe vantage point. After observing the ambivalence of Eros, that the passionate lover desires to unite completely, to devour, ultimately to destroy his beloved, Bonaparte considers sadomasochism in the inhibited or transformed shapes of moralization (the superego), the enquiring scientific spirit ("the surgeon reveals a certain regression, in this spirit, as actual penetrator of human flesh" (p. 188)) and art (Poe or Baudelaire). She ends on a sombre note, pointing to crimes of violence, blood sports and, above all, war as perseverating manifestations.

Margaret Brenman (1952) emphasizes that the masochistic character, as a complex phenomenon, serves many functions. It serves the id in gratifying instinctual drives, the superego in punishing or restricting pleasure as expiation, and the ego in providing a defense and even sometimes an adaptation to external reality. 'Specific' to masochism are an unusually strong need for love, resulting in aggression where the need is not met, and an unusually strong susceptibility to anxiety. The most typical ego defenses are denial, reaction-formation, introjection and projection.

Esther Menaker (1953) sees masochism primarily as a defense reaction of the ego to early oral frustration and emotional deprivation. Suffering is only its apparent, not its real, goal. Its function is as much self-preservative as libidinal—that of "maintaining a vitally needed love relationship to a primary object" (p. 208). If the mother fails to provide the loving affirmation necessary for the child's ego to develop normally, the demands of the developing ego become a source of pain and deprivation, and the self grows to be hated. The feeling of powerlessness is created by the mother's neurotic attitudes, yet she is regarded as the only hope of pleasure and survival long after this is biologically justified. For fear of being abandoned, the self is devalued and the mother idealized. Self-depreciation is at all levels—a submissive attitude, no faith in own faculties or judgment—in order to achieve passive oral gratification. Such a weak ego could have no life of its own, and to maintain the symbiotic bond, the mother's unloving attitude must be denied. Since no bridges have been built, the masochist's world is "divided into two antagonistic camps: children and adults" (p. 218) with the masochist as one of the children, entirely dependent and rendered helpless by the powerful adults. The masochistic reaction is even to be seen as the ego's defense against psychosis, "against loss of the outside world, since at this level of development the mother represents the total world outside the ego" (p. 220). The case history presented by Menaker is that of a young and attractive woman, whose development was mangled by being used for her mother's own narcissistic gratification. Its outcome was a relatively happy one. Masochism can, however, present a rather different picture from this, with a different aetiology and a different outcome. Possibly the quantity of aggressive drive, both internal and external, which is involved may be a determining factor.

Norbert Bromberg (1955), in emphasizing the role of the parents in the development of the masochistic character, notes that the narcissistic mother is sometimes transferring to her child a residual ambivalence towards her own parent. She is in turn cruel, seductive and restrictive, and she makes the child feel that it will obtain most love when it is suffering.

Rudolph Loewenstein (1957) divides Freud's 'phallic' phase into two stages, the earlier with passive aims of being looked at or touched, the later with aims of active penetration, the transition to which is often inhibited by castration anxiety. He identifies reversion or fixation to passive phallic aims as one of the prerequisites of masochism. The wish to be a helpless infant, taken care of by an all-powerful parent, is experienced as humiliating, but this is, in itself, also enjoyable.

The developing sexuality is beset by fears (of loss of the object or of its love, of castration, of the superego) and guilt, which demands suffering as the price of sexual pleasure, as a lesser evil than castration, or to expiate aggressive, incestuous impulses. The masochist anticipates actively what he fears may befall him passively. He devises his own torture so that he cannot be punished in an unexpected, uncontrollable way. (Horror films and books serve the same purpose.) In the case of a son's feminine wishes toward his father the fear of castration is alleviated by the substitution of a female figure who threatens and beats rather than penetrates him. Fixation to pre-genital, particularly anal, eroticism plays an essential part in the making of a masochist. He usually has screen memories alluding to traumatic events which involved a mixture of prohibition, seduction and reassurance. He seeks a specific form of humiliation and suffering, which must not be departed from or exceeded, and which is invariably the modified repetition of a childhood situation threatening castration. His sexual partner must play the prohibiting, threatening parent but, by participating in the incestuous gratification, annul the threat.

An anxious freezing into immobility at the moment of orgasm is sometimes connected with bed-wetting as a child, anticipating the mother's anger and threats. 'Bondage' may recall lying tightly tucked in a crib whilst a hated younger sib received attention, yet enjoying the suffering since violent resentment was safely curbed. Beating fantasies contain an element of hypocrisy which is the hallmark of a resexualization of morality.

Although Loewenstein refers constantly to Freud's writings on masochism, he does not accept the death instinct, only its aggressive aspect, and proceeds to talk it away by other Freudian concepts and mechanisms. (One cannot help wondering why Freud himself nevertheless firmly postulated a death instinct.) He terms one very early precursor of masochism 'the seduction of the aggressor', where every prohibition is turned into a game "to elicit the smile of the grownup, to create that affectionate complicity which undoes the prohibition and eliminates the danger of not being loved" (p. 214). Later this becomes "the seeking for situations that entail danger, fear and unpleasure, and their attenuation through a loving, erotic complicity of the threatening person" (p. 215). The unpleasure of the threat and the pleasure of its removal become closely linked. He points to another precursor in the fact that musculature and skin may give rise to both aggressive and libidinal gratification, both active and passive in form. Sometimes pain may be present before pleasure, as in itching or inflamed gums where scratching or clamping the jaws is simultaneously painful and pleasurable. Shutting the mouth to food or closing the anal sphincter may be prototypic masochistic behavior. The absence of a loving object relationship may lead to self-aggressive activity. Sulking, the complete ignoring of a hated person, is a form of 'passive aggression' which predisposes to masochistic character formation. The helpless child's anxiety over losing a powerful love object causes him to turn aggression inward. Later he seeks to "attenuate her anger into a domination precluding desertion" (p. 221). Guilt feelings may arise out of expectation of punishment, love and hate for the same object, or identification with the parent which enables the child to act in different roles at the same time. In masochism, instead of a surmounting of oedipal wishes, there is a regression to pregenital stages of development. "In this regression the genital involvement stems from the oedipal phase, the form and condition of the genital excitation—inflicting or undergoing suffering—from the earlier stage" (p. 222). The little girl, with her concave genitalia and lesser strength, learns to bend her aggression inward, to seduce the aggressor and be herself seduced by the threatening situation. (With 1950s' chauvinism, guilt is not thought to form much of her impedimenta!)

In choosing a love object, the masochist may form a slavish infatuation on the model of an early incestuous attachment or, at the other extreme, require only behavior which satisfies his condition for sexual gratification. This far end of the spectrum may involve a severe ego disturbance and verge on psychosis. There is a correlation between the masochistic character and paranoia, but Loewenstein does not believe in any general affinity between perversion and psychosis. One of the main functions of sadomasochism is to maintain object relations, albeit precariously, in the face of aggressions which threaten them or the individual himself. It permits a limited and precarious survival of genitality. Since he himself suffers, the masochist need feel no remorse that his suffering causes pain to others.

Isidor Bernstein (1957), in considering the importance of narcissism in masochistic character formation, observes that as infants his patients were "in the service of the parental narcissism and immature instinctual drives" (p. 376) and became masochistic to protect themselves from object loss. Unfortunately, the clinical material is served up with a briskness verging on incoherence and, since everything including the kitchen sink has been thrown into the pot, rather indigestible.

Bernhard Berliner (1940, 1947, 1958) attributes the masochistic character to punishment and humiliation from cruel, rejecting parents. Having never experienced normal parental love, the child later seeks similar treatment from others as a substitute for love, as the only form of love he knows. Masochism is a defense of the ego (as Esther Menaker also asserted in 1953) and serves to preserve object relations where the danger of loss causes overwhelming anxiety. Berliner's message is consistent and extreme: "There is a deep conviction in the masochist that he is not supposed to be loved and to be happy but that he has to meet the desires of those who hate him, to whom his existence or his happiness is unwanted" (1940, p. 327). "Masochism is the hate or the sadism of the object reflected in the libido of the subject ... Primarily it has nothing to do with the masochist's own sadism" (1947, p. 461). "Masochism is a defensive reaction, motivated by libidinal needs, to the sadism of *another person*" (1958, p. 44).

It is not his fault but his mother's that he is destructive—the masochist is given the benefit of the doubt, both in the case of the perversion and of moral masochism. What is Berliner's rationale for this wholesale exoneration? "In the beginning, all masochistic suffering was love—and the sadism of another person. One's own sadism vented upon the ego produces not masochism, but compulsion neurosis" (1947, p. 463).

Alex Blumstein (1959) outlines several cases where masochism is associated with self-preparation for a secure and physically gratifying union with an omnipotent figure. The particular path of incorporation depends on libidinal development. The wish to be eaten and the fear of being devoured belong obviously to the oral phase, but some individuals have fantasies of evaporating and being inhaled. One woman's fantasy concerned being prepared for sacrifice to the river gods, pushed down the river in a leaking boat and eaten by fish. This was not a punishment but a union with the gods and with her mother who had been drowned at sea. Another young man combined a tendency to overeat with a fear of cancer which dissolves the body. Both related to his dependency first on his mother then on his analyst, the one symptom a defense against and the other a self-preparation for being incorporated and protected by an omnipotent figure. In terms of the oral triad discussed by Bertram Lewin (1950), sadism and masochism are aspects of the wishes to eat and be eaten: "In the nursing situation, sadism finds its foreshadowing in the first active stage, masochism in the ensuing yielding and sleep" (Lewin, 1950, p. 116). Later phases of libidinal development may be regressively related to the oral phase. The sexual organ may be equated with the devouring mouth. One young man, suffering from premature ejaculation, would clutch the bed in his fear of falling into the woman, whom he identified with a pregenital, frustrating mother figure.

Blumstein sees the masochistic fantasy as a reversal of the wish to devour the object, a reversal due to feelings of guilt, to fear of retaliation or fear of losing the object. The basic objective is to maintain a bond with a frustrating, omnipotent figure.

Ludwig Eidelberg's (1959) paper on "Humiliation in Masochism" deals more in definitions of humiliation versus punishment than in insights into masochism. (It must be confessed that one is somewhat estranged on first reading by the fact that three of his five references are to his own publications, whilst he cites one of them after the admonition that "external punishment must be differentiated from what is *usually* referred to as external narcissistic mortification" (p. 275). The impression is not helped by wordings such as "... all individuals, *according to Freud*, are interested in achieving pleasure and in avoiding unpleasure" (p. 275), or "... this patient and some other masochists were *cured* after they had recognized that the defeat from which they had suffered was unconsciously self-provoked" (p. 281, italics added in each case).) However ... Eidelberg makes the initial point that 'the emotion of pleasure' only accompanies instinctual gratification if the object and means of discharging tension are acceptable to the whole personality. Anticipatory pleasure will change in time to unpleasure if end pleasure is not forthcoming. Another unpleasure, 'narcissistic mortification', is defined by Eidelberg as loss of control over reality caused by internal or external 'enemies', and related to both punishment and humiliation. External punishment may force an individual to refrain from certain actions or to do what the punisher wants, but it may also mobilize defiance. External narcissistic mortification may not necessarily be either a punishment or deterrent from trying again (for example, a lost game of chess or a failed examination)—it simply refers to a defeat or failure.

Although each humiliation represents a punishment, the converse is not true. Humiliation adds ridicule to punishment and represents an abstract condensation of various concrete images of people who would be considered as humiliated by some though not by others. The punishment sought by the masochist is a humiliating one, owing to exhibitionist tendencies, and it must be a consciously or unconsciously chosen one, in order to expunge a repressed memory of narcissistic mortification. This chosen punishment, which shows him as a failure and ridiculous, protects against humiliation which was not ordered or provoked by him.

If society can punish to protect itself, it can also increase the punishment by making it, in addition, a humiliation (as in the Middle Ages or the Nazi era) but the subject may or may not perceive the latter. A humble person may be difficult to humiliate. The best defense is self-humiliation or humility. An individual may prefer to be laughed at than ignored because in being laughed at he discharges exhibitionist wishes even though unpleasurably. However, if punishment seems unjust, the subject may refuse to humiliate himself. Where he acknowledges he did wrong (self-humiliation), he accepts punishment out of remorse and in the hope that by humbling himself he will eliminate remorse and undo the wrong, promising not to repeat it and begging forgiveness. He may, of course, be feigning contrition whilst planning revenge.

Those who humiliate usually wish to force a self-humiliation. Parents insist a naughty child should not only be beaten but acknowledge wrongdoing. The fact that punishment eliminates remorse may be advantageous to the individual but not to society, in the opinion of those who prefer guilt-ridden fellow-citizens. (By this time, the sensation of reading an 18th century treatise on moral philosophy is so strong that one becomes confused as to which side Eidelberg is on!) External punishment, calling up defiance, is deemed unfair because it does not accord with the judgment of the individual's own superego. Society must either find a punishment which is accepted by the criminal or prevent repetition by means such as capital punishment or life-imprisonment. It is surely preferable to adopt principles which appear reasonable to all or at least to the majority.

Eidelberg regards external humiliations as the masochist's aim. The pervert seeks genital discharge while being beaten, urinated upon or simply scolded. The moral masochist seeks to be humiliated by others in defeat. After a few rather garbled remarks about the reality principle, Eidelberg states that "the masochist is not interested in being able to accept pain or frustration in order to achieve a final victory after a long fight" (p. 280)—a statement which might well raise some doubt. He pursues his ruminations with a subtle distinction between external narcissistic mortification, where an external object forces us to abandon what we want, and external humiliating punishment, where we should never have had or disclosed the wish which led to humiliation. On slightly firmer ground, the masochist's unconscious guilt about immoral wishes is not eliminated by punishment because the repressed wishes are not repudiated, so the need for punishment is never satisfied. Infantile wishes persisting in an adult are not acceptable to the total personality and, as no distinction is made between wish and action, they produce remorse (?) and call for external humiliating punishment. The masochist buys permission to continue to sin and to discharge aggression by accepting unfair punishment and humiliation. He thus satisfies exhibitionist as well as aggressive wishes and retains his infantile omnipotence by always succeeding in provoking humiliating defeat.

In a short but extremely interesting paper 'On Teething', published in 1959, Otakar Kucera's point of departure is the Isakower (1938) phenomenon. This, he agrees, is a regression to an only slightly differentiated state of the psychic apparatus, but it may consist of several components—a mixture of tactile (mouth and skin), kinesthetic, vestibular, acoustic and visual perceptions. These perceptions are amorphous, both pleasurable and unpleasurable, and concern something that fills the whole of the mouth cavity but cannot be spat out. Kucera reports on a patient whose related sensations, mostly when lying awake at night, were of a smooth soft surface becoming torn, without any escape from the process, and who finally concluded himself that it was his first, preverbal memory of the eruption of his teeth. The psychoanalytic view is that this event is a dividing line between the first oral phase of sucking and the second cannibalistic phase of biting and tearing. The development of the aggressive instinct has, Kucera points out, mostly been considered as part of that of the libido. Both oral stages have been described as completed formations, but scant attention has been paid to the process dividing them, dentition. It appears when mouthing of the breast and other objects with the gums has fully developed, as have the muscles to execute aggression. Mouthing and gnawing are accompanied by crushing and squeezing with the hands. Both give unequivocal satisfaction until the eruption of teeth causes swollen gums. This new pain increases oral aggressivity but intensified gnawing only exacerbates the pain. The hands and other objects are put into the mouth, clutched and crushed with greater vigour for several days or even weeks. Dentition may cause raised temperature, loss of appetite, diarrhoea, irritability or sleeplessness which only subsides after tooth-eruption.

Increased neuromuscular excitability and increased intestinal peristalsis are distinct signs, the former discharging through the muscles of the mouth and hands, the latter giving rise to diarrhoea. Excitation of the oral zone can induce excitation of the maturing anal zone. The tension that cannot be overcome by gnawing or sucking the fingers is transferred to the digestive tract which has means of expelling irritating contents. Oral excitation is probably also a contributing factor to diarrhoea from malnutrition. Such early mechanisms may determine later functional disorders of the gastrointestinal tract.

Teething plays an even more important role, however, in the genesis of normal and pathological mental life. A usually pleasurable experience is suddenly disturbed by pain. The very activities by which tension was removed, sucking and gnawing, now produce more pain and tension, establishing a link between satisfaction of libidinal and aggressive drives on the one hand and painful experiences on the other. The connection is especially strong between aggression and pain, since pain normally mobilizes anger to remove its source through muscular activity, which here only intensifies it—in Kucera's opinion, the key organic foundation for primary masochism. The universal nature of teething would explain the universal basic quota of erotogenic masochism. There is a link to the skin, another organic basis of the masochistic component, by the hands touching, squeezing and scratching it. Nail-biting is derived from finger-sucking and -biting. The erogenous potential of the skin is extended by the libidinous cathexis of the anal mucosa, provoked by frequent cleansing of the buttocks. The masochistic component is variously influenced by individual circumstances, notably by the pattern of the Oedipus complex, but remains closely connected with the aggressive instinct through all developmental phases. Secondary masochism is nourished by aggression turned against the ego after frustration with external objects. The core of erotogenic masochism, created in the phase of dentition, may eventually be integrated in the personality as a subordinate part, converted into moral masochism, used in the faculty of objective thinking, deployed as so-called feminine masochism, incorporated in some neurosis, or developed as a sexual perversion. The outcome depends on three basic lines of development: that of the libido, of aggressivity, and of the ego. The quantity of primary erotogenic masochism, the trigger mechanism, is thought to be determined by heredity. This concept can be simplified into physiological factors, themselves often hereditary, such as the circumstances of teething (too soon, too late or too condensed) or the condition of the oral cavity itself (making tooth-eruption difficult). The facts might be looked for in systematic longitudinal research. The importance of the mouth as the primal cavity, the bridge between inner and outer perception, the organizer of further psychic development, will emerge in other connections, but dentition must play a key role in the aetiology of primary masochism. Kucera's arguments are persuasive in themselves and would seem to be supported by a simple personal observation made by the present author, that toothache and diarrhoea are frequent complaints of masochists. An original impression of long standing to this effect was confirmed by some of the biographical details collected in the course of the empirical study reported in Part 2 and mentioned in Appendix 3.

Charles Brenner (1959) defines masochism as "the seeking of unpleasure, by which is meant physical or mental pain, discomfort or wretchedness, for the sake of sexual pleasure, with the qualification that either the seeking or the pleasure or both may often be unconscious rather than conscious" (p. 197). (While a reasonable definition, this takes no account of the fact that masochistic practices may, of course, also be a mechanism simply for relieving neural tension. It is also debatable whether pleasure can be unconscious.) In summarizing Freud's theories, Brenner refers, rather unusually among the summarizers, to *Mourning and Melancholia* (1917*b*) where Freud deals with the mechanism of identification with a lost object which was both loved and hated, resulting in self-directed sadism, or masochism. (Brenner might have followed this through to the observation that the early death or divorce of parents does, in fact, figure largely in the history of many a masochist. Jules Glenn (1984*a*) describes how the disappearance of parents triggers masochistic defense behavior. Several sadomasochistic subjects participating in the present study spoke at length of the effect of early parental disappearance, death, or divorce (Appendix 3). Such early loss of parents obtained, of course, in the case of adopted subjects—no less than 5 of them in the sadomasochistic group of 48.) Passing from Freud's modified view (1924*a*) that pain, like any intense stimulus, causes concomitant sexual excitement in the infant and this later becomes 'the physiological substrate which is then covered by a psychic superstructure' to form basic erotogenic masochism, to Freud's hypothesis of the death instinct, operating independently of the pleasure principle, Brenner agrees with Fenichel (1945) that the validity of this hypothesis is a matter for biologists to decide. (Had Freud himself no scientific background, then?) Brenner reads (most would say misreads) Freud's (1924*a*) classification of masochism into erotogenic, feminine and moral as meaning that erotogenic, rather than feminine, masochism referred essentially to the perversion. He points out, in connection with the return of outwardly deflected aggression as secondary masochism, that in Freud's view, self-directed destructiveness and self-directed libido would have to fuse to some extent to account for *pleasure* in pain, since the discharge of destructive energies alone would not be accompanied by the subjective quality of pleasure. Finally, in close connection with oedipal conflicts, Freud related masochistic phenomena to the (Brenner omits to say 'sadistic') superego. After outlining the points of agreement and divergence in the work of analysts since Freud, Brenner attributes changes in technique and scope largely to ego analysis and superego analysis, "since the unconscious operations of the superego play such a large part in masochistic character formations" (p. 205). An appreciation of the defensive aspect of masochistic fantasy and behavior could only grow gradually after Freud (1926) had reintroduced the general concept of ego defenses in *Inhibitions, Symptoms and Anxiety*.

Proceeding to some formulations concerning the genesis of masochistic character traits, Brenner agrees with Reik (1941) that such traits are ubiquitous in so far as a need for punishment, be it conscious or unconscious, is a part of normal superego functioning. Oedipal fear of castration may engender a passive, feminine attitude to the father as a defense and, though normally becoming unconscious in the course of time, leave a need for penance and expiation—a subsidiary aspect of superego function referred to as remorse. The differences between normal and neurotic manifestations of masochism would seem to be quantitative rather than qualitative, with the resulting difficulty in separating the masochistic character diagnostically from various other pathological conditions, such as paranoia (Bak, 1946), obsessional neurosis (Fenichel, 1945), depression, conversion hysteria, phobia or addiction. One alcoholic patient's drinking bouts were a way of producing misery and helplessness from which he would be rescued by a loving father. Another bisexual patient with a phobia for ill-lit streets was tormented by an unconscious wish to be beaten and castrated by a man. There are many others with masochistic tendencies but no history of conscious beating fantasies or perversion, such as these two had. If in masochism the pathological differs from the normal only by degree, one may regard infantile factors as increasing or decreasing the tendency rather than look for a 'cause' in infancy of masochistic phenomena later in life. Why should masochism be universal, if indeed it is? One answer might be based on the dual instinct theory (Freud, 1920*a*): both the destructive and the erotic drives are self-directed in the neonate and this primary masochism, in view of the universal tendency to repeat an earlier state, may be reestablished in later life, at least partially, as secondary masochism (a somewhat garbled version of Freud's own account (1924*a*) since it omits the stages of instinctual defusion, projection and subsequent reintrojection of aggression, and regression). Another answer, reflecting clinical observation, might be that, given the instinctual drives and ego capacities of the child on the one hand, and its available gratifications and inevitable frustrations on the other, some degree of masochism is bound to occur in its psychic functioning. These two suggestions are not contradictory.

Also related to the ubiquity of masochism is the fact that sadistic and masochistic tendencies are always observed together. One expects behavior or fantasies to have a sadistic, hostile meaning as well as a masochistic, passive one. The relationship is not simply one of polarity or competition since each has a defensive function and each is a means of instinctual gratification. As Brenman (1952) emphasized, the multiple function of masochistic character formation means that it can best be understood by unravelling the interrelated functions of ego, superego and id. A single group of fantasies and behavior may serve various functions, as in the case of an unmarried woman suffering from anxiety and depression who was nevertheless able to continue responsible work, joylessly but uninterruptedly, for several years. As a child, her father spent every Saturday night drinking in the red-light district of their semirural community. In her fantasies, she was herself a prostitute and coitus was represented sadomasochistically as a violent fight between man and woman. On one occasion when her mother and father were quarrelling, the nine-year-old threatened to stab him with a fork. Although capable of verbal abuse, her mother's attitude was generally that of martyr, and in identifying with her, the child saw her own future as being abused and mistreated by men while striving to revenge herself on them. Her father died, vomiting blood, after a year's illness consequent upon his dissipations, when she was seventeen, and some years later her brother killed himself. The first event augmented her unconscious guilt, and the second confirmed her fear that her murderous wishes could actually kill. Self-punishment appeared instead of anger when men failed to respond to her with love. In analysis she manifested a negative therapeutic reaction and was often reproachful or silent. Brenner's interpretation is that, unconsciously, she was both expiating guilt for sadistic wishes and gratifying them. Her sulkiness duplicated her mother's behavior to her father. In her conflict with her superego, her suffering served not only as a submissive expiation but also as a defense against guilt, since it demonstrated that she was the meek victim of a cruel analyst. In every masochistic character, one is likely to find an unconscious need for punishment and atonement, but other motivating factors vary. Separation anxiety played a minor role in this girl's case but in others may play a major role in the genesis of masochistic traits. In emphasizing some particular genetic factor, authors have probably erred in what they have omitted to mention as motive or function in these traits. For instance, Berliner (1940, 1947, 1958) and Menaker (1953) concentrate only on object relations, and a similar emphasis is discernable in Bernstein (1957), Brenman (1952) and Bromberg (1955). Certainly masochistic fantasies and behavior may function as a defense against fears of losing an object or its love, but these are not the only fears. Fear of castration and fear of the superego also call up defense. In the boy who needs his father's love as a guarantee against castration, in the girl who equates possession of a penis with being her parents' favourite, the fear of loss of love and the fear of being without a penis are barely distinguishable.

Turning to problems of treatment, Brenner cites first the negative therapeutic reaction, due to an unconscious need to be punished. According to Eidelberg (1934; Panel, 1956), "the problem of the recognition and final elimination of the infantile omnipotence is of decisive importance". The masochist uses his ability to produce failure and to provoke punishment as proof of his magical control of the environment. One must focus on these manifestations of his fantasy of omnipotence, particularly in the transference, and then convince him that "to stop being masochistic does not mean that he will become the helpless slave of the environment" (p. 215). Of course, he must first see that his suffering is not in spite of himself but self-induced.

Freud was pessimistic about the success of treatment, except where the origin of a patient's masochism lay in an identification with a masochistic parent, and many since Freud have shared his pessimism. Brenner does not, however, regard masochistic character traits as unanalysable and believes that a masochistic transference reaction should be analysed, like any other resistance, by directing attention to it, viewing it objectively, discovering its role as a defense, a gratification, an expiation or a punishment, and by communicating understanding of its genesis and its role at an appropriate time. All patients use 'reality' to relive infantile conflicts and desires, and sadomasochists are no exception. From Brenner's experience, it is necessary, first, to avoid unconscious participation in sadomasochistic behavior through becoming angry or defeated, and second, to perceive the various meanings and purposes behind masochistic behavior, however well rationalized—in short, to handle the masochistic patient as one might "a sulky, stubborn, provocative child" (p. 224).

Victor Smirnoff (1969) looks at the life of Leopold von Sacher-Masoch himself, and at its curious parallel in *Venus im Pelz* (known in English as *Venus in Furs*), in terms of 'the masochistic contract'. Smirnoff's paper has some compelling insights but is uneven in comparison with Gertrud Lenzer's (1975) study, reviewed below. Besides commanding a better prose style and besides dealing in depth with much more of her subject's literary output, Lenzer is scrupulous in mentioning any doubts surrounding dates and events, whereas Smirnoff has no such tentative approach. This makes one uneasy.

Smirnoff glances briefly at previous contributions to the study of masochism: Reich (1932) on primary versus secondary masochism, Nacht (1938) on guilt, Reik (1941) on moral masochism and Lagache (1961) on aggressivity, the 'narcissistic masochistic position' and the 'search for submission'. This emphasizes the position of the masochist in the masochistic relationship and launches Smirnoff on his main theme. *Venus im Pelz*, he points out, must have been based partly on Sacher-Masoch's liaison with Fanny Pistor for (he believes) it was published at least a year before Sacher-Masoch met his wife, Aurore Rumelin (alias Wanda von Dunajev). Even more, it is a work of fantasy which he attempted to actualize. His wife, Wanda, reported to him the criticism that his novels were monotonous with their single female stereotype. "You shall have to mistreat me," was his response, "and I promise that all these cruel females will disappear for ever from my books." The most important characteristic of the contract in both life and fiction is the immutability of the arrangement. Wanda von Sacher-Masoch records in her (1906) *Confessions* that he did indeed give up flogging scenes in his subsequent novels but, conversely, forced her to repeat his initial formula with ever more elaborate whips, making her task 'as painful as possible'. For Smirnoff this is the real meaning of the masochistic contract: "to render the executioner's task more oppressive" (p. 666). Just as the sadist does not want a willing victim, the masochist does not want a consenting accomplice—there is thus no true complementarity between the two. The masochist treats his tormentor as an employee, specifying a uniform, the required setting, the rules. Neither the physical nor the moral suffering defines the specificity of the masochistic pleasure as much as the 'casting'. Alexis Papadopolis, the Greek, administers the final flogging in *Venus in Furs* much to Severin's disgust and dismay. Alexis is a real sadist, enjoying his role, not coerced into it, and therefore not part of the contract.

The pleasure, described by Sacher-Masoch as *übersinnlich* (Smirnoff renders this as 'beyond sensuality'), may incorporate vision, touch and pain, but it lies chiefly in the interplay between victim and executioner. The concept of *victima*, immolated to appease the gods, adds sacrifice to pain and pleasure. The iconography of martyrdom always portrays a basic component of ecstasy: the mystical trance, the languid tortured body, the orgasmic posture and expression--the same elements as are found in pictorial representations of masochism. The suspended sacrificial gesture, as when Abraham's knife hovers over Isaac or Agamemnon's over Iphigenia, is the equivalent of the decisive moment in the choice of a fetish (Freud, 1927): "it is as though the last impression before the uncanny and traumatic one is retained as a fetish" (p. 155). As a boy, Sacher-Masoch witnessed the adulterous relations of his aunt, Countess Xenobie von X, being interrupted by her husband and her ensuing rage. Young Leopold was dragged from the wardrobe and horsewhipped, with admitted pleasurable excitement. The whip and his aunt's fur-lined jacket become the fetish, just before the feminine image is shattered, at the moment when the guilty sexual relations and the voyeuristic pleasure are related to violence. This traumatic scene is nevertheless regarded by Smirnoff as a screen memory, with an already established symbolic network lying behind it.

In the masochistic ceremony, everything is settled by strict rules, in advance. The masochist can only be the victim of a reluctant executioner. He must bear witness to his victimized status by the evidence of his wounds. He must be branded, but not destroyed, and not by the absolute power of the executioner but by the power conferred by himself, a power forced on the executioner by contract, only to be exercised at the victim's order. Masochism is defiance, expressed through apparently passive behavior, through compliance in pain and humiliation. The executioner, obliged to play the role of master, is in fact a slave, a creature of the masochist's desire.

Smirnoff emphasizes the dual feminine ideal of the masochist. In her *Confessions* (1906), Wanda reports that her husband's mother represented for him 'the noblest and highest of all women, unattainable in her perfection and her pureness'. He believes that women are degraded by social conventions and, even worse, 'they do not realize their own falseness and mental deformity'. Given the unattainability of the ideal, he must make do with its opposite, the evil woman who at least admits to her brutality and egotism. On the one hand, the burning image of a callous and rejecting woman, on the other, the cold and empty image of purity, two sides of the same coin, the projection of the split ego on the primary love object (Freud, 1940*b*). The dual structure of the object is preserved throughout *Venus in Furs*, clothes, rather than the physical core, determining which role is to be played according to the masochistic contract. Both roles must be played by the same woman, the masochist's wife or mistress, so clothes and accessories become indispensable for keeping the roles apart. Were they to coalesce and nullify the ego defenses, delusion might take over. At first Severin thinks Alexis is a woman in disguise. When this 'hermaphrodite' has maltreated him, Severin thinks himself cured by too much pain and humiliation. What he has actually been deprived of by the sadistic Greek is his ascendant masochistic position and his fantasy of a phallic Venus. Wanda deserts him, laughing, in her vulgar furs, and there is no secret fantasy left. Further disavowal is useless—he must confront the fear of castration without the masking panoply of masochism. Smirnoff urges a redefinition of clinical forms of masochism: not pleasure in pain but the actualization of a contract regulating the relationship in the masochistic performance.

Gertrud Lenzer (1975) introduces her excellent paper on the character and writings of Leopold von Sacher-Masoch with some biographical details. (If aware of Victor Smirnoff's (1969) paper dealing with his life from the standpoint of 'the masochistic contract', she makes no mention of it.) Born on January 27, 1836 (or according to Magnus Hirschfeld (1930), on January 7, 1834), in Lemberg, von Sacher-Masoch studied law in Prague and Graz, became a *Privatdozent* in history but abandoned an academic career for writing. His short stories and novels are mostly unread and unobtainable, but their essence has survived in the concept of 'masochism', coined by Krafft-Ebing (1886), in which the "individual affected is controlled in his sexual feeling and thought by the idea of being completely and unconditionally subject to the will of a person of the opposite sex; of being treated by this person as a master, humiliated and abused. This idea is associatively suffused with sensual pleasure; such an individual revels in phantasies, in which he creates situations of this kind and often attempts to realize them" (pp. 94–95). Sacher-Masoch died on March 9, 1895 (or according to James Cleugh (1951), was committed to a mental hospital in Mannheim on that date, dying there only in 1905), but Krafft-Ebing's term and definition, despite Hirschfeld's suggestion of a more impersonal alternative, algolagnia, have continued to influence both scientific and popular writers. Krafft-Ebing defined a phenomenon which until then had remained undifferentiated; inadvertently he demonstrated the historical limitations of consciousness, for once the boundaries of interpretation are trespassed, they are subsequently revised. Masochism was soon linked with its supposed opposite, sadism, by Freud, Stekel and others. Freud made a distinction, sometimes overlooked by more recent writers, between latent and manifest perversions, the former occurring much more frequently than the latter. Beside those who seek satisfaction in reality are those content to imagine that satisfaction, who need no real object since it can be replaced by phantasy. Though de Sade and von Sacher-Masoch were prisoners of their phantasies, they made a step toward their objectification, externalizing them by verbalizing them. To Krafft-Ebing the content of masochistic phantasies constituted masochism—the symptoms of the disease constituted the disease—whereas to Freud these phantasies emanated from hidden impulses and ideas which they sought to mask and to fortify. Lenzer's own study was undertaken in the context of an investigation of the cultural and political climate which culminated in Nazism. She was struck, she says, by the quantity of German publications, from the latter part of the 19th century to the 1930s, on women, perverse sexuality and criminality. These subjects were the preoccupations of historians, philosophers and doctors alike. Not perhaps by chance was psychoanalysis itself created during this period.

A recurrent theme in these scholarly investigations was the superiority of women and their dominating influences upon men, whilst just as frequent was the countertheme that women were inferior in various respects to men. The idea of the cruel, dominating woman underwent considerable formal variation, and its persistent treatment was not only scholarly but, equally, pornographic. The homogeneity of the phantasy and the formal heterogeneity of its appearance suggested to Lenzer that it was a shared or collective one, meriting detailed examination. She chose the works of Sacher-Masoch because they presented the phantasy components with little elaboration and lacked rather than possessed the literary qualities to which their author aspired. He permitted his phantasies such associative licence that they clearly reveal the 'primary processes' at many points. They are endless variations on the one theme of the cruel woman in her relations to men who enjoy submitting to her domination and wantonness. The incomplete revision that his phantasies undergo facilitates their interpretation, precisely because of the hybrid (pseudopornographic, pseudoliterary) form of their presentation. It soon emerged that they covered, besides masochism (as initially conceptualized from them), what would later be categorized as fetishism, voyeurism, transvestism or latent homosexuality. These perversions were isolated in the course of evolving psychoanalytic theory rather than in the subject matter now again under scrutiny.

Although Sacher-Masoch is thought to have written some piously religious works under the pseudonym C. Arand (Lenzer is too cautious to point to the invariable masochistic trait of hypocrisy), most of his stories and novels are repetitions of the themes which predominate in *Venus im Pelz* (dated 1870 by Hirschfeld). Here as elsewhere, he employs the device, frequent in pornographic fiction, of a 'framing action', an account told through a diary or a series of letters. Severin von Kusiemski's 'Confessions of a Supersensualist' are given in trust to a nameless friend who takes tea at his estate. The stylistic device serves as a defense, to distance the main action from the author (again evidence of hypocrisy). Before his afternoon visit, the friend has in fact had a dream which not only introduces the larger action but outlines it: Venus, the ideal of female beauty, faces him across the massive fireplace, her marble body curled cat-like in a huge sable fur. She complains of the coldness, both physical and emotional, of the Germanic North. They agree that in the immutably regulated game of love, man and woman are natural enemies, uniting briefly, before renewed alienation. "Whichever of the two fails to subjugate will feel the foot of the other on his neck only too soon." The more devoted the woman, the cooler and more domineering the man; the more wanton and cruel she is, the more passionate and worshipping he becomes. Woman has the advantage since man is the one who desires.

In the 'Confessions,' the friend's dream is transposed to a sort of reality. Severin von Kusiemski's diary tells of his youth in a park-encircled house in a Carpathian spa, where he has fallen in love with a stonily smiling statue of Venus. At night he kneels and presses his face against the cold stone beneath her feet, but he also worships a reproduction of Titian's painting depicting Venus in sables. One day his stone and painted images come to life when he encounters Wanda von Dunajev, the twenty-four-year-old widow who lives in the rooms above his. She seeks "the serene sensuousness of the Greeks, pleasure without pain" and could only remarry a man who would subjugate her, before whom she would have to kneel. Severin, however, explains: "Whenever it is a matter of choice for me of ruling or being ruled, it seems much more satisfactory to be the slave of a beautiful woman." Wanda, with her 'demonic' red hair and 'diabolic' green eyes, agrees to her role-change and, as his ideal of the cruel female despot, finds pleasure in abusing and flogging him, always wearing the mandatory furs. They go to Florence, noted for homosexuality, having 'sanctified' (again hypocrisy) their liaison with a contract by which Wanda is given the power of life and death over her slave (now renamed Gregor) provided she perpetrates her cruelties in furs. He significantly renounces "all his rights as her lover" and follows "at a repectful distance of ten paces" when they go out. The disastrous climax is reached when, lashing the horses of their carriage along the promenade, Wanda is arrested by the god-like Greek, Alexis Papadopolis, on his small black horse (the farcical element in masochism is strongly implied but never made explicit by Lenzer). She now finds 'Gregor' only boring and he attempts suicide, pulling himself out of the Arno with a convenient willow to threaten instead to stab her. Wanda confesses she only meant to mislead him with her cruelties and faithlessness and really wants to be his wife. Soon reverting to cruelty, however, she contrives a final ritual beating

('Gregor' is now Severin once more) at the hands of the Greek, who enters suddenly through the bed-curtains. Half-dead and deserted, Severin awakens from his dream, returns to his father and employs himself about their ancestral home. There in due course, as lord of the manor, he can conclude: "The cure was cruel, but radical, and the main thing is: I have been cured." The bizarre moral of the tale, in reply to the friend's query, is that woman can only be man's enemy, his slave or his despot, never his companion, so long as she has no equality with him in education and work.

Lenzer points to the repetition of themes and images throughout Sacher-Masoch's writings. Even the paintings, statues, mirrors depict the cruel woman, the submissive man, neglect, tortures and passions. This preoccupation with a single cluster of ideas, the obsession to repeat, is characteristic of pornographic phantasies. Sacher-Masoch also displays a need to rationalize and systematize, as if his prime concern were to reveal the general laws governing relations between the sexes. His power conflict does not leave room for Plato's idea of male and female craving reunion as the single being they once formed. His affinity is with 'la belle dame sans merci' of the *Minnesang*. Physiology has ensured her victory since man's sexual drives are stronger and make him her slave, but he elects to be cruelly treated, and this is his pleasure. The female is the cruel, overpowering principle to which the male submits, not only because he is weaker but also because he wishes to be so. The theory thickens in complexity to the point of total confusion when woman's natural cruelty is revealed to be really a response to man's, in demanding of her "faithfulness without love, and submission without pleasure". Against her nature, she thus brews the love potion of cruelty which alone will bind him to her. The application of the theory carries similar contradictions: Wanda wants a man who will dominate her but readily agrees to dominate Severin, complying with his will yet often demonstrating her own innate cruelty, maintaining at one point that she is only play-acting. Is the cruelty of Sacher-Masoch's ideal woman genuine or simulated, inborn or acquired? Two types emerge from his stories—those who are intrinsically cruel, like Lola who tore the wings from flies as a child, or Drama-Dscheuti who roasts and eats her husband in an excess of love, and those who revenge themselves after being betrayed, like Anna Klauer in 'The Hyaena of Pussta', though even before she is deserted by Baron Steinfeld, "this obstinate, self-willed, imperious creature was only born to bring other people under her feet". In Sacher-Masoch's 'witch-algebra' the two types are only apparently different.

Lenzer next considers his style and points out that often ideas are not linked logically but associatively, that the premises on which conclusions are based are in the unconscious where contradiction is tolerated and logic suspended. Thus, in spite of his attempts at systematization, he can neither conceal nor escape from the realm where furs and cruelty are meaningfully related, in short, the primary processes. His writing constructs elaborate defenses which are constantly broken through from within, the very elaboration a measure of the strength of the opponent to be both warded off and submitted to. (This, of Lenzer's many telling observations, is well worth dwelling upon for it illumines what one half-notices again and again in masochistic mental functioning, if not in the perversions in general, namely the extraordinarily large, infantile contribution of the primary processes.) Sacher-Masoch's characters and situations leave an impression of *déjà vu*, emptiness and banality. Lenzer gives a literal translation of the passage introducing the painting of Venus in furs, and therefore of dramatic importance. She comments on the clichés and stereotypes, the ready-made formulae which have lost their power of expression and become shorthand notation which can stand for a range of referents but no concrete particular instance. Language has ossified and can no longer represent individualized content. The reduction of meaning thus achieved serves to hide the author and to assure certainty. The stereotyped stylistic elements form larger stereotyped units—the development, the action, the characters. Sacher-Masoch's heroines, however painstakingly delineated, reduce to a single phenotype: "this woman with the sphinx eyes ... the body of a tiger". Whether her hair is red, black or blond, it is always a symbol of domination. Her foot, which man kisses, always ends on his neck. And always she has fur, this second skin essential to her beauty, about her. This figure is the prison from which his phantasy cannot escape.

Sacher-Masoch's fetishism is so prominent that he even perceives it himself and attempts to explain it 'scientifically': "Furs have an exciting effect on all highly strung natures ... Science has recently established a certain relationship between electricity and warmth." However, it was left to psychoanalysis to understand the fetish as the maternal phallus. Foot, hair, eye and fur, not generally recognized as sexual symbols, are not socially censored and Sacher-Masoch's work has therefore not been exiled to the realm of pornography. His screening devices are not confined to the fetish—the blind Titus, woman as machine or electric battery, the whip, the slipper are recurrent clichés, fulfilling their functions while concealing their sexual connotations. The work of defense and disavowal is carried out repeatedly on all levels, the cliché preventing communication, but these secondary processes are often disrupted by the primary ones. If Sacher-Masoch's attempt to construct a coherent narrative out of such disparate stereotyped elements can be regarded as analogous to secondary revision in the dream work, his theories about the natural laws governing relations between the sexes can be understood as a form of tertiary revision. Both secondary and tertiary revisions are revealed in his descriptions of male characters. These are defined only in their relations to women and treated in a dichotomous manner, either dominated (voluntarily or involuntarily) by women or dominating, deceiving and deserting them, either Severin von Kusiemski or Alexis Papadopolis.

The three stereotypes may, at first, be thought to represent the oedipal situation: Wanda the mother, Alexis the father, and Severin the son. The first names of many of Sacher-Masoch's heroines are assonant with 'mama' and the oedipal scenario is repeated obsessively throughout his work. Nevertheless, it is not the whole story. In the novella *Don Juan von Kolomea*, there is sibling rivalry—it is his wife (mother) Pana's preference for their children which ruins the marriage and drives Don Juan to infidelity (and indeed Lenzer might have noted that ambivalence, rooted in rivalry, towards children is a common masochistic trait). There is also a recoil from genital sexuality, which is always only latent, hidden behind symbols. While Sacher-Masoch is fascinated by the female breast, his descriptions of women's bodies are denials, metaphors of which the prototype is the Sphinx. Lenzer points first to fixation to the mother, then to castration fear, and its disavowal for his women are adorned obligatorily with phallic symbols. Alexis, the Greek, is not only the father, strong, cruel and daring—"what makes him so peculiarly beautiful is that he is beardless. If his hips were less narrow, one might take him for a woman". Like Wanda, he is cruel and he wears a short fur coat. They are only nominally of differing sex: "It is a man as well as a woman". (Again Lenzer succeeds in actually casting light on two neglected characteristics of the masochist, an almost prudish distaste for genital sexual relations and a curious vagueness with respect to gender, often leading to puzzling mistakes in pronouns and possessives—a personal observation which I have made repeatedly in the course of everyday conversation, where no doubt could attach to the gender of the person or animal under discussion. The observation was confirmed by some of the interviews with masochistic subjects reported in Part II; for instance, a 42-year-old male subject, speaking of his mother and her boyfriend, said: "I think when he asked her to marry her she got very—she got cold feet about it." My impression has been that these instances are not simple slips of the tongue but, in so far as they extend beyond linguistics to gender-associated behavior, reflect a general vagueness concerning gender.) Within all the rigidity of Sacher-Masoch's style, plots and characters there is simultaneously an instability which appears as role-playing, transvestism and switching of sexual identities. Surely, Lenzer concludes, the ambiguous, androgynous being to which he submits is both the phallic mother and the phallic father, in other words the still undifferentiated phallic parent with whom he once experienced a state of oneness and blissful omnipotence.

Thomas O'Donnell's (1977) study of T.E. Lawrence, though exhibiting literary scholarship, has nothing new to say about its subject. It is not only hostile, it is appallingly shallow by comparison with John E. Mack's (1976) thorough and sympathetic examination of Lawrence's life and character to which O'Donnell has the gall to refer with tempered approval. Wholeheartedly espousing Wilhelm Stekel's (1929) and Erich Fromm's (1973) depiction of sadomasochism, he concentrates on the homosexual and sadistic components and gives scant recognition either to Lawrence's sufferings or to his extraordinary gifts (Turner, 1991). To attribute the stereotypes of sadomasochistic pornography to *Seven Pillars of Wisdom* or *The Mint* requires a truly monstrous animosity.

Mervin Glasser (1979) points initially to the crucial distinction between true perversion and perverse elements in a disturbed or even a normal sexuality, where they may appear as foreplay. He defines perversion as persistently chosen sexual deviance involving the whole personality. He then proceeds to define the 'core complex' of which aggression is a major element: a longing for union which is so complete that it threatens permanent loss of self, causing 'annihilation anxiety', flight into narcissism, isolation, and a return to the vicious circle of the core complex, which was fixated in the pervert at a very early stage of development. The 'object' is thus the mother or her surrogate.

The next distinction made is between aggression and sadism, the former aiming at the destruction or 'negation' of the object which threatens psychic homeostasis, the latter aiming at causing the object to suffer. Merging with the mother, a serious threat to psychic homeostasis, provokes an intense aggressive reaction yet also fear of losing her. This conflict can only be dealt with by primitive mechanisms, such as projecting aggression onto an engulfing, intrusive mother, or splitting the internal representation of her so that part of her can be loved and part attacked. The aggressive feelings can later be displaced onto the father but initially only directed against the self as 'somatic displacement'. Internalized aggression may result ultimately in generalized 'numbness', in loss of the ego's basic functions of perception and synthesis, in suicide. In infancy, the negligence, rejection or, conversely, the 'smothering' of the mother exerts enormous influence on the core complex. In perversion, the ego attempts to resolve conflicts by sexualization—aggression is converted into sadism—thus preserving the mother though hurting and controlling her, and achieving a certain stability through this binding and organizing force. If it breaks down, sadism may revert to aggression.

Crucial to sadistic pleasure is that the object should be experiencing what the sadist wants, both absorbed in the same situation. The object must not wish to suffer, but be ultimately carried away, whilst the sadist revenges himself (on the mother). Glasser parts company with Freud in that he does not regard sadism as part of the sexual drive itself.

He refers to ego-functions subserving a perverse sexual aim, citing a patient who developed eye symptoms through the 'penetrating, phallic' activity of looking. (He does not, however, cite Freud's brief 1910 paper 'The psycho-analytic view of psychogenic disturbance of vision'.) He notes that the superego of perverts is characteristically sadistic, reflecting object relations at the time of its formation. The mother often relates to her child narcissistically, now overattentive, now neglectful, occasionally even stimulating him sexually (cf. Berliner, 1940, 1947, 1958). Her inconsistency determines his later need to control the object sadomasochistically. Where she was remote or not there at all (an institutional upbringing), vicious sadism may ensue.

The masochist, as master of operations, determines strictly what he will suffer. With the reassurance that his aggressive impulses are controlled, his faults must be noted and punished to the satisfaction of his superego. He moves towards or away from the object as the anxieties of annihilation or abandonment alternate, often preferring to masturbate after he has left her rather than lose control of the situation in her presence. If his specified forms of pain and humiliation are departed from, he reacts against them. He makes the aggression in himself and in the object innocuous: he is not attacking so the object cannot be destroyed, whilst her anger is attenuated so she will not desert him (cf. Loewenstein, 1957). There are always elements of deception, contempt and cryptic dominance in masochism as in any perversion, since sadomasochism features in all, the fundamental motive for deception being survival in terms of the core complex.

Individuals only become true perverts after adolescence, when their psychopathology is established. They passed through the 'prism' of the Oedipus complex, but this prism was distorted sadomasochistically by the core complex: the father was not to be destroyed or castrated so much as humiliated or denigrated (sadism rather than aggression), and fear of castration was dealt with masochistically through beating fantasies. The mother was often the predominating, castrating figure, the father simply convenient for the displacement of drives split off from those directed towards the mother. To negate her seductiveness, she might be idealized and devoid of sexuality, whilst all her dangerous attributes were transferred to the father. The latency period is often characterized by minor delinquencies, seductions by older relatives and deliberate masturbation. The unresolved conflicts of the core complex and, later, the Oedipus complex permit the instinctual life no rest. At puberty, the intense desire for 'merging' with the mother causes severe annihilation and abandonment anxieties and an extreme aggressive response which may be sexualized and displaced onto the father or onto the subject's own body (narcissism), or remain as antagonism towards the mother. When aggressive feelings threaten direct expression, the perversion is used to contain them, perhaps even averting suicide from fear of losing control of the body which is regarded as an instrument of destruction.

At the Fall Meeting of the American Psychoanalytic Association, New York, December 1979, Arnold Cooper, in the chair (Panel, 1981), expressed the hope that current knowledge of the separation-individuation process, early object relations, self-esteem regulation and affect development might cast new light on masochism. (Sadly, he proposed no limit for the use of psychoanalytic jargon!) The first speaker, Arthur Valenstein, on 'The Psychoanalytic Concept of Masochism', tracing its evolution through Freud's writings, observed that Freud's speculative theory of life and death superordinal drives lay outside the mainstream of psychoanalytic practice. It left the dubious question of an innate primary masochism, developmentally transformable into sadism directed outwards, and set a historical precedent for subsuming all shades of pain that fulfill a need for suffering under the concept of masochism. It was important, however, to distinguish between subjective experience of pain and masochism. He illustrated the distinction between preverbal, preoedipal attachment to pain and masochism as an erotic phenomenon with the case of a thirty-year-old woman. Beneath her obsessional defensive organization and depression was a sadomasochistic masturbatory fantasy life, arising from fixation at the anal stage. She had been locked into a symbiotic power struggle with her overwhelming, widowed mother and "had internalized these pain-ridden *but* fulfilling experiences within the context of the mother-self representation" (p. 675). She had always had a pain-and-struggle orientation to objects and their internal representations.

Arnold Cooper's presentation, 'The Masochistic-Narcissistic Character', enquired into the pleasure in masochism. Painful experiences may be libidinized defensively and cause ego distortion in which self-directed aggression becomes sexually exciting. Physical perceptions of pain, particularly through the skin, serve not only to avoid injury but also to form the self-image, to defend against the anxiety of identity diffusion, and to promote separation-individuation. Mastery, not avoidance, of pain is a major achievement in self-development, and it may imply the capacity to derive satisfaction from a certain measure of self-inflicted pain. When threatened with the narcissistic humiliation of passivity and helplessness in the face of external danger, the infant reasserts control by making suffering ego-syntonic, but the repair mechanism may miscarry in extreme cases. The object is perceived as excessively cruel, and gratification from disappointment becomes the preferred mode of narcissistic assertion, the aim not reunion with a loving mother but control over a damaging mother. The ultimate clinical picture may seem more narcissistic (charm, preening, ambition) or more masochistic (depression, humiliation, failure), but in either case there is a deadened capacity to feel, muted enjoyment, oscillation between grandiosity and humiliation, no satisfaction in relationships or in work, envy, the conviction of being hardly treated, and an endless capacity for provocation.

Jules Glenn pointed out how masochism and narcissism are interrelated. In narcissism, the self-representation is libidinally cathected, while in masochism, fused aggressive and libidinal energies are directed against the self-representation. This first appears during the preoedipal period when narcissism is dominant over object love.

Charles Kligerman's main thesis was that some masochists suffer from a fragility or vulnerability in self-cohesion. They try to fill the deficit by merging in fantasy with an omnipotent self-object or reminding themselves through pain of the body-self to counteract a feeling of deadness. To illustrate this, Kligerman reported the case of a man with a masturbation beating fantasy which was walled off from the rest of his personality by a well-integrated ego. However, the core problem, lack of a firm sense of self as a centre of initiative, remained. He had formed, in Heinz Kohut's (1977) terms, a 'vertical split'. In most of his activities, he was effective but in sexuality he felt deficient and had to invoke his 'dominatrix' figure. Later he only needed to invoke her in nonsexual contexts, when he was feeling fragmented. When in a good state of narcissistic balance he could ultimately feel at ease in sexual relations. The fantasy was used to fill the deficit in his self-cohesion, to give him a painful sense of autonomy when threatened by narcissistic enmeshment with a maternal self-object. It was also a screen for anal penetration by a powerful father. Kligerman ended with the suggestion that many masochistic perversions attempt not only to fill a deficit but to complete the internalization process and achieve structure formation through a fantasized self-object.

Newell Fischer, in summing up the contributions, emphasized that masochistic phenomena, though mystifying, are universal. Masochism is multiply determined and serves multiple functions. Its relation to narcissism was the focus for this Panel, but Kligerman approached narcissism from Kohut's self-psychology, including issues of self-fragmentation or cohesion (a separate line of narcissistic development), whereas Glenn's more classical concept related to shifts in libidinal cathexis from object-representation to self-representation (an intermediate stage along a single line of libidinal development from autoerotism to object love). Fischer suggested also that the preoedipal seeking of pain might be a precursor of masochism, but pain itself served an important role in development.

In the ensuing discussion Glenn pointed out that 'fixation' could refer to a weak spot in development to which there is a return in the face of later anxiety or it could refer to developmental arrest which causes an intense distortion in the oedipal experience. Cooper insisted that masochism arises in the resolution of issues that are primarily narcissistic rather than derived from the development of the sexual instincts. Like narcissism, masochism can have normal as well as pathological developmental aspects. Silverman (from New Jersey) and Valenstein agreed that the masochist may derive narcissistic gratification from self-induced isolation and suffering which he sees as noble and romantic. Isidor Bernstein (of New York City) saw masochism as a compromise formation, a perversion of the synthetic function of the personality, combining opposing tendencies. The mothers of the patients reported were involved in obtaining their own instinctual gratification through their children (cf. Bernstein, 1957). Harold Levitan (from Montreal) pondered whether prepubertal experiences of orgasm were felt as painful. Masochistic perverts are often overstimulated. They are compulsive masturbators. Perhaps this leads them later to associate pain and sexuality. Cooper felt that masochism, like narcissism, is there from the beginning, before the full development of a psychic structure.

Selma Fraiberg's (1982) paper, published posthumously, on pathological defenses in infancy makes harrowing reading. It reminds one, if any reminder were necessary, that more masochists are made than are ever born, and made at a very early age. The disturbed children she describes are between three and eighteen months old. Their defenses are drawn, she believes, from a biological repertoire. Before the formation of an ego, pain can be transformed into pleasure or expunged from consciousness. A symptom can stand in place of an original conflict. The paper was read, as the René A. Spitz Lecture, before the Denver Psychoanalytic Society, April 1981, and opens with a tribute to her mentor's work with institutionalized infants (Spitz, 1945).

A defense mechanism, such as reaction-formation, cannot be postulated in the case of an infant but, if the infant is old enough to perceive danger or a threat to his functioning, he will react with behavior which serves as defense. Biological modes on the model of 'flight or fight' may, of course, be precursors of later defense mechanisms (Hartmann, 1950; Spitz, 1961). What happens to an infant of less than a year-and-a-half when his human protectors fail him and he is exposed to repeated and prolonged helplessness and pain? When his mother is associated only with pain, disappointment and even abuse? Fraiberg points to four main types of behavior she observed in such infants: avoidance, where the baby will not only avoid all eye- or voice-contact with his mother but even edit her altogether out of his surroundings; freezing, where complete immobility can be maintained until it causes physiological pain and disintegrates into screaming, disorganized collapse; fighting tantrums during the day which give place to terror at night; and transformations of affect where, for instance, bottle-feeding has been turned into a sadomasochistic game between infant and mother. The mother is often repeating morbid experiences from her own childhood. The child's aggressive intent is masked by smiling through clenched teeth, or by giddy, theatrical laughter. Grief as well as anxiety can be transformed in infancy. One sixteen-month-old girl who was not permitted to cry when her mother left her each morning at the nursery would stand rubbing her tearless eyes silently and persistently.

Finally, Fraiberg confirms the observations made by Spitz and Cobliner (1965) on even younger children, that aggression is frequently turned against the self. The child will bang his head against the floor, collide with pieces of furniture, fall from heights, all without showing pain, without crying or even wincing—another cutoff mechanism in these biological defenses against intolerable pain.

At the 1982 Annual Meeting of the American Psychoanalytic Association, Jules Glenn examined the influence of a child's early separation from parents on depression and masochism. His subsequent paper (Glenn, 1984*a*) defines depression as reactive depression, endogenous depression, mourning, grief or melancholia, and masochism as a clinical condition in which pain is consciously or unconsciously sought and associated pleasurably with sexual fantasies, even in moral masochism.

Three of the cases described by Glenn were originally reported by others; the fourth was his own four-year-old patient, Andy, who had been separated from his parents for a week at the age of three, looking sad and not recognizing them for a while on their return. His behavior became provocative and had all the hallmarks of masochism: irritating his parents until his father slapped him, teasing his sister and getting her to squeeze his penis painfully and at the same time pleasurably, teasing his elder brother until hit by him, playing with dolls and wanting to be a girl with no further castration anxiety. His oedipal attachment appeared to oscillate between his father and mother. When they quarrelled, he identified with each of them. He could only obtain satisfaction from his father, himself suffering from an only child's resentment of any surrogate sibling, by provoking his anger. His mother transferred a sadomasochistic relationship with her younger brother to Andy. They were both negligent and insensitive to the child, making him take a hot bath when he was badly sunburnt and share a bedroom with his dying grandfather.

As factors in the etiology of depression Glenn enumerates longing accompanied by a buildup of physical tension, grief, attacks on the self when no object is available for attack, or when the object must be protected from attack, or when the object has been introjected, attacks from the superego due to guilt, poor self-esteem and affects associated with helplessness. An older child can tolerate absence as long as the missing parent's image is libidinally cathected, but after superego development, loss of object may be regarded as punishment.

The ego tries to cope with painful situations by denial, by decathecting the object representation, by avoidance, by repression, or by repetition in an endeavour to control the pain. If it has been precipitated, it feels less severe and it can be turned off. It can be diminished by cathecting the painful representation with libidinal energy.

Painful preoedipal experiences, when self and object are undifferentiated, may be a basis for masochism. Traumatic and painful illness in the oedipal stage may likewise. Glenn concludes that early object loss with attendant depression may cause a child to seek masochistic gratification by libidinizing the pain itself, by reproducing the painful situation either by self-attack or by provoking attack in order to gain mastery. When parents are the source of pain, the child will seek pain-producing objects in order to imagine their presence. The means of self-punishment will later reflect the relative importance of depressive or masochistic mechanisms.

Glenn (1984*b*) also reports on the central role of early psychic trauma in the case of three adult masochists, all of whom underwent surgery. The traumatic experience is defined as "one in which the individual is subject to such severe internal or external stimulation as to render him unable to utilize his usual defenses adequately" (p. 357). It is recreated in later attempts at mastery, using reversal and injuring rather than being injured. Another defense is erotization of the traumatic event or its associated anxiety. The trauma may also be regarded as punishment for forbidden oedipal or preoedipal gratification. Regression to narcissistic, symbiotic states may enhance masochism.

Glenn's first patient contracted scarlet fever when he was six and an ensuing retropharyngeal abscess was lanced without anaesthetic, causing him to faint. During latency, he would stab at pictures of heads in magazines with a scalpel. At twenty-three he had a masturbation fantasy of placing his penis into the mouth of a worm whose sharp teeth cut it on withdrawal. He identified both with Prometheus and with the bird daily tearing his liver.

The second patient had a tonsillectomy when she was three, screaming as the 'poison gas' was administered, habitually retaining bowel movements after the operation. At twenty-eight she was taking valium on account of anxiety dreams which had started after an appendectomy when she was nineteen. She had one masturbation fantasy in which her husband withheld sex and another in which she was being raped. She also withheld associations and payment from Dr. Glenn!

The third patient had been operated upon by his uncle for mastoiditis, undergoing anaesthetization sixteen times between the ages of two and eight. As a forty-year-old dentist, he identified with his patients and feared giving them anaesthesia and drilling their teeth. During Easter, he identified with Christ who had also been betrayed, crossing one foot over the other as in a crucifixion, but rising ultimately to be united with the Father.

Each case contains much more material which Glenn subjects to classic Freudian interpretation, but the psychic trauma, he insists, remains pivotal in the development of both masochism and narcissism. Each patient became the active reduplicator of the event in disguised form in an attempt to gain mastery. The first used the word 'titrate' when he described how he regulated the degree of his provocation and thereby the danger. They all imagined their sexual partners as dangerous, dominating but controllable. Their sadism appeared as identification with the aggressor became eroticized, but was disowned in a second reversal, identifying with the victim and adding to the masochism. Glenn points to different mechanisms of erotization: defensive sexualization of a traumatic event, with consequent fantasies and object relations; the erotization of anxiety itself, making it pleasurable as well as painful (cf. Reik, 1939); libidinization caused by excessive parental stimulation, constitutional hypersexuality or deficient restraint mechanisms. He makes the further observations that under surgery the patients were forcefully restrained and they were deprived in other ways of the possibility of mastery through action, that the surgical procedures were seen as punishment for forbidden sexual activity, and that regression to oral-narcissistic-symbiotic as well as anal libidinal stages occurred. (All three patients experienced the Isakower (1938) phenomenon.) Confirming the findings of earlier authors, Glenn mentions the symbiotic mother–child relationship, toilet-training, and teasing games with parents as virtually universal factors in protomasochism. Illness, surgery or separation from parents enhances a feeling of deficiency and leads later to a desperate seeking for completion, for union with a powerful person, but seeking this object will involve seeking painful stimulation associated with the object.

Otto Kernberg (1988) proposes a classification of masochistic psychopathology for diagnostic, prognostic and treatment purposes. 'Normal' masochism is the price exacted by the superego of the average individual, restricting a full enjoyment of life. It consists in self-criticism together with the sublimatory endurance of pain to achieve future reward, and the residues of polymorphously perverse infantile sexuality (cf. Freud, 1905, p. 191), the sadomasochistic dimension representing a primitive synthesis between love and hatred. The condensation of physical pleasure and pain leads to a predisposition to experience a similar psychological condensation in the accusations and attacks of the superego.

The depressive-masochistic personality disorder presents a well-integrated ego identity (good anxiety tolerance, impulse control and sublimatory capacity), an excessively severe but well-integrated superego, and an ability to establish object relations in depth. There is a tendency to be solemn, reliable, concerned about work performance and responsibilities, overconscientious with extremely high standards and harsh judgments. This leads to indignation with others, depression with the subject's own performance, and the unconscious creation of circumstances that perpetuate a sense of being mistreated or humiliated. Abnormally vulnerable to disappointment and slights, he goes out of his way to obtain sympathy and love and is, typically, able to respond with deep gratitude. However, he tends to be demanding, to make others feel guilty and ultimately to reject him. He becomes depressed instead of angry. 'Faulty metabolism' of aggression, generating unconscious guilt, means that a 'justified' attack is followed by overly apologetic, submissive behavior, then a second wave of anger. This personality structure may be accompanied by an actual masochistic perversion or masochistic masturbation fantasies.

Sadomasochistic personality disorder manifests as alternating cruel and self-demeaning behavior toward the same object and usually presents severe identity diffusion, ego weakness, part-object relationships and primitive defensive mechanisms such as splitting and denial. 'The help-rejecting complainer' fails at work and in his social life. The corruption of superego functions is in marked contrast to their rigid integration in the depressive-masochistic personality.

Primitive self-destructiveness goes together with a severe lack of superego integration, of the capacity for experiencing guilt. Typical of this borderline personality organization are individuals who obtain nonspecific relief of anxiety by self-mutilation or suicidal gestures carried out in rage not from long-standing depresssion. These gestures are an effort to reestablish control over the environment by making an offending partner or parent feel guilty. When chronic, this behavior can be seen as 'malignant narcissism'. There is no dependency, rather aloofness, and attacks of rage occur when pathological grandiosity is challenged. The self-destructiveness is overtly sadistic. A history of bizarre and cruel suicide attempts points to a possible psychotic syndrome. All these self-mutilating individuals derive a sense of power as they seek to destroy love, gratitude and compassion in themselves and others. They are scarcely masochists, strictly speaking, since neither unconscious guilt nor the erotization of pain is present. Moving towards this extreme of the spectrum, Kernberg notes a decrease in superego participation, an increase in aggression, primitivization of object relations and defense behavior, together with a fading out of erotism.

Under his heading 'syndromes of pathological infatuation,' Kernberg points out that the masochistic personality selects an object who does not respond to his or her love, though the pervert may simply require sexual gratification through pain or humiliation. For the most part, these patterns do not coincide. The all-consuming infatuation for the unavailable (sometimes sadistic) object represents submission to the ego-ideal projected onto the object, and the lover is filled with narcissistic pride as 'the greatest sufferer on earth'. Stable relations with friends and other interests may, however, be maintained simultaneously. Where impossible infatuation is narcissistically rather than oedipally determined, Kernberg discerns "an unconscious effort to consolidate a symbolic integration within the grandiose self of the characteristics of both sexes" (p. 1016).

Masochistic perversion, defined as the restrictive, obligatory use of physical pain or humiliation to achieve sexual excitement and orgasm, presents several levels of severity. At a neurotic level of personality organization, it takes the form of a 'scenario' enacted in a 'safe' object relation. Oedipal conflicts require the denial of castration anxiety and the assuagement of a cruel superego to obtain sexual gratification with incestuous meanings. Identification with the opposite sex and with a punishing incestuous object also figures in this play-acting, which may represent a 'primal scene', such as the oedipal triangle in the form of a *ménage à trois*. The masochist must watch a rival making love to his object before he can do so himself. Masochistic fantasies may accompany masturbation or the individual may bind and hurt himself in front of a mirror to achieve orgasm. Usually the perverse scenario is determined in detail by the masochist himself, and its repetition is reassuring against unconscious anxieties as well as sexually gratifying. Situations leading to mutilation or even accidental death arise only with a borderline personality organization, often narcissistic, and a severe pathology of object relations. Other cases which break out of the play-acting frame are those masturbatory procedures which have an undisguised anal, urethral or oral content, giving them not only a masochistic but a regressive, pregenital quality. (One might feel some unease with this distinction. Is not masochism, in general, and very obviously in the case of the perversion, a regressive phenomenon?) Superego structure, object relations and sex differentiation deteriorate jointly as primitive aggression becomes predominant. Kernberg interprets chronic, erotized self-mutilation as "a triumph over life and death, over pain and fear, and, unconsciously, over the entire world of object relations" (p. 1021). It has, he states, a poor prognosis for psychotherapeutic treatment but he does not ascribe any physiological basis (such as the addictive release of endogenous opioids through pain) to account for this.

In summing up, Kernberg notes that "at milder levels of masochism aggression is recruited at the service of erotism; at severer levels of masochism, erotism is recruited at the service of aggression; at the most severe level of masochism, erotism fades out altogether" (p. 1022). The quality and degree of superego integration, the level of ego organization (whether neurotic or borderline-psychotic), the type of narcissism (whether 'normal' or pathological) and the extent of integration of infantile sexual components codetermine the level of masochistic pathology.

Steven Berglas (1989) introduces a new clinical perspective on what Freud called 'moral' masochism with his exposition of self-handicapping behavior. He sees its true function as helping an individual to deal with a threat to self-esteem by structuring the context within which an evaluation will be made. "The self-handicapper controls impressions by getting into situations or circumstances that may look painful or problematic but, paradoxically, sustain a lofty image of competence" (p. 268). Timing differentiates self-handicapping from other self-protective strategies: it occurs following a success which is deemed noncontingent, and it is "a proactive coping strategy initiated in anticipation of losing his or her favorable but fragile competence image" (p. 269). Snyder (1990) argues that most people may experience such a tenuous, positive self-image but that "it is the uncertainty of subsequent success that is the key to understanding the self-handicapping phenomenon and its effects" (p. 111). He goes on to examine the effects of self-handicapping on self-esteem, affect, competence and control and reaches the conclusion that it is a tactic chosen by many facing the uncertainty of future success, "one tactic, among several in the reality-negotiation armamentarium, for coping with the larger existential fight with our inevitable fallibility" (pp. 144–145).

SUMMARY AND CONCLUSIONS

The ideas presented in the papers reviewed above fall into three main categories: the aetiology of masochism, its characteristics, its dissection into other entities.

Various aetiologies are put forward. (a) The withholding of infantile sexual pleasure is a plausible one. Stimulation and satisfaction give rise to love in the infant, whereas deprivation arouses hatred, and both these are linked with being helpless in the power of a stronger person (Menaker, 1953). Unsatisfactory breast-feeding, weaning, dissuasion from masturbation are all likely to constitute a basis for masochism (Sadger, 1926;

Lewinsky, 1944). (b) Where a mother is associated only with disappointment and pain, an infant's grief and anxiety may be expressed as head-banging, avoidance, freezing or transformed affects. Biological modes of defense on the model of 'flight or fight' may be precursors of later defense mechanisms (Fraiberg, 1982). (c) A desire for union with an omnipotent, protecting figure may alternate with fear of incorporation and loss of self (Blumstein, 1959; Glasser, 1979). (d) Masochism is frequently seen as the turning of sadism upon the self, with the interaction of aggressive, self-punitive and erotic components (Menninger, 1938; Reik, 1939; Brenman, 1952), but a residue of primary erotogenic masochism may also be present (Lewinsky, 1944). (e) Masochism serves the function of maintaining some relationship, however tormenting, with a damaging but vitally needed mother (Menaker, 1953; Loewenstein, 1957; Berliner, 1940, 1947, 1958; Blumstein, 1959). (f) As well as being a defense reaction of the ego, i.e., a matter of survival, masochism may gratify the instinctual urges of the id and the demand for expiation of the superego (Brenman, 1952; Brenner, 1959). (g) The female child in particular may adopt the defence of 'seduction of the aggressor', whereby the loving complicity of the threatening person is engineered and every prohibition is turned into a game (Loewenstein, 1957). (h) An intergenerational cycle of ambivalence may establish itself (Bromberg, 1955; Fraiberg, 1982; Glenn, 1984*a*). (i) The influence of erotogenic zones of the body on early sexual development is considered with respect to orality (Lewin, 1950; Kucera, 1959), to anal fixation and skin erotism (Lewinsky, 1944), to reversion to a passive phallic phase (Loewenstein, 1957). (j) Masochism may arise out of the psychic trauma of surgery in early childhood. The experience is recreated in later attempts at mastery (Glenn, 1984*b*).

There is some agreement on certain characteristics of masochism. (a) The coupling of anxiety and pleasure is a frequent observation, in particular, the prolongation of erotic forepleasure and the use of anxiety as a substitutive gratification (Laforgue, 1930; Reik, 1939). (b) Masochism and sadism are always observed together (Brenner, 1959), but there is no true complementarity between a sadist and a masochist since both require unwilling partners (Smirnoff, 1969; Glasser, 1979). The masochist has an endless capacity for provocation (Panel, 1981). (c) The importance of fantasy lies in producing sexual tension. Fantasies will only be modified when they lose their effectiveness in generating sexual excitement; otherwise, themes and images are rigidly repetitive (Lenzer, 1975). (d) The theatricality serves to 'synchronize' the course of masochistic ritual with sexual arousal and satisfaction (Reik, 1939). The partner must undertake, by contract, conflicting roles, and clothes and accessories serve to keep the roles apart (Smirnoff, 1969). (e) Insistence on specifying the punishment is linked with psychic preparedness for displeasure, in other words, a flight towards suffering in the future (Ferenczi, 1925, 1926; Reik, 1939; Lewinsky 1944; Loewenstein, 1957; Eidelberg, 1959). Punishment permits sexual release. (f) The exhibitionism of the masochist is provocative. Whether it should also be regarded as narcissistic is disputed (Reik, 1939, versus Lewinsky, 1944; Eidelberg, 1959; Panel, 1981), but exhibitionism is still present in the desexualized forms of masochism, as exemplified by the voluptuous suffering of religious or political martyrs, by great characters in art. (g) Castration threats abound in masochistic fantasy and ritual but only in order to annul such a perceived threat, emanating originally from the oedipal situation, in reality (Lampl-de Groot, 1937; Fenichel, 1945; Loewenstein, 1957). (h) The masochist's incessant demands that he should be loved, that the environment should minister to his desires is partly to reassure himself that he exists (Horney, 1935; Lewinsky, 1944; Panel, 1981). (i) He retains an infantile sense of omnipotence, of magical control of his environment (Eidelberg, 1934; Brenner, 1959). His mentation is frequently invaded by the 'primary processes' of the unconscious where contradiction is tolerated and logic suspended (Lenzer, 1975).

Much ink has been spilt in search of a precise definition of masochism. (a) The most frequent, and indeed irrefutable, observation emerging from its dissection is the universality of masochistic impulses and masochistic character traits (de Monchy, 1950; Reik, 1941; Brenner, 1959; Glasser, 1979; Panel, 1981; Berglas, 1989; Snyder, 1990). (b) It is difficult to separate the masochistic character diagnostically from paranoia (Bak, 1946), from obsessional neurosis (Fenichel, 1945), from conversion hysteria, phobia or addiction, above all, from depression (Brenner, 1959, Glenn, 1984*a*). (c) As a perversion, masochism often presents features which psychoanalytic theory isolated and categorized as fetishism, voyeurism, transvestism or latent homosexuality (Lenzer, 1975). (d) Distinctions are made between aggression, which aims at destroying the object, and sadism, which aims at causing it to suffer (Glasser, 1979), between subjective experience of pain, where suffering may become ego-syntonic, and masochism, where gratification from disappointment becomes the preferred mode of narcissistic assertion (Panel, 1981). (e) For diagnostic purposes, masochism may be more usefully analysed as faulty metabolism of aggression, severe identity diffusion, or lack of superego integration, such as characterizes a borderline personality organization. Chronic self-mutilating behavior may be seen as malignant narcissism (Kernberg, 1988).

The most obvious conclusion to be drawn from these expositions is that masochism, if not only a blanket term, at least refers to an extremely heterogeneous phenomenon which transmutes every time one attempts to grasp it. Another equally obvious conclusion which might have been drawn but which does not, in fact, appear to have been drawn in this literature is that the masochist's sexual attitudes and patterns of sexual behavior do not enhance his chances of reproducing himself biologically.

In compiling this survey in chronological order, a general impression has formed, with notable exceptions of course, that moving forward through time is accompanied by an increase in jargon and a decrease in substance. One reason for this is not hard to perceive. As the rock face fills up with birds, the squabbling increases, and available niches get smaller. Another less obvious reason is that a scrutiny in depth of the particular is usually more fruitful than a sweeping glance at the general.

Whilst piecing together, laboriously enough, this picture of masochism from the post-Freudian literature, I have inevitably been aware of another based on personal observation. Most of the bells of recognition have rung in the course of my reading but not all. The question of the etiology of masochism, of even the masochistic perversion, has, I find, been inadequately addressed, particularly by later writers who seem chiefly concerned to dissect masochism conceptually out of existence and press their academic seal with some satisfaction upon the vacuum: "the matter remains unclear".

CHAPTER 3

REVIEW OF EMPIRICAL STUDIES ON SADOMASOCHISM

"I have no faith in anything short of actual Measurement and the Rule of Three."

CHARLES DARWIN

"General impressions are never to be trusted. Unfortunately when they are of long standing they become fixed rules of life, and assume a prescriptive right not to be questioned. Consequently those who are not accustomed to original inquiry entertain a hatred and a horror of statistics. They cannot endure the idea of submitting their sacred impressions to cold-blooded verification."

FRANCIS GALTON

To hypothesize is more enjoyable than to provide supporting evidence—the one a flash of insight, an exhilarating flight of the imagination, the other a painstaking gathering, interpretation and presentation of information.

To criticize is easy—to do is difficult. Any attempt to investigate the sadomasochistic deviance on an empirical basis therefore deserves the preliminary acknowledgement that a valiant effort is being made to tackle an almost impossibly difficult problem. That said, serious general grounds for criticism are not lacking, and they are, of course, equally applicable to my own imperfect efforts in the following section.

(1) Method

Most empirical studies are based on questionnaires designed by investigators with varying degrees of psychological and statistical background knowledge (and—dare one say it?—with varying endowments of natural insight and common sense). These questionnaires are answered by highly selective samples of sadomasochists—one might say, the tip of the iceberg. Even more seriously, they are answered by people with a vast, life-long potential for fantasy and self-deception. If it were not for what Theodor Reik (1939, 1941) pinpointed as the 'demonstrative feature' of the masochistic personality, they would be lucky to be answered at all.

(2) Interpretation

In analysing the results of such studies, a distinction is often made between heterosexual and homosexual respondents. This totally ignores the strong vein of homosexuality running through all sadomasochism, which can only be understood through its etiology. It also ignores the bisexual element innate in all human beings, if not in all sexually reproducing organisms. Wilhelm Fliess, in his preoccupation with this, may have finally incurred Freud's criticism when he advanced it as the regulating factor of repression, but Freud never doubted the truth of the basic observation, and indeed, what physiologist, anatomist, zoologist, anthropologist or psychologist since Freud would seek to refute it? Thus the division of sexual orientation, which is relative, into cut-and-dried categories, on the strength of certain behavior, for purposes of statistical presentation, constitutes a distortion.

This is not the only distortion likely to be introduced by the necessity to categorize. Where is the dividing line to be drawn between masochism and fetishism? between masochist and sadist? between masochistic pleasure and pain? Analysis of empirical data does not easily accommodate ambiguity or paradox. Masochism is a highly amorphous problem.

(3) Inherent limitations

There are quite inevitable limitations to the empirical method itself, as generally understood in the academic field. Firstly, it is quantitative, not qualitative. The strength of a salt solution can be measured, but there is no method of measuring the taste of salt. Psychological problems are, in many ways, particularly insusceptible to quantitative, as distinct from qualitative, examination. It is doubtless for this reason that empirical studies on psychological phenomena are predominantly descriptive, with little attention paid to the question 'how' or the even weightier question 'why'. True, behavioral phenomena can be quantified and analysed statistically, and conclusions can be drawn from the results. For the most part, they furnish supportive evidence for something already observed, deduced or hypothesized without recourse to measurement—they provide a rather unstimulating confirmation. Results *disproving* a generally accepted assertion are, on the whole, more interesting but they have, after all, a negative value. To underline this initial point in respect of the masochistic perversion, there have been several painstaking studies aimed at statistical presentation of masochistic behavior, its variations and its prevalence, but none of these can convey the fundamental, all-pervasive, invincible, 'Screwtape Letters' quality of masochism.

Secondly, it should be recalled that the academic definition of 'empirical', concentrating on measurement, is by no means the only definition, or even the general definition. Observation and experiment, as opposed to theory, are not necessarily linked to quantification and statistical presentation. To be empirical, rather than theoretical, it is only necessary that observation is concrete, sufficiently established and unambiguous. The close, first-hand observation of masochistic patterns of behavior (including verbal behavior), rigidly repetitive and predictable as they are, can be termed 'empirical' equally with responses to a questionnaire. In both cases the observer stands between the subject and the observation as presented.

Thirdly, it should be borne in mind that the word 'empirical' carries connotations of objectivity—an aspiration achieved to varying degrees. What is crucial to an understanding of masochism, where reality is richly stood on its head, is not objective but subjective observation, and this is impossible unless the investigator happens to be an entrenched masochistic pervert himself. In that unlikely event, and assuming an even unlikelier gift for honest introspection, the presentation of such observations would be invaluable. It would, without doubt, be very different from that of the average empirical study.

By way of illustrating these general remarks, I propose to open this survey of the empirical literature with an examination of one substantial paper in some detail, and thereafter to review papers comparatively under headings.

Andreas Spengler (1977) presents a study of 245 West German males who completed a questionnaire anonymously. They were approached either because they had placed sadomasochistic contact advertisements or because they belonged to sadomasochistic clubs. Spengler justly points out that this limits his sample to those prepared to share their deviance with others and of this unspecifiable proportion of all sadomasochists only 27% were prepared to cooperate in his study, presumably the most open and self-confident. He states that he found hardly any women in the clubs or advertising who were not prostitutes and he therefore confined his investigation to males.

Spengler's first table presents the percentages of heterosexuals, bisexuals and homosexuals constituting this 'definitive' sample (of 244 rather than 245 in this table) on the basis of a self-rating. There are, of course, 'pros' and 'cons' to this method of assessment. Who should know better, it might be argued, than the *anonymous* individual himself whether he is heterosexually or homosexually orientated? However, since sadomasochism is often, amongst other things, a defense against and a denial of homosexuality and since it later emerges that only 10% of these individuals have ever sought psychological advice, which might have uncovered latent homosexuality, the proportions given by Spengler can be noted with interest but not accorded unreserved credence. He divides his sample into 30% heterosexuals, 31% bisexuals and 38% homosexuals, the latter two groups finding outlets for their deviance more easily than the first group who mostly had recourse to prostitutes.

With respect to demographic characters, the upper age groups are, he says, overrepresented (one might perhaps expect sadomasochism to manifest itself most conspicuously in middle age), but unfortunately his tabulation does not present equal units of time. Not altogether surprisingly, also, his respondents were often well educated and well paid in their professions, having more disposable time and money to pursue their deviance and possibly more interest in participating in the investigation. Their divorce rate was above average—16% among heterosexuals, 12% among bisexuals, and 5% among homosexuals (presumably above the West German average). This information is introduced cautiously by what may be regarded as somewhat of an understatement: "the deviant desires are frequently incompatible with the interests of the wife" (p. 444), but no comment is made on the possibly confounding effect of homosexuality or bisexuality *per se*.

After a courageous effort to present potentially useful information on secrecy (in percentages since each category has a different total and absolute numbers presumably overlap), from which it seems that most care is taken to conceal deviant behavior from fathers and from colleagues, Spengler examines success in finding a partner. He seeks to demonstrate on the basis of three complex criteria that homosexuals are considerably more successful than heterosexuals in this respect but, again, does not state absolute numbers, only percentages (the '*p*' values given probably pertaining to χ^2 tests) and he does not consider the possibly greater promiscuity of homosexuals in general.

Next he turns to participation in the subculture, as evidenced by association with like-minded persons at parties or privately, through correspondence or by purchasing sadomasochistic magazines. Since his sample was obtained by these means, the quoted '*p*' values of 0.001 are not unexpected, but he underlines his point that heterosexuals have a less fulfilling prospect than bisexuals and homosexuals, having to rely more on pornographic literature than direct contact. Sexual relations, in which active sadistic and passive masochistic activities usually occur interchangeably, are characterized by low frequencies, particularly for heterosexuals, and frequent change of partner, particularly for homosexuals. Most heterosexuals practise their deviance passively with prostitutes, sometimes sustaining a parallel non-sadomasochistic relationship with a wife or other steady partner. Such parallel loose and firm partnerships can also be found among homosexuals. Spengler raises the interesting question of whether men may be accepted as sadomasochistic partners simply as a substitute solution, in default of acquiescing women, but he does not attempt to answer it.

The investigation gains psychological interest when he examines the degree of self-acceptance of his subjects. As he himself expected, the vast majority viewed their deviance positively, and 70% ('*n*' values necessarily fluctuate in every table) would not change it even if they could. Their rate of suicide attempts (9%, again of an unknown total) was less than that found by Dannecker and Reiche (1974) for homosexual men in West Germany "We found a number of significant correlations," Spengler continues, "which indicate that subcultural integration (defined by the frequency of participation in sadomasochistic parties) and the possibility of realizing the deviance in a partnership context are associated with self-acceptance" (p. 450).

With respect to role preference he tabulates active/sadistic, passive/masochistic and three degrees of 'versatile' against his main three categories of orientation. The *n*-values for heterosexuals, bisexuals and homosexuals differ slightly from table to table, so percentages are given and *p* is stated as nonsignificant. It might be expected, from this complex psychological and statistical situation, that 'bisexuals' would tend to be 'versatile,' but this was not so: "The fact of assuming an active or passive role with a partner is, therefore, of no decisive consequence for the realization of this deviation" (p. 451). However, having shifted (with percentages presumably reflecting the regrouped absolute numbers) to these 'active', 'versatile' or 'passive' categories in order to analyse the degree of dependence on sadomasochistic practices or fantasies in achieving sexual satisfaction, "there was a somewhat stronger fixation on these practices by the passively orientated persons" (p. 452).

As to the practices themselves, the more extreme and dangerous occurred with minimal frequency, in contrast to flagellation, bondage or fetishism, which occurred without appreciable distinction between heterosexuals and homosexuals. There was likewise no distinction in frequency of masturbation, which was as high as Dannecker and Reiche (1974) found for 'common homosexuals' in West Germany, and highest in those practising sadomasochism most frequently with a partner, thus indicating an independent parallel activity rather than a substitute satisfaction. No mention is made of a fantasized partner in the case of the 28% reporting self-bondage, self-beating and other self-torture accompanied by masturbation, nor any allusion to these autoerotic practices being stepping-stones or rehearsals for deviant activity with a partner. The difficulty that fantasy is so prominent, so interwoven, in all sexual relations of sadomasochists that it can become impossible, strictly speaking, to extricate a discrete phenomenon 'masturbation', is perhaps a consideration lying outside the scope of this study and of most empirical studies, including my own as reported in Part II.

First awareness of sadomasochistic desires was reported as occurring at a later age by bisexuals and homosexuals than heterosexuals. Positive reactions to this awareness predominated, especially amongst those actively integrated in the subculture. "I wanted to do it again" was the most common reaction to this original 'coming out' (69%, $n = 245$), as it was also 'after sadomasochistic sex' (this earlier table states 85%, $n = 220$). In reporting this result, Spengler does not consider the possibility of physiological addiction (for instance, an addiction mediated by endogenous opioids which are produced in response to pain).

He concludes tentatively with the suggestion that the differing prospects of finding a partner which exist for heterosexuals, on the one hand, and homosexuals or bisexuals, on the other, together with the differing characters of their respective subcultural groups, might be explained by the fact that there are so few women who are prepared to enter the subculture "in the mode of behavior that manifestly sadomasochistic men seek" (p. 455). Nearly all the heterosexual groups exist, therefore, in cooperation with prostitutes, often maintaining the fiction that they are like-minded, genuinely passionate 'sadists'. (Of course, the point has been made by Victor Smirnoff (1969) amongst others that there is no genuine complementarity between sadist and masochist since they both really prefer to coerce or persuade an unwilling partner.)

It is churlish to pick holes in the design and statistical presentation of Spengler's study, since it must be laid to his credit that the approach is in many respects careful and painstaking. Relevant definitions and control data are often supplied, assumptions and reservations are often stated, sources of bias are admitted and the scope of the investigation is an ambitious one, on a large sample. He states initially that it is "an exploratory and primarily descriptive study" (p. 442). That, of course, points to the most serious limitation of empirical studies in general—tables, for all their statistical support, may furnish little further insight into the nature of sadomasochism.

STATISTICAL NONSENSE

In embarking now on a comparative review of the empirical literature, a few words need to be said at the outset about statistical nonsense, which is occasionally encountered in this literature. To avoid boring to the point of extinction, they can then be regarded as said and done with. One or two examples will suffice to delineate the category:

When Spengler (1977) states that heterosexual sadomasochists had on average 3.3 contacts with 2.8 partners in the 12 months preceding his study, he is stating a statistical possibility. When he continues: "homosexual sadomasochists by contrast had 5.7 contacts with 7.0 partners", he is presenting a physical impossibility, and leaving the reader to deduce that in both cases he probably means "contacts with each partner".

Norman Breslow *et al.* (1985), in examining 'means of first exposure' to sadomasochism, give a p value of 0.001 for the 63.9% of males who had a 'natural interest from childhood' but of the 61.8% of females who 'were seemingly introduced to sadomasochism by another person', they remark that 'no significant results were found'. They conclude their examination of the matter with the formulation: "Pornography, although a factor, is not a significant issue"—by which they presumably mean that males (21.3%) and females (17.6%) showed little difference in quoting it as an introduction to their deviance. The same authors state initially that they decided to exclude (10) male and (12) female prostitutes from their analysis of 130 male and 52 female respondents to their questionnaire, but they report 45 females in their first table with respect to education, and one notices that their percentages in the same table with respect to income sum to 73.3. In their later tabulation of sexual orientation, they make no comment on their surprising report of 0% male homosexuals.

One can well understand how such improbable reports arise. When faced with the challenge of extracting and analysing data from a pile of hard-won, erratically completed questionnaires, the temptation is to regard statistical procedures as tokens of scientific rigour. However, leaving aside the occasional inaccuracy of the investigator, if the data are not adequate to start with, elaborate statistical analysis can become—sometimes manifestly—unconvincing.

SAMPLING PROCEDURES

The crucial issue of how data are obtained for empirical studies of sadomasochism is also a thorny one. The method of sampling is usually by questionnaire—but where and to whom? For instance, Breslow *et al.* (1985)

placed a questionnaire in two U.S. digest-type magazines, one monthly, the other yearly, catering to sadomasochists. They apparently took no account of the differing statistical probabilities of monthly versus annual publications being read, nor of their respective sales, subscriptions and circulation figures, since both magazines were produced by the same publishing company, the only one (out of 16) agreeing to assist in the investigation, suggesting therefore a comparatively more intellectual readership. They also sent their questionnaire to approximately 300 advertisers in a sadomasochistic contact magazine "chosen because of its relatively low number of ads placed by prostitutes and its high number of ads placed by single females and couples" (p. 306). By this method of sampling, of course, they found the nonprostitute females they were looking for. A 'small number' of questionnaires were deposited in shops and one club. In addition to the 40 questions relating to demographic factors and participation in the subculture, there was an invitation to complete a further questionnaire consisting of 21 'in-depth' structured questions and several others based on answers to the original set. Approximately half of the original 182 respondents opted to continue, but only half of these actually returned the second questionnaire.

Charles Moser and Eugene Levitt (1987) arranged for a 'survey form' to be printed in the *S/M Express*, an American magazine with photographs, drawings, articles, stories and advertisements catering specifically to sadomasochists. The editor, who claimed a circulation of 20,000, recommended the survey and republished it in his December 1977 issue. It was also handed out, after a short explanation as to its importance for Charles Moser's doctoral dissertation, at 'support' meetings of the Janus and the Eulenspiegel Societies. Self-definition as a sadomasochist was adopted as the basic criterion for the inclusion of respondents in the study, since it was deemed the least biased—as mentioned previously in connection with Spengler's (1977) use of self-rating, a debatable but reasonable assumption.

Robert Litman and Charles Swearingen (1972) obtained the cooperation of the editors of the *Los Angeles Free Press*, an underground weekly newspaper with a circulation of about 90,000, in order to make contacts for their study on 'bondage and suicide'. An illustrated article entitled 'Whips, Chains and Leather' and an advertisement elicited 30 responses, 15 by letter and 15 by telephone, which led to interviews with 9 men and 3 women.

Neil Buhrich (1983) based his study of 'erotic piercing' on an examination of advertisements appearing in a magazine produced by Gauntlet Enterprises of California, which also supplied gold, silver or stainless steel rings or studs up to 2 cm in diameter. These were figured, inserted through nipples, scrotum, perineum or penis, in the many photographs of *Gauntlet Magazine*'s 1000 subscribers. Founded in 1977, the magazine carried an insert, *PFI (Piercing Fans International) Quarterly* consisting of contact advertisements. These were sifted from 1977 onwards: 138 were excluded because no specific interest in piercing was stated or because the sex of the subscriber was uncertain; 71, placed by couples, were excluded because it was unclear whether the advertiser was 'speaking on his own behalf, on behalf of the partner, or both'; a small number offering professional services were also excluded. Buhrich himself points to the limitations of this method of collecting data: "Some of the advertisements may not be genuine, some may fulfill the subscriber's fantasy rather than indicate his or her practice, and some may be placed by the same person in a different format in subsequent issues. In addition, it is not possible to ascertain whether subscribers are using the publisher's recommended code terms to represent similar sexual deviations" (p. 168). There are, however, other pros and cons of this method, as against a questionnaire, which he does not mention. Most advertisements are aimed at direct satisfaction of deviant desires and, to the extent that they are more basic, may yield more reliable indications of the deviance than any self-conscious responses to the questions of an unknown investigator, or, even more, to the questions of a 'sympathetic' but nonetheless prying interviewer. On the other hand, the amount of information which can be extracted from each brief advertisement is very much less and, such as it is, subject to the judgmental errors of the analyst. There are many more advertisers than respondents to questionnaires but, with respect to a sample of sado-masochists, it may well be the difference between the tip of the iceberg and the tip-of-the-tip. Buhrich is of the same opinion as Richard Green (1975), investigating sexual identity, that it is permissible to collect information from any available source and to draw conclusions from an overview of the relevant published literature, given the extreme difficulty of obtaining any unbiased sample of sexual deviants—a difficulty underlined by Frederick Whitam (1977) in his investigation of male homosexuality: "... how does one obtain a random sample of homosexuals or heterosexuals, the parameters of which are not known ... it is possible that ... matching homosexuals and heterosexuals according to occupation serves to confound rather than to clarify ..." (p. 91).

COMPOSITION OF SAMPLE POPULATIONS

Turning now to matters of substance, there is a basic difference between the two fairly large sample populations reported by Spengler (1977) and Breslow *et al.* (1985) ($n = 245$ and $n = 182$, respectively). Unlike Spengler, who found almost no women apart from prostitutes in the West German sadomasochistic subculture, Breslow *et al.* received responses from 52 women, only 12 of whom were allegedly prostitutes and excluded from their analysis. One cannot help wondering whether this discrepancy reflects any real difference between the general cultural climates of Hamburg and California, respectively, or whether one of the concerns from the outset of the American study was to challenge the German findings on some basic controversial issue. Historically, Germany has hardly lagged behind in sexual deviance. Moser and Levitt (1987) are equally insistent on the presence of some women in the American sadomasochistic subculture, but they do not report in the same detail on their 47 female as on their 178 male respondents because of the small size of the sample and the "difficulty in comparing it to any other sample of women involved in variant sexual behavior" (p. 333).

As to other demographic findings on age, education and income, the three studies are in agreement that the majority of their respondents were aged over 30, well educated and well paid. The American authors note that, on the whole, males achieved a higher level of education and earned more than females. Both Spengler and Breslow *et al.* record the finding that sadomasochists have a higher divorce rate than that of the general population. Breslow *et al.* consulted the 1981 Bureau of the Census figures and found that their subjects tended to marry later and less often. They challenge Hunt's (1974) hypothesis that "individuals engaged in sadomasochism are personality disordered and unable to engage in meaningful relationships" (Breslow *et al.*, p. 308), with the suggestion that they may do better with partners who share the same sexual interests.

Litman and Swearingen (1972), on interviewing their 12 selected respondents, decided to retain only the 9 men and exclude the 3 women from their study since they judged that "for each of them, the involvement in bondage was transient or secondary to a wish to please the sadistic needs of a man" (p. 83). Most of their male subjects, as in the three larger studies, were middle-aged, financially successful and either single or divorced.

Buhrich (1983) selected a final sample of 160 advertisers interested in erotic piercing: 154 males and 6 females. One of the females stated that she was bisexual, two that their interest was in tattoos, none stated their age. The ages stated by 102 of the males ranged between 23 and 55 years, with a mean age of 40.

DEVISING A QUESTIONNAIRE AND SCORING RESPONSES

Of equal importance with sampling procedures is the structure of the questionnaire and/or interview on the basis of which the sample population is investigated. Moser and Levitt (1987), for instance, used "57 major items as multiple choice, one word fill-in, or checklist questions" (pp. 326–327). These related to demographic characters (11 items), sexual identity or behavior (16 items), attitudes or responses to sadomasochistic behavior (7 items) and general attitude to sadomasochism (4 items). The remaining 19 items apparently elicited nothing suitable for presentation in their 1987 'exploratory-descriptive study'—one unspecified item was largely ignored by their respondents. A psychological functioning inventory, 'implanted' in the questionnaire and similar to that used by Weinberg and Williams (1975) for male homosexuals, indicated that the two distinct samples functioned equally well. Unfortunately, "problems with comparing slightly different versions of the inventory, size of the sample, and inability to match subjects on all demographic criteria make statistical analysis inappropriate" (p. 327). They do, however, present a comparative tabulation of Spengler's (1977) data on 'first awareness' of deviance and their own on 'first experience' and 'coming out'. The questionnaire devised by Moser and Levitt also listed specific deviant practices, with space to indicate any others which had been overlooked. No novel practices were in fact reported. The form was completed by most respondents in about 15 minutes. In scoring their heterosexual-homosexual orientation, as perceived by themselves, Moser and Levitt used the classical 7-point continuum of Kinsey *et al.* (1948, 1953) and found that they were largely heterosexual. The same scale of 0 to 6 applied to dominant-submissive role preference showed that they were, for the most part, 'switchable'.

Miles Shore *et al.* (1971), since there are four of them, might well have troubled to get Sacher-Masoch's first name and some of their references right before publishing their empirical study of patterns of masochism. Most clinical papers report the defensive and adaptive functions of masochism but Shore *et al.* consider they are breaking new ground in distinguishing and objectifying these defensive functions systematically so as to delineate behavioral patterns. They decided to look at (1) object relations, (2) defense against aggressive impulses, (3) enjoyment of pleasure, and (4) narcissism, by devising a questionnaire, interviewing some 'highly masochistic' subjects for one to two hours, and comparing their questionnaire scores with their classification of interviewees into subtypes. The 100 true–false statements were put to 300 heterogeneous in- and out-patients of the New England Medical Center Hospital and the results analysed using a principal factor rotation system. Interview protocols on 26 individuals "with a high density of masochistic characteristics" (p. 61) were summarized by the research team and mounted in subcategories on a large chart—seven 'Victims', five 'Doers', three 'Somatizers' and eleven transitional or defying categorization. The Victims were fearful of hurting others but felt free to vent hatred on their respective sadists and to enjoy sexual relations if coupled with pain. They feared their fathers, felt their mothers let them down, and had oral-hysterical, passive personalities. The Doers were self-sacrificing and prone to reaction-formation. Aggression was proscribed except in defense of someone else, pleasure was confined to cooking for others, sex was a duty. They had obsessive-compulsive personalities. The three Somatizers had obtrusive, mysterious ailments, were excessively demanding and not above terrorizing their children. Their mothers were cold and their fathers seductive but strict over sexual matters. The statistical analysis of the questionnaire scores reflected these three groups of interviewees to a substantial extent provided one introduced the Suspicion factor, the Balancing factor, the Compulsive factor, the Negative Fun factor and Factor X expressing stoicism and forgiveness. "The purpose of this study," Shore *et al.* state, "was to clarify confusion in the literature and in clinical practice about the nature of masochism" (p. 65). Unfortunately sophisticated statistical handling of data does not guarantee success in this endeavour.

Claude Crépault and Marcel Couture (1980) undertake a more complex investigation in French Canada of men's erotic fantasies. Their methods merit discussion here, partly because their introductory assessment of the nature and various functions of erotic fantasy is eminently sound and partly because they found three main themes: confirmation of sexual power, aggressiveness and masochistic fantasies. Their 94 unpaid volunteers, recruited by poster and newspaper advertisement, were interviewed for approximately two hours then asked to complete a two-part questionnaire. This consisted of a list of 46 erotic fantasies against each of which the subject was to indicate whether he entertained it 'often', 'sometimes' or 'never' during heterosexual activity with his regular partner (first part) and/or during masturbation (second part). The 46 fantasized scenarios, culled from clinical literature and the authors' previous research (Crépault *et al.*, 1977), are tabulated in order of their incidence (i.e., popularity), giving the frequency ('often' or 'sometimes') of each and its 'rank according to average score'. The average score was calculated from the data of frequency of occurrence, 'often' scoring 3, 'sometimes' scoring 2, and 'never' scoring 1. Crépault and Couture also undertake a sophisticated factor analysis (like Shore *et al.*, 1971—Varimax rotation with Kaiser correction) on the basis of fantasy content, identifying six principal factors: (1) assertion of sexual power, (2) aggression, (3) masochism, (4) maternal fixation, (5) exhibitionism, (6) oral eroticism. However sceptical one's attitude to factor analysis as a statistical procedure, one has to grant these investigators considerable psychological penetration and clever use of interrogation on an extremely slippery subject. Their success in arriving, after combining written and verbal information, at some interesting concrete conclusions (for instance, that men engaging frequently in fantasy can control the timing of ejaculation during coitus) probably derives initially from the simple, clear-cut design of their questionnaire.

CATEGORIZATION AND GROUPING

Categorization hinges on definition, the most fundamental definition being, of course, that of (sado)masochism itself. Spengler (1977) states, reasonably enough: "We define manifest sadomasochistic deviance as a specialization of a type of sexual behavior where the interaction between the partners is concentrated on inflicting and receiving physical and psychic pain, or on ritualized submission and dominance" (p. 442). In other words, his study deals with the overt masochistic perversion, not the masochistic character, that is, it deals with what Freud (1924*a*) categorized as erotogenic and feminine masochism, not moral masochism. It has no means of reporting on cryptic as distinct from overt sadomasochistic practices, since these are usually hidden from the subjects themselves, though constituting an important and never-ending part of their behavior. Breslow *et al.* (1985) introduce their report with a glance at different perspectives (they misquote Freud as asserting that women's natural state was one of moral masochism), but they do not give their own definition of sadomasochism. Breslow *et al.* largely and deliberately follow Spengler's groupings in their analysis. Their sample population is divided into heterosexuals, bisexuals and homosexuals and, despite their finding that 57.9% of their female subjects ($n = 38$) were 'heterosexual'/'usually heterosexual' and 39.5% were 'bisexual'/'forced bisexual', we are told that "females tended to lean toward bisexuality" (after being informed that a 'forced' bisexual enjoys homosexual relations only when bound or commanded by a sadist), whereas "males tended to be predominantly heterosexual". As to the success of the latter in finding an outlet for their deviance, they disagree with Spengler (and, incidentally, misrepresent him). He found that 85% of his male heterosexual subjects had no sadomasochistic relations (actually the percentage referred only to participation in sadomasochistic parties) during the preceding year, whereas their finding is that "only 13.3% of the male heterosexual respondents in this survey reported no encounters".

Both these studies examine the 3 categories: 'dominant/active/sadistic', 'submissive/passive/masochistic' and 'versatile'. They both note that the majority of their subjects adopt sadistic or masochistic roles flexibly and opportunistically, though Breslow *et al.* report 48% of males and

37% of females as inflexible. Of course, neither study makes the crucial psychological comments that the sadist's pleasure is also masochistic (vicariously, by the mechanism of projective identification), that the masochist's suffering or humiliation is also a sadistic enactment (by intended role reversal, as a stage in the etiology of masochism, and often in everyday life, straightforwardly following the formula "I must suffer and you must suffer"). Litman and Swearingen (1972) report that half their male subjects were willing to play a sadistic role occasionally, but with reluctance and only in order to satisfy a partner.

In attempting to examine the question of first awareness of sado-masochistic tendencies, Spengler employs the categories 'heterosexual', 'bisexual', 'homosexual' and various age groupings. Breslow *et al.* tabulate 'male' and 'female' against different units of time. So detailed comparison of their respective findings becomes virtually impossible. Spengler comments that homosexuals experienced this 'coming out' later than heterosexuals. Breslow *et al.* report (at the end of their paper): "Males realized their sexual interests in sadomasochism considerably earlier in life than females. Males seemed to discover sadomasochism on their own, whereas females tended to be introduced to it by a sexual partner" (p. 316). However, Breslow *et al.* also make two comments in connection with their tabulation which (as possibly the most psychologically interesting in the paper) deserve quotation: "A belief exists within the subculture that sado-masochistic interests are 'natural ones' from childhood, that is, that they are the earliest sexual thoughts that can be remembered ... Although the males did feel that their interests were natural ones, the issue becomes clouded by the manner in which different men defined *childhood*. Older men (those in their 50s and beyond) tended to extend childhood to include their mid-20s, while younger men tended to restrict childhood to the teenage years or younger" (pp. 309–310). An observation which underlines the general problem of categorization of psychological data!

Both studies agree that their subjects show a high level of self-acceptance and then proceed to a tabulation of deviant practices—each in a different manner. Spengler divides 'sadomasochistic practices' from 'fetishistic preferences'. Breslow *et al.* compare the interests of females with those of males, recorded 'in descending order' in percentages, but since we are given no *n* values, we have no means of knowing the amount of overlap between categories, nor whether the percentages refer to numbers of individuals actually engaging in the specific practice or to averaged 'ratings' by individuals whether or not they pursued the activity (the text is ambiguous). However unclear the attempts at quantification, the lists of deviant practices are of concrete interest. Both studies agree on the relative rarity of the more extreme or dangerous practices and on the importance of fetishistic elements. Breslow *et al.* note that their female subjects were more interested in 'bondage' than their male subjects and—a somewhat naive observation, perhaps—more interested in erotic lingerie, boots and shoes! An interest in rubber and leather was shared equally by males and females. Although the fantasies submitted, presumably in response to the follow-up, 'in-depth' questionnaire, had dwelt much upon the feminization of males, "only a few respondents indicated an interest in either transvestism or 'petticoat punishment' (a form of transvestism in which the male is made to look ridiculous instead of feminine)" (p. 315). Since they give *The Economic Problem of Masochism* (Freud, 1924*a*) as one of their references, one wonders idly whether this observation, so reminiscent of 'dressing up', actually recalled to Breslow *et al.*, or not, Freud's remarks on "the superimposed stratification of the infantile and the feminine" in masochistic fantasy and practice.

Litman and Swearingen (1972) also report of their 9 male subjects: "In this group transvestite elements were surprisingly infrequent" (p. 85). Since their paper deals specifically with 'bondage and suicide', their categorization (they present only one table) is on an individual basis and gives information on the age, occupation, sexual orientation, masochistic behavior, special fantasy, use of pornography and psychiatric history of each subject. Most of these men were homosexual or bisexual. There was a trend toward increasing homosexuality with age, probably because gratification through bondage was more easily obtained in homosexual circles than with women. As the sample is a small one, and as one would expect in the *Archives of General Psychiatry*, the authors are able to make much more psychological comment, some of it quite telling: "Each man had his own special most desired combination of components and could adjust to less optimal circumstances to different degrees. Nearly always the fantasy is more important than the actions, as if the sexual experiences and sexual partners are felt as fragments of experiences and fragments of people held together by imagination like tiles in a mosaic" (p. 85). The paper is a harrowing one and though it may not refute the statistical finding of Spengler and Breslow *et al.* that the more extreme and dangerous deviant practices are comparatively rare, it goes some way towards doing so, and certainly provides a corrective counterweight to their view. According to Litman and Swearingen, deaths by hanging or asphyxiation "do not represent medical rarities or forensic curiosities". From coroners' reports in Massachusetts, Virginia, Texas and Los Angeles itself, they estimate that there are about 50 'bondage' deaths in the United States per year. Two cases, one certified as an accident, the other as a suicide, both leaving written material which is quoted at length, serve as an extremely sombre introduction to the investigation.

Since Neil Buhrich's (1983) study is based only on a selection of advertisements and, like Litman and Swearingen's, is concerned with a special category of sadomasochistic activity, 'erotic piercing', one might anticipate that there is not a great deal of further categorization or grouping left open to him. He does, however, undertake some rudimentary analysis of his sample of 154 male advertisers. His single table is headed 'Sexual deviations of 154 male erotic piercers' and presents percentages (necessarily overlapping) for a mixture of groupings: 'homosexual or bisexual' (49%), 'sadomasochism' (44%), 'tattoos' (41%), 'bondage and/or discipline' (18%), 'fetishism' (10%), 'urolagnia' (8%) and 'other' (10%). This ultimate category "includes six subscribers who advertised an interest for coprophilia, three for chastity or antimasturbatory devices, three for transvestism, and four for castration, penilectomy, or genital mutilation" (p. 169). Well, at least he states absolute numbers, and they do indeed form 10% of his sample, so let us hastily avert any slide into flippancy—under any interpretation ill-becoming—and look at what else he says. He explains that subscribers were classified as homosexual / bisexual if they stipulated male contacts (only 24 stated specifically that they were heterosexual), as sadomasochistic if they sought dominance or submission, as fetishistic if they expressed an interest in leather, Levis (jeans) or boots. In *Gauntlet Magazine*, the code 'BD' coupled 'bondage' and 'discipline'. Commenting on the fact that three times as many subscribers specified a homosexual rather than heterosexual contact, Buhrich notes that Kinsey *et al.* (1948) reported a prevalence of homosexuality of 5% in the adult male population and that 22% of males were sexually excited by sadomasochistic literature.

GENERAL, UNCATEGORIZED FINDINGS

Common to most empirical studies, 'popular' as well as 'scientific', is the finding that overt masochism is a widespread phenomenon in developed urban centres (Hamilton, 1929; Kinsey *et al.*, 1953; Hunt, 1974; Stein, 1975; Sue, 1979). In Los Angeles, Litman & Swearingen (1972) report a dozen stores trading profitably for years in flagellation, bondage and torture pornography, with many other bookshops adding a 'bondage nook' as police attitudes relaxed. These authors also emphasize the loneliness, and frequent boredom, of the male masochists they interviewed. None of these intelligent, articulate volunteers accepted the payment on offer for expenses. They revealed no consistent pattern of pathological family interaction or sexual abuse in childhood. With increasing age, there was a trend away from autoerotic activities toward partnership. Some joined sadomasochistic clubs, where the inhalation of amyl nitrite was a common practice "to prolong masochistic activity and endure more pain". They all seemed deeply depressed and death-orientated, fending off suicide by their perversion, as described by Weisman (1967). The erotization of helplessness in the face of danger led through endurance and survival to eventual triumph and orgasm. Even when engaging in deviant activities with others, they remained preoccupied with their own fantasies, their own scenarios.

Most empirical investigators of sadomasochism accord some importance to pornography—necessarily, since it was usually the means of setting up their studies. Litman and Swearingen (1972) confirm the view of Stoller (1970) that there is a pornography corresponding to each form of perversion. About a third of their subjects stated that they had discovered aspects of their perversion through pornography and had been strongly influenced by it. Several had expensive collections. They would become bored or ashamed and dispose of them only to purchase afresh at a subsequent date.

Chris Gosselin and Glenn Wilson (1980), comparing the anonymous responses of 133 male sadomasochists, 125 rubber and leather fetishists and 269 transvestites to a questionnaire, conclude that 35% were interested in all three deviations and that fetishism mediates between sadomasochism and transvestism. They chiefly compare aspects of personality and fantasy content between the deviant groups.

Moser and Levitt (1987), whilst largely confirming Spengler's (1977) findings, supply some unusual references in a brief historical overview. Their introduction asserts that sadomasochistic behavior can be traced from nonhuman primate and primitive human communities, through ancient Egyptian, Indian, Oriental and Arab cultures, to the present. No doubt the assertion is broadly correct, though assertions as broad as that must surely have a limited value.

EMPIRICAL INVESTIGATIONS OF OTHER TYPES

Judson Brown *et al.* (1964) conducted an experiment on rats with a view to examining masochism in terms of behavior theory. They first trained them to escape from an electrified starting box along a straight passage to a safe goal box at the end. When the habit was established, control animals were given 60 'extinction' runs on which no shock was administered, whereas experimental subjects encountered shocks of moderate intensity in the passage between the two boxes, giving them the option of staying in the safe starting compartment or traversing the electrified passage to the safe goal box. Surprisingly, many persisted in running to the goal box in spite of the 'punishing' shock, and this behavior was described as 'masochistic-like'. In order to answer objections to the application of this term to rats rather than humans, Brown (1965) decided to review "the broader problems of how masochistic behavior might be defined or recognized, of how the painful or aversive attributes of a stimulus situation should be specified, and of how to resolve the paradoxical assertion that the masochist finds 'pleasure in pain'" (p. 65). Having pointed out that a stimulus cannot be judged noxious, neutral or pleasant on the basis of its physical properties, since "one man's meat is another man's poison", but only on the basis of the recipient's behavior, he presents a table of 'Pairs of behavior items defining masochism or hedonophobia'. The first item of each pair categorizes a situation or object as noxious, the second as pleasant or at least neutral. Thus, in behavioral pair number one, we have an object rejected by most individuals but accepted by Individual A; in pair 2, an object rejected by Individual B but accepted by Individual A; in pair 3, an object rejected by Individual A at one time but accepted by him at another time; in pair 4, an object rejected by him verbally but accepted by his nonverbal acts. The behavior categorized in pair 3 would correspond to that of the 'self-punitive' experimental rats. Brown asserts that any organism, at any time, may be used as a reference subject provided one adopts a completely relativistic position in defining aversiveness and nonaversiveness. "The outcome is relativism, to be sure, but not anarchy or confusion" (p. 66). The psychoanalytic conception of masochism emerged from a preoccupation with 'mental life' as opposed to overt behavior. The former easily accommodates ambiguity and internal contradiction, the latter immediately highlights the paradox of pleasure in pain: "if the pleasant and painful qualities of the situation are defined, respectively, in terms of approach and avoidance reactions, then the masochist is in the unique and impossible position of approaching and avoiding at one and the same moment" (p. 67). Whilst asserting on the behaviorist platform that approach and avoidance cannot occur simultaneously, Brown explains the anomaly of pair number four in his table with the example of a man who says 'this coffee tastes dreadful' but who nonetheless swallows it: "We may, however, emphasize the behavior that defines the coffee as noxious and yet place some credence in the opposite behavior pattern by stating that the subject is a masochist" (p. 68). Yes indeed, for what Brown is not willing to grant explicitly is that such irreconcilables as simultaneous approach and avoidance are of the essence—one might say, the stock-in-trade of masochism. "Yes, no" is a not uncommon utterance, quite literally, from a masochist.

Brown's (1965) paper is, however, closely argued and substantial despite its succinctness. It encompasses hedonophobia, the complement to pain-seeking, which, Brown justly remarks, might well receive more attention in the study of abnormal behavior. It also reviews some mechanisms by which masochism might be understood: a high pain-receptor threshold (or a low one in the case of the hedonophobic who might be irritated by stimuli which most people would experience as pleasantly mild or neutral), a fatigued effector system which might prevent expression of an avoidant reaction (or a low effector threshold which might account for hedonophobic hyperreactivity), or a third mechanism, conditioning, so as to produce "reactions of opposite polarity to a single set of physical conditions" (Pavlov, 1927; Guthrie, 1935; Masserman, 1946; Miller, 1960; Melvin & Brown, 1965) or so as to produce a vicious circle of flight into danger, initiated by fear (Mowrer, 1950). As Brown was then writing before the definitive isolation of endogenous opioids (Hughes *et al.* 1975), he could not, of course, relate them to his rat experiment though, had he not been so firmly committed to the behaviorist camp, he might have read, rather relevantly, in *Civilization and its Discontents* (Freud, 1930, p. 78): "it is a fact that there are foreign substances which, when present in the blood or tissues, directly cause us pleasurable sensations; and they also so alter the conditions governing our sensibility that we become incapable of receiving unpleasurable impulses. The two effects not only occur simultaneously, but seem to be intimately bound up with each other. But there must be substances in the chemistry of our own bodies which have similar effects ..." How many hapless rodents have since been tortured to confirm this hypothesis!

Of course, such torture (admittedly an emotive word)—up to 400 volts—was blithely undertaken by Neal Miller (1960) and his co-workers (one is tempted to say acolytes) on 100 hungry Sprague-Dawley rats, in three experiments, not to test any such far-reaching, immensely important hypothesis as Freud's, just mentioned, but to 'induce an approach-avoidance conflict' and to provide data in support of the following rather obvious expectations: (1) Hungry rats habituated to gradually increasing shocks run into pain for food more swiftly than those suddenly shocked for the first time. (2) A series of similarly graded shocks outside 'the rewarded conflict situation' does little to improve rats' resistance to stress above that of nonshocked controls. (3) Additional training runs for rats who have already become adept at reaching their food pellets, reduce rather than increase their resistance to disruption when shocks are introduced. (This unremarkable finding was actually contrary to Miller's original expectation. One can almost picture him holding up a forefinger darkly as he advises (p. 145): "Although widely advocated, mere overtraining may not always be helpful preparation for subsequent stress.") His final conclusion (4) is that "it should be feasible and profitable to analyse further at both the animal and human level the laws governing the learning of resistance to stresses such as pain, fear, fatigue, frustration, noise, nausea, and extremes of temperature" (p. 145). One can only feel relieved that he was not employed at Auschwitz.

But to return (explicitly) to the theme of sadomasochism on the human level, Marks *et al.* (1965) report successful aversion therapy in the case of a 34-year-old married man who had suddenly become impotent three months before admission to the Maudsley Hospital. For all the sophistication of their methods of assessing the treatment, certain features of their paper strike one as simplistic. We are informed, for instance, that from nine years old he had a fetishistic interest in high-heeled shoes and rubber boots, associated from 12 years old with daily masturbation, from nineteen years old he had fantasies of being kicked by men or women wearing the fetish, of being beaten to death, that he "actually slapped his genitals with boots", however: "The longstanding masochistic desires or fantasies surprisingly ceased after the two operant procedures preceding admission, and only recurred a few times momentarily" (p. 255). We are told that he married at 21 and urged his reluctant wife to kick or stand on him, once leading to a broken coccyx, but that this was the only source of friction "in an otherwise happy marriage". The operant conditioning procedure (Skinner *et al.*, 1954; Lindsley, 1956) consisted of measuring the rate at which he moved a lever with his right hand before and after treatment. Before the treatment, this stabilized at 70 movements per minute over several control periods but increased to 85 whilst he was holding the fetish in his left hand. He was then warned that he might receive faradic (most people would find 'faradaic' the more common adjectival usage) shocks to his left forearm, though not that they were designed to occur when the response rate exceeded 70. (How long would it take to deduce this, one wonders!) Soon after they started, his movements decreased below the control rate even whilst holding the fetish, and a second day's testing confirmed that he was trying to avoid shocks whether the situation was sexually arousing or not. His masochism was evidently restricted to a sexual context and to certain stimuli only, not electric shocks, so Marks *et al.* felt justified in admitting him for a fortnight's aversive treatment. He filled in a 16-page 'semantic differential' booklet (Osgood *et al.*, 1957) before the treatment, two days then one week into the treatment and finally on being discharged from the treatment. His attitude to the control concepts of 'women', 'my mother', 'my father' and 'myself' did not change; 'boots' and 'shoes' became markedly devalued, 'psychiatrists' were scored as less friendly and 'sexual intercourse' (in agreement with clinical observation and the testimony of his wife) as more satisfactory. The operant conditioning procedure confirmed that the fetish was no longer arousing after treatment. So what was the treatment? For up to an hour twice daily, he was asked to visualize his favourite boots and signal the visualization by tapping a pencil. (One is immediately uneasy about this. My own view, and one which a simple trial will confirm, is that it is impossible to daydream to order. 'Visualization' must therefore have been on a very superficial level, with no development into emotionally charged fantasy, though Theodor Reik's observation (Reik, 1939, 1941) that every masochist has a long history of fantasy preparation and only requires a trigger, must be taken into account. An interesting discussion of the question is provided by Crépault & Couture, 1980.) A shock was immediately given which dispelled the image (cf. McGuire & Vallance, 1964). After one or two minutes' respite, the process was repeated. The latency period increased until finally the images could no longer be produced at all, though since the latency curves corresponding to various sessions started at roughly the same point, this was deemed to reflect 'suppression' rather than 'extinction'. 'Fantasy aversion' was then combined with shocks given whilst he was actually wearing the boots and until he took them off. Booster treatments were arranged to prevent any relapse. In their 'Discussion' Marks *et al.* report: "the masochism disappeared unexpectedly rapidly, before the fetish object itself became neutral; this suggests that it was a secondary phenomenon. Normal intercourse became more enjoyable" (p. 258). It would seem unlikely, however, in view of the protean nature of masochism, that it could disappear overnight and doubtful whether it should be called 'a secondary phenomenon'.

EMPIRICAL STUDIES WITH A BEARING ON SADOMASOCHISM

Inge Lunde *et al.* (1981) present physiological data on 17 male victims of torture, of whom 29% subsequently experienced reduced libido and erectile dysfunction. These 17 Greeks were 'randomly' selected from a larger group subjected to torture for political reasons. Aged 21–50, they had been tortured by beating (sometimes prolonged, on the soles of their feet), electric shock, suspension by their feet or hands, dripping water, solitary confinement or mock execution. They had in some cases been deprived of food, fluids and sleep, and had been forced to watch the maltreatment of their relatives. These events occurred between 1967 and 1974. In June 1976 and June 1977 blood samples were taken between 8 and 10 am to determine plasma concentrations of luteinizing hormone, follicle-stimulating hormone, prolactin and testosterone. Control samples were taken from 11 healthy Greek males, aged 32–46, though no enquiry was made into the sexological history of these men. The sexual dysfunction of the tortured subjects, classified as (1) reduced libido, (2) erectile dysfunction or (3) retarded ejaculation, was investigated by a 29-point questionnaire, presented and explained in Greek. Premature ejaculation was not considered a dysfunction, and fertility was assessed on the pregnancies of the subjects' partners—somewhat naively perhaps, since the majority had an academic background and may well have been familiar with techniques of birth control. Three men reported less coital activity subsequent to imprisonment but still sufficient to be satisfactory to themselves. Five others were classified as sexually impaired, but no relation was found between the development of dysfunction and the length of internment (ranging from 5 months to 6 years) or torture (ranging from 2 to 47 days)—no effect relating to the type or severity of torture, the exposure to head, genital or multiple injuries. Levels of pituitary and gonadal hormones were within the same range as the Greek control group and also that recorded as normal for Danish men of the same age. Lunde *et al.* do not, however, consider the possibility that they were testing the wrong hormones and that assays of neuronal hormones under other circumstances might have resulted in a different picture (Olson *et al.* 1980–1987). They simply comment: "Plasma concentrations of gonadotrophins, prolactin, and testosterone were all within normal limits, making it less likely that any major hormonal disturbances were the cause of the sexual dysfunctions described" (p. 31). Their incidence (29%), similar to that (30–75%) found in men with 'the concentration camp syndrome' (Kral, 1951; Kral *et al.* 1967; Helweg-Larsen *et al.* 1952; Ström, 1968; Thygesen *et al.* 1970), suggested to Lunde *et al.* that malnutrition might not be a major factor, as the Greek victims had not suffered any severe weight loss, but that internment *per se* might account for the similar sequelae to some extent. There is, of course, no discussion of the psychological effects of torture so no consideration of any psychological mechanism which might shed light on the sexual dysfunction. Guarded references to hypothalamic and limbic system injury, to possible 'psychogenic action upon the gonads', are as far as Lunde *et al.* are prepared to venture in this direction. The possibility of any modification of sexual aim, of the blocking and rechannelling of psychosexual function, was presumably not explored in the questionnaire, though a masochistic attitude has often been attributed to survivors of the Holocaust. The biochemical data, though tabulated with scientific exactitude, may not be the most relevant to an investigation of the physiological effects of torture. One is reminded of the famous six monkeys at their typewriters who might, in the course of millennia, happen to type out Shakespearian sonnets!

There have been numerous investigations of the possible correlation between depictions of sexual violence in 'male sophisticate' magazines and violent assaults on women—Donnerstein (1980), Burt (1980), Malamuth & Spinner (1980), Malamuth (1981), to mention but a few. For the study by Joseph Scott and Steven Cuvelier (1987) eighteen luckless undergraduates, half of them male and half female, were recruited in 1984 to thumb through every issue of *Playboy* magazine from January 1954 to December 1983, rating cartoons and pictorials as sexually violent if they portrayed rape, sadomasochism or 'exploitative/coercive sexual relations'. Not surprisingly, in view of the instruction to be conservative in rating and discount ambiguous material, depictions of violence, both sexual and nonsexual, were found to be rare and, in any case, after increasing somewhat during the '70s, were decreasing during the '80s. *Playboy* magazine had a 1983 circulation of over 4 million, correlating with rape rates by American state more than any other 'adult' magazine, but Scott and Cuvelier conclude that "such correlations cannot be accounted for by violent sexual depictions ... or, for that matter, by violent depictions in sexually oriented magazines" (p. 287). The logical alternative explanation of their findings, namely that an environment conducive to violence is likely to harbour both *Playboy* magazine and potential rapists and potential perpetrators of other forms of physical assault, who will indeed be likely to purchase the magazine, goes unstated. One would also like to ask these many untiring investigators of the possible influence of pornography, after all, how they think such habitual reading could fail to influence a human mind in some way.

WHAT HAS THE EMPIRICAL LITERATURE TAUGHT US?

In so far as they are well directed, accurate and large enough to go beyond individual differences, empirical studies may, in principle, permit general inferences to be drawn and essential characteristics to be identified. The investigator is likely to confine himself to the possible, to precisely formulated and not overambitious hypotheses which may be upheld or refuted without ambiguity. Different studies in the same field can be seen clearly to support or to undermine each other's findings, to add or to detract from the validity of a specific theory. These scientific rewards become possible through measurement.

In the present survey, the ideals of empirical research are present but in danger of disappearing over a distant horizon. There is an obvious deduction to be made from the fact that percentages—regarding sexual orientation, let us say—vary widely from study to study: the samples must have been recruited in different manners or from different populations. In other words, almost anything can be demonstrated provided the appropriate sample has been selected—sampling or ascertainment is of paramount importance.

Nevertheless, the studies have information to offer, chiefly of a demographic nature, and on this information they are in reasonable agreement: (a) sadomasochism is a widespread phenomenon in urban centers; (b) fewer women than men are involved in it; (c) most subjects willing to participate in research are over 30, well educated, well paid, the men more so than the women; (d) they have a higher divorce rate than the population average.

General agreement continues on somewhat more specific issues: (a) the majority of practitioners are able to switch between dominant and submissive roles opportunistically or if required to do so; (b) there is a high level of self-acceptance amongst those overtly pursuing their deviance; (c) the importance of fetishistic elements and pornographic reading matter is well attested; (d) the commonality of certain practices is determined. The more dangerous practices are mostly recorded as of rare occurrence.

The occasional shaft of psychological insight comes in the investigation of fantasy, but it is worth noting, in concluding this survey of empirical studies on sadomasochism, that whereas it would be quite possible to review the psychological literature on the subject under headings relating to different aspects of the deviance, such a method would be fruitless, if it were even possible, in the present case. This is because so very little light is shed on the etiology and the essential nature of masochism by the average empirical investigation. Lists of deviant practices are a far cry from an illumination of the phenomenon. One fact is, however, highlighted, and it is a fundamental one: there is no such thing as masochism, strictly speaking—there is only sadomasochism. At least empirical investigation establishes that almost immediately.

CHAPTER 4

AN INTEGRATED PSYCHODYNAMIC MODEL OF MASOCHISM

What is masochism? A defense against depression? Should it be linked primarily with the vicissitudes of the sexual drive or with the personal relations we carry in our minds? What it is not is an inoffensive, inconsequential, passing kink.

The model of masochism proposed is a multicomponent system based largely on psychoanalytic theory but having physiological as well as psychological aspects. The personal observations communicated are noticeably harsh. It must therefore be emphasized that personal observations cannot be assumed to be objective or of general application. Even when accurate, they are apt to be stated in forceful, if not exaggerated terms. They refer to 'the masochist' in so far as he is a masochist. But masochism, though exceptionally pervasive, cannot be the whole of a human being any more than a crippling disability is the whole of the person afflicted with it. Masochists come in all shapes and sizes, have other qualities besides deviance and sometimes considerable talents or skills, as in the case of Gesualdo (Gray & Heseltine, 1971, pp. 50–52; Watkins, 1991, pp. 73–91), Musorgsky (Turner, 1986/7), Dostoevsky (Freud, 1928), C.S. Lewis (Wilson, 1990), T.E. Lawrence (Turner, 1991) and Yukio Mishima (Yourcenar, 1986), to mention but a few.

In any investigation of masochism, a crucial difference of behavior must be expected between the masochist actually engaging in overt sadomasochistic practices and the masochist to whom these rituals are denied.

The latter is likely to pursue a course of unremitting provocation (Panel, 1981), not surprising where fulfilment of sexuality, however deviant, is frustrated. The former may present a more likeable and reasonable personality *outside a sexual context*, to the extent that sexual drives have been satisfied.

In masochism, I believe, there has been a very early and fundamental distortion of developmental processes connected with (1) ego versus object libido (Lewinsky, 1944), (2) pleasure versus reality principle (Lenzer, 1975), (3) expression versus control of aggressive instincts (Kernberg, 1988), (4) helplessness versus mastery (Freud, 1920*a*), (5) union versus individuation (Glasser, 1979).

It seems likely that this process of developmental distortion is started by very early trauma. If *severe* enough, this may be enough in itself to account for the all-pervasive ultimate distortion. More likely, it is reinforced, confirmed, consolidated by succeeding and similar traumatic situations which gradually become self-engineered.

The nature of the trauma may vary from individual to individual—it may be predominantly physical (early injury, illness or stress), predominantly psychological (maternal rejection, parental loss) or a combination of both (corporal punishment, hospitalization)—but common to all masochists are the elements of fixation and regression.

Lewinsky (1944) linked masochism with narcissism, a link which had been strongly refuted by Reik (1939): "the narcissism of these masochistic persons is deranged in the deepest levels" (p. 58). Whether one prefers to call it egocentricity, whether one argues that it is primary or secondary, there is little doubt that the narcissism of the masochist is monumental and malignant. It is usual for a person's interest to be caught initially by something which relates to himself. The difference in the case of the masochist is that he cannot extend that to a more general interest in the person or subject (it might be a painter or a scientific theory) that originally attracted his attention by seeming relevant to his own life, his own inner world. He remains imprisoned in his own egoism (Lenzer, 1975), taking note only of the few elements which coincide with his own circumstances, forming a grossly curtailed and distorted picture of whatever or whoever has impinged upon his consciousness, giving a garbled account of it. This inability to extend exploratory feelers into the world beyond himself only increases his isolation—the real isolation which was doubtless in part the cause of the imprisoned condition and, in its turn, was caused by a withdrawal of libido into the ego, itself so battered and weak.

In desperation, the wounded ego may take its own body as the safest libidinal object. Although I believe that an inverted oedipal attachment to the father (Freud, 1919) is frequently at the root of the latent or overt homosexuality almost invariably present in the male masochist, I also endorse the observation of Thomas Szasz (1957/1975) concerning "the misleading impression that the notion of 'homosexuality' creates—namely, that the patient is (sexually) interested in another person who is of the same sex. Observation often shows that the patient is interested only in his own body. An ego orientation to the body might readily appear to be homosexual to the observer, particularly if it is in a manifestly projected form" (p. 141). 'Petticoat punishment', a ritual where the effect of the female garments is ridiculous not feminine, is not only a sought-after humiliation for the male masochistic deviant, it is also, by implication, a derogation of women. It is a Lacanian-type trickery. The ambiguities of Jacques Lacan, particularly his exposition of 'the phallus' (Lacan, 1958), and the whole complex issue of gender and sexual difference are considered in depth by Frosh (1994).

It is my conviction—and I become increasingly persuaded of it—that the masochistic perversion, besides being a psychosexual deviation, is also a physiological addiction involving the pain- and stress-produced endogenous opioids (Turner, 1991, pp. 412–416).

I believe that the sadomasochistic perversion is predominantly a deviance of the male for three reasons. First, quite simply, it has a much higher recorded incidence in men (Spengler, 1977). Second, the male has constitutionally a stronger aggressive drive than the female. The possession of an extra Y chromosome (the XYY male) has even been used as a legal defense in cases of criminal violence. Third, I believe that male sexuality is more fragile in general, and female sexuality more robust in that it is anchored through child-bearing to the survival of the species. The sexual behavior of a male masochist does not well serve the biological function of reproduction. Is masochism simply less obvious in a woman? Yes, that I would grant—and less obviously disruptive. In sexual relations, it could easily remain hidden and even gratify a partner. It might often be classified as hypochondriasis, 'the martyr syndrome' or 'the clinging-vine syndrome', for instance. Only perhaps when a woman assumes the sadistic role does her deviance become strident and attract attention. However, when those who simply oblige male masochists out of pity or for money are excluded, these 'super-bitches' (Gosselin & Wilson, 1980) are the rare exception which proves the rule. The women, mostly in their teens or early twenties, who cut their arms with razors or broken glass or burn themselves, do so almost invariably to obtain relief from psychological distress, not for sexual satisfaction (Babiker & Arnold, 1997). These views are somewhat uncontemporary—not to put too fine a point on it, old-fashioned! There is currently a marked increase in lesbianism. Competition, sometimes amounting to overt hostility, between the sexes, the fear of AIDS and exhortations to 'safe sex' have seemingly conspired to liberate not only the bisexuality always present but also infantile, polymorphously perverse components (Freud, 1905), leading to an increased, 'trendy' interest in sadomasochistic games, even perhaps by a few women. Well, what usually ensues on the swing of a pendulum is a swing in the opposite direction and, meanwhile, I think the masochist can still justifiably be referred to as "he".

Descriptively, I would single out the following characteristics. They are, of course, well-worn for the essential picture of masochism is not susceptible to much change (Freud, 1924*a*). They are, however, likely to vary according to the degree of self-knowledge of the individual and his reactions to it. At some points, they reflect the paradoxical nature of masochism itself. Lastly, it must be underlined that they are, to a considerable extent, the product of personal observation and subject to the *caveat* placed at the beginning of this chapter.

(i) RIGIDITY

As with other sexual deviations, there is a dismaying rigidity in the masochistic personality. One first becomes aware of it in habits and tastes. One notices stereotypes and clichés. One encounters an implacable obstinacy, a trait which lends support to Freud's suggestion that obsessional neurosis is the negative of which the sadomasochistic perversion is the positive.

Rigidity manifests as the compulsion to repeat at its most ineluctable—to repeat the same situations, the same dreams, the same ideas, the same phrases. Novick and Novick (1972), in their report on children treated at the Anna Freud Clinic, London, found that "the beating fantasy in this group of disturbed children was crude, monotonous and repetitive ... the fixed fantasy seemed impervious to years of interpretive work and in cases where follow-up evidence was available, the beating fantasy persisted after termination" (p. 240). Whatever new situation chance throws up for the adult, perhaps an exceptional opportunity for happiness, it will be drawn into the same inexorable mill and ground in the inevitable, dismal pattern until it is the same as the one before it, and the one before that. Round and round in the same situation—no use is made of feedback, so there is no learning from experience. Reactions are totally predictable. Nothing changes, except to deteriorate.

There is a point of fixation in his early development to which he is involuntarily drawn back. The subject of his conversation, the focus of his thoughts and feelings, the manifest content of his dreams consist largely of things, places and people from his childhood. These come up again and again.

(ii) FANTASY

Novick and Novick (1972, p. 238) define fantasy as conscious daydream. If you ask a masochist what he has been dreaming during the night, he will often report a fantasy. It becomes clear from his account that he had it, not whilst asleep, but whilst dozing after awakening. In my view, his mental functioning is habitually, and to a large extent, at the level of the primary processes (Freud, 1911; Lenzer, 1975). He can fall asleep with astonishing ease. Where worry or agitation would prevent a 'normal' person from sleeping and leave him tossing and turning with tensed muscles, the masochist can go to sleep with no difficulty. It is as if sleep, rather than action, were the way of relief. Recurrent masochistic dreams (for instance, beatings which usually have the character of escalations) are akin to masturbation fantasies. They may in fact be fantasies rather than dreams, or something between the two, for the twilight fantasy world of the masochist with the 'pleasure' ego reinstated on his throne, has misty, shifting borders with the realm of sleep. In short, Novick and Novick's (1972) definition is a useful one, but for the masochist there may be no clear distinction between fantasy and dream.

Many investigators, most notably Theodor Reik (1939, 1941), have identified fantasy-production, fantasy-dependence, as a quintessential characteristic of masochism. Many have portrayed masochists as lonely, usually self-isolated people. Litman and Swearingen (1972) wrote: "We feel that these volunteer subjects were motivated by loneliness" (p. 82) ... "The outstanding impression created by this group of subjects was that of pervasive loneliness and isolation" (p. 84). Not much has been said, however, about the relation existing between the two observations. In fact, they may well constitute a vicious circle. Immersed in fantasy, preferring it to the ardours of real human interaction, the masochist is perforce cut off from others and imprisoned in a haunted solitude, in autoerotism. Isolated, lonely, ever more socially inept, as described in the DSM-III-R Diagnostic Criteria for Self-defeating Personality Disorder set out in Appendix 1, what other recourse has he but to fantasy? (The qualification in parenthesis of DSM-III-R criterion 5, "despite having adequate social skills", I would challenge on two counts: (a) it is internally inconsistent with the criteria enumerated; (b) I have personally observed the contrary in most masochists I have encountered during the present study and over twenty years before it was undertaken, i.e., a lack of social skills proportionate to the penetration of masochism into the personality.)

The more hopeless the situation, the more estranged from reality does he become—further and further from reality with less and less incentive to turn back to it and face it. He is not prepared, possibly not even equipped, to make the necessary efforts to change it. As an infant, he hallucinated gratification, and as an adult, he prefers fantasy to reality. Typically, he will escape from the dreariness and drudgery of life into science fiction or the occult. It is unlikely to be an accident that the costumes, make-up, hair-styling, accessories and overall appearance of the *aficionados* depicted in sadomasochistic magazines are so strikingly similar to those of science fiction comics, paperbacks and films. Many of the sadomasochists I interviewed in the course of this study explicitly mentioned comics and/or science fiction as early formative influences. As might be to some extent expected in association with fetishism (the word 'fetish' comes from the Portuguese *feitiço*, meaning 'charm' or 'sorcery'), there was also a fascination with the occult. One twenty-five-year-old, for instance, actually attibuted his sexuality to his sign of the zodiac, whilst one sixty-four-year-old insisted his childhood bungalow was haunted. The masochist prefers the safety of the synthetic, the artificial, as Sacher-Masoch fell in love with his statue of Venus.

(iii) INFANTILISM

An eighty-four-foot diplodocus with a brain the size of a hen's egg constituted a menace—so does a middle-aged man fixated at the age of two. The masochist has an indomitable drive to return to childhood. His provocations are partly a method of reinstating childhood situations, partly a resentful protest against present situations and the person blocking the regression to childhood. Remorselessly he tries to force his partner into the role of 'dominatrix'/mother. Whatever he undertakes, usually after maddening procrastination, he bungles or handles inadequately (DSM-III-R diagnostic criterion 6 for Self-defeating Personality Disorder; Appendix 1), so that she has to intervene and take over the matter. In the end, she is apparently an officious, domineering scold, doing all the work; he is a downtrodden, aimiable bumbler, sucking sweets, doing nothing whatever!

Many investigators, such as Bernhard Berliner, Esther Menaker and Kerry and Jack Novick, have made the intrusive, immature or neglectful mother responsible for her child's masochism. As his earliest caregiver, she is likely to be the main culprit when it comes to infantilism. It is extremely likely that her ambivalence was perceived and passed on as a dominant character trait. It is for her betrayals that he is ceaselessly revenging himself, yet he has an overwhelming desire to return to the helplessness of infancy, with its freedom from responsibility, from effort, a need which has been profitably catered to by so-called adult baby clubs such as the Hush-A-Bye Baby Club in Gravesend. Those who practise 'bondage' aim at utter helplessness, in which they can triumphantly obtain their satisfaction.

Most of us must occasionally experience a dim longing to behave spontaneously, tactlessly, regardless of ruffling feathers. The masochist demands to be accepted however repugnant he makes himself—as if he were testing a relationship to the limit: "I will be loved for myself alone, whatever I do, however badly I behave, however unpleasant I am. Unless you will put up with anything at my hands, I will not trust your love. I must have the ultimate proof of it."

Very characteristic is the masochist's belief in the 'omnipotence of thoughts' (Panel, 1956). He attributes blame to himself for mishaps and even family disasters over which he had no control because he feels that, in fact, his repressed malevolence brought them about. Childish omnipotence (Brenner, 1959) leads him to interpose himself in the discussion of a subject about which he knows virtually nothing. This brings a bonus in that, whilst his other listeners take him seriously, his partner must endure the irritation of a conversation which she knows will end in embarrassment.

Like a child, his appetites must either be appeased instantly or, conversely, he will stubbornly deprive himself. Like a child, he is adept in sulking and 'dumb insolence'. His bodily functions, apart from the sexual, are childishly uncontrolled. He must urinate or defaecate instantly (Menaker, 1953), he will vomit over the floor, his sneeze is an explosion (possibly combining mess-making with substitutive orgasm!).

(iv) HYPOCRISY

Rudolph Loewenstein (1957) wrote: "We see here what Freud called a regressive resexualization of morality. Morality is upheld, but with a transparent and unmistakable hypocrisy which invariably is the hallmark of this sexualization and aggressivization of morality" (pp. 205–206). A masochist *has* to deceive himself. He *cannot* look straight at what he is and what he has done or omitted to do.

In explaining what he identified as 'the suspense factor' Reik (1939) wrote: "In cases of advanced masochistic attitude there results … that characteristic vacillation between the pleasurable and the fearful … 'to eat his cake and have it' " (p. 41). And not merely in overtly sexual activities does the masochist want to have his cake and eat it. He wants to lose control and to retain it. He wants to destroy and to be prevented from destroying. With respect to his own body, he will persistently damage it, making sure that his partner will make every effort to stop him. Her remonstrances are, of course, defiantly ignored (and she is portrayed to the world as bossy and interfering) as long as the self-destructive situation is still retrievable.

A split in the personality (the ego) of a masochist, particularly when frustrated, manifesting as a truly remarkable capacity for self-deception is easily observable, but even if it were not so patently evident, it could be inferred with confidence on theoretical grounds. The masochist may assert that his sexuality, if a little different, is nonetheless 'natural' and that he is content with it, he may obstinately present a brave face of self-acceptance, but somewhere in the remnants of his regressed, contorted superego there remains an awareness that the sustained torture and destruction of another human being is not an acceptable way of obtaining sexual satisfaction. Tormentor, destroyer, is not an acceptable self-image. His only escape must be into self-deception; he can only disavow this, continually and in every way. "Pain is, among other things, a currency with which we repay damages done unto others" (Szasz, 1957/1975). *He* is the one who is suffering, and that makes it all right. His partner *enjoys* the dominatrix role, or ought to, and loves him in spite of everything. *What* harm has he done, *what* devastation has he wreaked? He keeps it out of consciousness, in his reservoir of guilt, to refuel the vicious circle of guilt, punishment, satisfaction, more guilt.

Curiously, if a masochist learns of the cruel behavior of someone else, he will click his tongue and wonder how anyone can be so inhuman. It is difficult to decide whether this is 'double-think', i.e., stemming from a split ego, or hypocrisy, for the observed cruelty, of commission or omission, is often so strikingly similar to, if not identical with, his own that it is well-nigh inconceivable that he does not recognize the parallel. The traditional psychoanalytic wisdom on the subject is exemplified in Norbert Bromberg's (1955) formulation: "Anxiety is warded off by the mustering of the defenses of denial, projection, displacement, reaction formation and rationalization, in abundance" (pp. 805–806). In terms of the more recent constructionist concept of 'the dialogical self' expounded by Hubert Hermans *et al.* (1992), there is fantasy in superabundance, at best a "polyphony of voices" (p. 27), but no inner dialogue. The last thing the right hand wants to know is what the left hand is doing. On a more down-to-earth level, it is, of course, true that we all tend to judge others by their actions and ourselves by our intentions.

The distinction made at the outset must be underlined at this point, for we have been describing the masochist to whom sexual gratification through masochistic ritual of his own prescribing has been denied. The ruthlessness of the frustrated masochist may be explained by two mechanisms: (1) A large portion of his masochism is secondary (Freud, 1924*a*), that is sadism turned against the self, which when thwarted in this reintrojection resumes the form of outward directed sadism. (2) One goal of the desired masochistic practice was always the vengeful torture or humiliation of the object by projective identification, and when overt, primitive satisfaction is denied, the sadistic gratification will simply become covert and more sophisticated. The object will be tortured or humiliated in a multitude of ways, but preferentially and most satisfyingly in a sexual context. To these two mechanisms, the first hingeing on the projection or introjection of the destructive instinct, the second on the mode of gratification of the sadistic drive, must be added a simpler reaction of the thwarted infant—he will provoke and provoke until he obtains what he wants. The sustained provocation becomes ruthless and cruel—even if fleetingly admitted, that is the partner's fault, of course, and would all be different if he had his own way! Before leaving it, let us really try to come to grips with this hypocrisy. Many masochists are of high intelligence and keen intuitive potential. It is therefore impossible that they should never, at any moment, glimpse the real consequences of their destructive and self-destructive behavior. But the reality must be intolerable to them—if it were not, they would almost certainly be straightforward sadists rather than masochists. They are consumed with sensuality yet prudish in their projected attitudes. How is one to explain this puzzle? At an early stage some impairment or defensive alteration of information-processing took place (Bowlby, 1980, chapter 4). Most probably this was the only available defense against unbearable trauma in infancy or childhood (Fraiberg, 1982). With time, the malformation and dysfunction of cognitive processes are not only cumulative but they develop. Logic is more and more stubbornly shunned in favour of wishful interpretation (illusion, magic, 'omnipotence of thoughts'); reality is more and more ignored in favour of fantasy. By adulthood, not only has a stringent censorship been established, suppressing and distorting incoming perceptions which might disrupt the masochist's narcissistic fairyland, not only are his erroneous and tendentious memories of past events and people frozen, as in a glacier yet still exuding their poisonous influence, not only are his attitudes and habits set in granite, but he has also lost, to a large extent, the very capacity for logical thinking. Logic itself should tell him, as a general principle, that a course of relentless self-damage can only spiral downwards to self-destruction, but he is the god of his fantasy universe who has decreed that defiance will ultimately triumph. Those he damages on the way can be the objects of his 'love' and 'pity' in some other sealed compartment of his mind. Thus can he remain the mildest and most inoffensive of people. In cybernetic terms, there is a profound malfunction of *feedback* (Bowlby, 1969).

(v) PASSIVITY

Novick and Novick (1987, p. 368) distinguished between passivity and receptivity, pointing out that masochists are very active in their pursuit of pain and failure, whilst highly receptive to external stimuli. (I would qualify this—to *certain* external stimuli. This is part of the overlap with fetishism.) They feel guilty about asserting independence. Striving for autonomy is felt to be disloyalty (usually to an overprotective mother). On this I would only comment that day-to-day behavior seems rather to reflect a paradoxical amalgam of *passive* faithfulness with disloyalty where action is required.

One of the most baffling aspects of a masochist's behavior is his seeming inability, amounting to paralysis, to take actions to improve his very low self-esteem. He will watch another person working hard to improve a garden he also uses but he will not take a hoe, a rake or a wheelbarrow to help, even though his contribution would permit him to share and enjoy the garden so much more. He will complain of his ignorance and lack of skill with respect to household equipment but never take any steps to learn how to use it. He will bewail the fact that he cannot read something he wants to understand because it is in a foreign language but never make any effort to procure a translation or to learn the language. He is frozen. He is worthless, but his omissions *shall* not be remedied, for even-lower self-esteem is what he is aiming at. At rock bottom there is peace, there is invulnerability, there is victory in defeat. This was a perception set down by T.E. Lawrence, a practising masochist who combined 'the demonstrative factor' identified by Reik (1939) with a rare gift for introspection. He continues in the same Chapter 103 of *Seven Pillars of Wisdom* entitled 'Myself': "Many things I had picked up, dallied with, regarded, and laid down; for the conviction of doing was not in me" (Lawrence, 1926, p. 582).

The active sexual role requires cathexis to be directed away from the self and onto an object. This constitutes, in the short term, a loss of narcissistic libido. The masochist, fearful and insecure, is preoccupied with his own sexual performance. In the terminology of Thomas Szasz (1957/1975), his is a 'one-body', not a 'two-body' experience. If he senses that he is losing control there is panic, cold sweat, even sobbing. The physical efforts involved may be considerable, but he is often a pathologically lazy person. His energy is sapped by the never-ending process of keeping so much material out of consciousness.

(vi) TENSION

The masochist is carrying an enormous load of nervous tension. He is not easily startled by something sudden and frightening. It is as though he were neurologically prepared. He deals in anxiety and suspense (Reik, 1939). In his relationships he lives on a knife-edge. He provokes until the thread might snap at any moment; tentatively, he toys with what might well be the last straw. He engineers humiliations for himself and permits himself no discharge of anger. As Freud (1924*a*) puts it: "the true masochist always turns his cheek whenever he has a chance of receiving a blow" (p. 165). If he essays 'normal' sexual intercourse, he produces and inflicts an agony of suspense and anxiety (Reik, 1939) until the pleasurable goes over into the unpleasurable, until pleasure has become torture—and still with no discharge of tension. With such long-term abuse of the autonomic nervous system, it is hardly surprising if, as has been claimed, he is prone to high blood pressure, strokes and heart conditions (Menninger, 1938).

The tension of the masochist builds up as a result of conflicts on many levels of functioning. Karen Horney (1935) was right in observing that the masochist "needs constant signs of attention and affection, and as he never believes in these signs except momentarily, he has an excessive need for attention and affection" (p. 252). Hilda Lewinsky (1944) was right, too: "Being loved would include a demand for loving in return, for actions and feelings which the masochist does not want to give or cannot give" (p. 154). He perceives no more need for reciprocity than a spoilt child. On the contrary, the frustrated deviant is relentlessly repelling, with his provocative behavior, the love he so badly needs. Where a loving relationship is initially, and as a piece of rare good fortune, offered to him, he systematically disfigures, distorts and destroys it. He is thus in a state of perpetual emotional conflict and anxious tension.

Theodor Reik (1939) was right in conveying his 'demonstrative feature': "a shameful or degrading exhibitionistic display of bodily or psychic awkwardness" (p. 51). He finds social gatherings an ordeal but makes an exhibition of himself, feeling the embarrassment keenly and wallowing in it. (Several of the fantasies recounted by the sadomasochists interviewed in the course of this study were concerned precisely with situations of intense embarrassment.) He is totally self-centred, yet has low self-regard and no self-confidence. He commits himself to impossible tasks, *half*-knowing at the time that he cannot succeed in them. The conflict of narcissistic grandiosity (Kohut, 1971) and defeatism creates more tension.

The very nature of his deviance, attempting the impossible combination of suffering and satisfaction, is the very bedrock upon which layer upon layer of tension is laid down. As Norbert Bromberg (1955) put it, "the need to wrest control in a situation is incompatible with the need to become its pitiable victim" (p. 808). Tension is habitual and cumulative, a way of life. Everything must be precarious—books are piled so as to be on the verge of toppling, the teapot must be right on the edge of the table, gas taps not quite turned off. Necessary preliminaries are delayed to the last moment so that every task, if it is fulfilled at all, is fulfilled late and under stress. But until the body, after amazing endurance, finally succumbs to the perpetual abuse, tension is sought and stored, for tension is unpleasure. There is also the alluring prospect of a 'blow-out'.

An ejaculation, an explosive catharsis of aggressive and erotic drives, is presumably what is sought in sadomasochistic rituals, the intensity being akin to the wild release of tension with the down-drop of a roller coaster. Typically, on a physiological level, the 'nonpractising' masochist is likely to carry a background load of undischarged tension. There is a qualitative difference between the release of nervous tension through discharge (e.g., through orgasm) and its relief through diminution (e.g., through inhibition of neuronal transmission by stress-produced endogenous opioids; Turner, 1991, pp. 412–416). This fact cannot be ignored since everyone knows it from his own experience. On an emotional level, it is the difference between positive pleasure and the mitigation of stress. But this qualitative, as distinct from quantitative, difference must be the result of two differing physiological mechanisms. In an electrochemical process—and it is long established that the nervous system functions electrochemically—discharge removes the load whereas inhibition of transmission only 'freezes' it. When the masochist has reached the stage of sexual impotence, what he obtains physiologically may be a form of numbness or anaesthesia with a persisting background load. Certainly, on the level of personality, he is anhedonic and may be relied upon to cast a blight over any enjoyable activity (DSM-III-R diagnostic criterion 5 for Self-defeating Personality Disorder; Appendix 1).

To return to our original questions, the masochist was almost certainly both helpless and depressed in his childhood. His strategy was to *choose* to suffer, to specify how and when the pain he might well regard as inevitable (Seligman, 1974) should come upon him. However negatively, he would thus assume control: not "how can I escape?" but "*I* shall design my prison", not avoidance but doggedness. In John Gedo's opinion (Panel, 1984, p. 605) "masochistic perverts tend to become psychobiologically depressed when the opportunity to practice their perversion is lost … eroticism is often used effectively as an antidote for childhood depression."

Given the infantilism which is so prominent in masochism, given that masochism permeates the whole personality and exerts such a basic influence on behavior, an investigation of the primary family relationships of early childhood (or their absence) would seem likely to throw significant light on its development. The following section is devoted to an empirical study of these issues.

Part II

AN EMPIRICAL INVESTIGATION OF SADOMASOCHISM

SUMMARY

Forty-eight index cases were compared with 35 controls with respect to their early family relationships, whether they were currently depressed or not, and their performance on a computer-driven color-naming task, followed by free recall of words just viewed. Subjects were debriefed after each task, and biographical details were ascertained informally. Additional information, specific to sadomasochism, was collected from all index subjects by means of 3 questionnaires and, in some cases, by a further open-ended questionnaire, by further correspondence, or by further interview on subsequent occasions.

INTRODUCTION

Any study of sadomasochism, in so far as it attempts to go beyond behavioral statistics, ascertained by questionnaire, is bound to be largely descriptive. It is difficult to provide more than plausible speculation when seeking causes. However, as concluded at the end of Chapter 4 of the previous section, there are two fields which appear likely to shed light on the etiology of sadomasochism: depression and early family relationships. An overlap between depression and sadomasochism is to be expected but so is the emergence of differentiating features. The main hypotheses adopted for testing in this Section were (1) that sadomasochistic subjects, more than controls, be they depressed or nondepressed, would display discrepancies between their general characterization of their early family relationships and their episodic memories of specific interactional events, where these memories were forthcoming at all; (2) that these index subjects would have achieved less integration of painful experiences (less containment within consciousness), less understanding of why mother, father or sibling treated them thus (theory of mind), less often a whole picture of these figures (a 'singular', coherent working model), more often a split and conflicting one ('multiple', incoherent models (Main, 1991)), inciting revenge; (3) that certain etiological factors would emerge repeatedly in the case of male masochists, who were expected to present themselves for interview in greater numbers than females. The recurrent factors anticipated were (a) an idealized father, often absent, who proved to have feet of clay, (b) a rejecting or inadequate mother, (c) a favored younger sister, (d) a tormenting elder brother, (e) a parent lost before mourning was possible, (f) parental divorce, (g) long separations. Lastly it was proposed to test the etiological significance of (A) corporal punishment, (B) lonely, unhappy schooling, (C) prolonged physical pain or stress.

Design

The recruitment of index and control groups had a certain symmetry, in that index subjects were reached through the two subculture periodicals, *Skin Two* and *Forum*, whilst controls were reached through *New Statesman & Society* and *The Spectator*, selected for their predominantly male readership, the one slightly left, the other slightly right, of center politically. Cards aimed at recruiting SM subjects were displayed in appropriate clubs and shops, and questionnaires probing 'Morale' (actually the Beck Depression Inventory, BDI, Beck, 1967), aimed at recruiting controls, were left in several London libraries and museums, but only one further index subject was obtained in this way.

Subjects

The basic demographic composition of the index and control samples is shown in Table II. 1.

In accordance with the requirements of the Joint UCL/UCH Ethics Committee (University College London/University College Hospital), all subjects were healthy adult volunteers. All but one were Caucasian, and all but two had English as their first language. The sex, age, marital status, total Beck Depression Inventory (BDI) score and overall Adult Attachment Interview (AAI) classification of each subject are set out in Table 5.1.

TABLE II. 1. Composition of index and control samples with respect to sex and marital status (Actual numbers of subjects with percentages in parentheses)

	Index group ($n = 48$)		Control group ($n = 35$)	
Male	43 (90%)		26 (74%)	
	Married	Unmarried	Married	Unmarried
	25 (58%)	18 (42%)	14 (54%)	12 (46%)
Female	5 (10%)		9 (26%)	
	Married	Unmarried	Married	Unmarried
	3 (60%)	2 (40%)	6 (67%)	3 (33%)
Married (Males + females)	28 (58%)		20 (57%)	
Unmarried (Males + females)	20 (42%)		15 (43%)	

'Married' status has been given to subjects who are (a) at present married, or (b) remarried, or (c) who were at one time married, or (d) who have a permanent partner; all others have been classified as 'Unmarried'.

The editor of *Skin Two* obligingly inserted, at no charge, the following line advertisement in issue no. 14, appearing at the end of 1993:

"ACADEMIC RESEARCH. Could you spare an hour of your time to take part in a serious academic study? I am researching the influence of early family relationships on the development of personality. If you have SM interests, I believe your contribution would be valuable and interesting. It would, of course, be confidential. So, if you have time to come and talk, please write to… (Department of Psychology, University College London). Your name is not necessary, but please give an address for correspondence."

The editor of *Forum* was similarly obliging, in that she included, also without charge, a notice of almost identical wording in the editorial section of Vol. 27, No. 4 of 1993.

Of the 82 respondents, 48 came with alacrity for interview, answered the Beck Depression Inventory, completed the 'emotional' Stroop task and answered the three questionnaires relating specifically to sado-masochism. They were, in fact, extremely cooperative and, as expected, nearly all men (only 5 women). It might be argued that their readiness to come forward was due to their commitment to the research topic but another explanation, and one supported by their increased interest and arousal when finally questioned directly about their sexuality, might be their need to reveal themselves, in other words, might confirm Theodor Reik's 'demonstrative factor' (Reik, 1939). These self-declared sado-masochists were predominantly middle-class and most of them created an overall impression of above-average intelligence. They met the criteria (summarized in Appendix 1) laid down in the Diagnostic and Statistical Manual of Mental Disorders (Third Edition—Revised) of the American Psychiatric Association (DSM-III-R) on pages 286–288 for sexual sadomasochism: over a period of at least six months, recurrent intense sexual urges and fantasies involving real, not simulated, suffering or humiliation, which have been acted upon or which cause marked distress. In some cases, they also met the criteria described on pages 369–374 for sadistic and self-defeating personality disorders: a pervasive pattern of cruel or self-defeating behavior in a variety of contexts. (It is underlined in the Introduction (p. xxiii) that DSM-III-R classifies disorders not people, but one of its astonishing blind spots, probably a result of the very endeavor to classify itself, is that it does not appear to recognize, or very barely recognizes (p. 286), what Freud recognized, what linguistic usage has recognized for so long, and what all *aficionados* certainly recognize, namely, that sadism and masochism are two aspects of one entity, sadomasochism. One other, rather less important, point on which I would take issue with DSM-III-R (p. 374) is that the masochistic personality retains, in any usual sense of the words, "adequate social skills and the capacity for pleasure". Personally, as stated in Chapter 4, I doubt this.) More detailed information concerning the chronicity, practice and motivation of these subjects' sadomasochism is given in Chapter 8.

As a preliminary to this investigation of attachment in early childhood and its effects in later life, the main plank of this research, I completed a pilot study, chiefly to gain expertise in conducting the Adult Attachment Interview (AAI, Main & Goldwyn, 1985–1994). My pilot study had prepared me for the difficulty of obtaining a control group containing mildly depressed individuals. Approaching professionals in the field for assistance in finding subjects was not fruitful. Twelve thousand copies of the Beck Depression Inventory were therefore launched on an unsuspecting world: 10,000 stapled into the centre of *New Statesman & Society*, distributed in London and the South East of England on 22 April 1994, and 2000 inserted in *The Spectator*, distributed in its plastic envelope on 21 May 1994. Both papers charged for the service. In response to this invitation to take part in a serious academic study, 189 were returned completed, and 35 of these respondents could be persuaded to come for interview and complete the Stroop task! The control group thus constituted with considerable (one might be tempted to say 'disproportionate') effort, consisted of 20 subjects scoring 14 or more on the Beck Depression Inventory and 15 scoring less (26 men and 9 women).

One might first ask why it should be so difficult to obtain controls. Several possible factors come to mind in seeking an explanation: (a) controls are notoriously difficult to obtain randomly—the norm is an elusive entity; (b) people are now bombarded with questionnaires and 'junk mail'; (c) the Beck Depression Inventory is not a very appealing piece of reading matter—several respondents remarked on its "negative, downbeat bias"; (d) there is perhaps a reluctance to become entangled with psychological investigations amongst the intelligent English middle class who may prefer their inner world to remain private; (e) of those who replied, many were not willing to enclose a stamped, self-addressed envelope, thereby revealing their identity and whereabouts; (f) many respondents could not spare the time and effort to attend for interview—indeed, some lived too far afield; (g) low scorers living out of London were simply congratulated on the state of their 'morale' and not invited for interview since I was seeking a sample with a significant proportion of mildly depressed subjects.

The next question requiring to be addressed is how representative this control group of 35 subjects is of the general population. Depressed individuals are overrepresented but this is inevitable, both for purposes of meaningful comparison with sadomasochistic subjects and, that given, for practical considerations (the procedures employed in the investigation were extremely time-consuming for every subject). The fact that BDI low-scorers lived in the London area would not seem to make them seriously different from the general population of southeast England. As readers of *New Statesman & Society* or *The Spectator*, the 35 individuals finally forming the control group might not be considered representative of the general UK population with respect to education or socioeconomic status, but neither could they be regarded as belonging to an eccentric cult! The two papers yielded more men than women and this certainly makes the control group unrepresentative of the general population, but far better matched to the index group, with respect to gender.

The final question must be what are the limitations of the control group employed in this study. The following short-comings must be clearly admitted: (1) at 35 individuals, it is small, so conclusions drawn from comparisons with the index group should be treated with appropriate caution, particularly when the groups are subdivided; (2) self-selection is not a random method of recruitment (it can be seen from Table 7.1 that 34% of the 189 respondents to the Beck Depression Inventory were indeed depressed) but, given the aim of examining the difference and the overlap between depression and sadomasochism, it is probably the next best thing in that the sample has not been tendentiously manipulated by the investigator; (3) the high proportion of depressed individuals might suggest a certain vulnerability associated with the 189 people who returned the questionnaire, and such vulnerability might, in turn, increase the number of 'insecure' individuals with respect to attachment. However, if this were the case, it would be likely to diminish the differences from the sadomasochistic group and would therefore pull in a conservative direction in contrasting the two groups. In the event, 'secure' (F) AAI primary classifications predominated in the control group and were absent in the index group (Figure 5.1).

INSTRUMENTS

The three main instruments used in the investigation were (a) the Adult Attachment Interview (Main & Goldwyn, 1985–1994), (b) a variant of the classic color-naming task (Stroop, 1935), often referred to as 'emotional' Stroop, and (c) the Beck Depression Inventory (Beck, 1967, revised 1971–1979). These are presented separately as Chapters 5, 6 and 7. Chapter 8 reports on the 3 questionnaires completed by all 48 index subjects, and on the fourth open-ended questionnaire ("Requesting your opinion") which 15 out of 20 returned by post. The exact wording of all 4 questionnaires is given in Appendix 5.

CHAPTER 5

THE ADULT ATTACHMENT INTERVIEW

Many of the most intense emotions arise during the formation, the maintenance, the disruption, and the renewal of attachment relationships.
(Bowlby, 1987)

SUMMARY

Without exception, sadomasochistic subjects (n =48), unlike controls (n =35), are found to have developed insecure internal models of personal attachment, as a result of childhoods which were all problematic in one way or another. Their capacity for metacognition and their coherence of mind are found to be, on average, less than that of controls.

INTRODUCTION

John Bowlby (1969) observed that a child was constantly concerned to maintain proximity to his mother for protection. He postulated that these efforts stemmed from an attachment behavioral system which was shared by some birds, most mammals, all primates, and which had evolved as a mechanism of safety and survival. In adopting the evolutionist position, he made two important *caveats*: (1) "The two lines of animal evolution that led ultimately to birds and to mammals have been distinct since the days of the early reptiles, and it is therefore nearly certain that attachment behavior has evolved independently in the two groups. That, and the fact that brain structure in birds is very different from what it is in mammals, make it more than probable that the behavioral mechanisms mediating attachment behavior are also very diffferent for the two groups" (p. 183). (2) "It may, in fact, be that all parts of man's behavioral equipment are well adapted not only to man's primeval environment but to all his present-day environments also. But it may not be so, and certainly cannot be assumed to be so" (p. 60).

Conceptualizing the proximity-seeking of the human infant, according to attachment theory rather than dependency theory, Bowlby (1987) emphasizes (1) its specificity: "Attachment behavior is directed towards one or a few specific individuals, usually in clear order of preference"; (2) its duration: "An attachment endures, usually for a large part of the life-cycle"; (3) its engagement of emotion: "Threat of loss arouses anxiety, and actual loss gives rise to sorrow; while each of these situations is likely to arouse anger. The unchallenged maintenance of a bond is experienced as a source of security and the renewal of a bond is experienced as a source of joy" (p. 57).

Bowlby believed that relationship patterns can be transmitted across generations. Patterns of interaction with mother, and indeed father also, are internalized by an infant. They guide the infant's expectations and assessments of experience. While they may be modified in the course of time, these internal representations continue to exert an influence on relationships not only throughout childhood but throughout the life of the individual and are even transmitted socially to the next generation.

On the basis of John Bowlby's attachment theory, Mary Ainsworth and co-workers developed their Strange Situation procedure (Ainsworth *et al.* 1978) to test an infant's attachment to mother directly. The child's behavior is monitored for 20 minutes in an unfamiliar room with an unfamiliar person. In particular, reactions to two brief separations from mother are observed and how the child greets the mother's return to the room during the two 3-minute reunions. Detailed study of video recordings then leads to a determination of secure versus insecure attachment. Certain types of behavior, such as the avoidance or freezing described by Selma Fraiberg (1982), would thus be given the insecure infant attachment classification of 'A' (Avoidant) or 'D' (Disorganized/disoriented), respectively.

Mary Main and colleagues at Berkeley, California, originally devised their semistructured Adult Attachment Interview (Main *et al.*, 1985) to examine the working model of attachment operating in the mother and father of the infant tested in the Ainsworth Strange Situation. Defending the Bowlby-Ainsworth approach, L. Alan Sroufe (1985) pointed out: "In accepting a relationship interpretation ... one does not have to abandon an interest in physiological factors. Attachment and temperament constructs refer to different domains, and there is no inherent incompatibility between relationship and temperamental concepts in moving toward a wholistic understanding of the child" (p. 12).

In the course of analysing many interview transcripts, four principal adult attachment classifications have been identified (Main & Goldwyn, 1985–1994; see Appendix 2). Each represents a state of mind with respect to attachment, and each has been related, empirically as well as theoretically to an infant attachment category. These states of mind are not determined so much by the history of childhood events recounted, as by the manner in which these are presented, i.e., discourse usage. Two important criteria are coherence and collaboration as defined by the linguistic philosopher, Grice (1975). Beneath the general principle of coherent conversation, which he termed the Cooperative Principle, Grice set out four maxims: quality (be truthful, and have evidence for what you say), quantity (be succinct, yet complete), relation (be relevant or perspicacious), and manner (be clear and orderly). The interview is judged either to adhere to these maxims or to violate them. Several other considerations, such as insistence on lack of memory, vagueness, unsupported positive description, play a part in identifying overall state of mind. (1) A subject is classified as Securely attached yet Autonomous when the portrayal of childhood experiences is internally consistent, clear, relevant and succinct, be they good or bad experiences. In a truthful and collaborative fashion, the focus of his attention can shift as needed between the questions put and the memories they evoke. (2) A speaker is classified as Dismissing when discourse is apparently aimed at minimizing attention to attachment-related experiences. He most typically violates the maxim of quality (have evidence for what you say) in that he describes one or both his parents in positive terms, which he cannot support with illustrative memories or even goes on to contradict. In other words, idealization and frequent insistence on being unable to recall childhood experiences often point to a childhood involving rejection. (3) In direct contrast, the Preoccupied subject appears to maximize attention to attachment, unable to move on in a timely way to deal with fresh queries. Whether angrily or passively entangled with smothering or role-reversing parents or caught up and overwhelmed by traumatic childhood experiences, the maxims of quantity, relevance and manner are frequently violated. (4) An interview is classified Unresolved-Disorganized on the basis of lapses in the monitoring of reasoning or discourse. The subject becomes disoriented whilst discussing loss of important persons, physical or sexual abuse. Because the lapses leading to an Unresolved-Disorganized classification are limited to certain areas of discussion and do not reflect a global pattern, such an interview is always given a second best-fitting alternative classification, for example, Unresolved-Secure.

A fifth classification, comparatively rare in 'normal' samples, also must be followed by second and even third best-fitting alternatives. This is the Cannot Classify category of transcripts, which either contain strong evidence of two mutually incompatible states of mind, Dismissing and Preoccupied, or are so lacking in coherence as to be ruled out of the Secure-Autonomous category whilst carrying no scores high enough to justify Dismissing or Preoccupied as a primary classification.

Since the Adult Attachment Interview (AAI) was brought into the public domain in 1985, it has been successfully applied in contexts other than the Ainsworth Strange situation, such as investigations of the peer-relations of adolescents (Kobak & Sceery, 1988), child and maternal behavior patterns during a tool-using task (Crowell & Feldman, 1988) and maternal attachment disturbances as a factor in infants' failure to thrive (Benoit *et al.*, 1989). It seemed eminently suitable and was therefore adopted for the present study for several reasons. (a) Its rating and classification system provides a means of testing the accuracy of the observations concerning sadomasochism recorded in Chapter 4. Passivity, for instance, can be measured on a 9-point scale by the application of precise criteria (Appendix 2). (b) It likewise enables hypotheses formulated at the beginning of this section to be tested, for example, the first hypothesis, that in the accounts of childhood given by sadomasochistic subjects, more than in those given by controls, discrepancies would become evident between semantic and episodic memory, between their general characterization of early family relationships and actual interactions with their parents, pointing to multiple and conflicting internal representations of attachment. The AAI addresses this issue with the 9-point scales for 'Idealization of Mother' and 'Idealization of Father' and the final assignment of a Dismissing (Ds1 or Ds3) classification (Appendix 2). (c) Certain questions put in the course of the interview, for instance, those asking subjects to reflect on why their parents had behaved in the way they had behaved, enable an assessment to be made of capacity to understand mental states, in other words, theory of mind. The AAI scales which reflect the capacity to 'mentalize' are those for Metacognition and Coherence (Appendix 2). (d) In probing actual events of childhood, recurring factors likely to influence development, particularly sexual development, could be identified. The hypothesis that sadomasochistic subjects would frequently have suffered serious illness, painful injury or prolonged stress, creating a physiological basis for their deviance, could be tested directly by the interview question regarding childhood illness. There is, of course, no 9-point scale to provide a standardized measure in this case, so the importance of illness, injury or protracted stress as developmental factors can only be assessed informally. Similarly, in the case of the the third hypothesis put forward at the beginning of this section, the possible aetiological factors of (a) idealization of father, (b) rejection or role-reversal by mother can be measured systematically by the respective AAI 9-point scales, whereas (c) envy of sister, (d) resentment of brother can again only be judged informally (Table 5.8*d*) from pointers occurring in the course of the interview. The AAI scale measuring unresolved loss relates to bereavement in general, but the same opportunity to make an informal assessment of the developmental importance of (e) the early loss of a parent, (f) divorce, (g) separation from parents can present itself as one of the advantages of a semistructured interview. The influence of corporal punishment is addressed to some extent by the rating scale for unresolved trauma, whilst that of schooling is likely to become apparent in the importance attributed to it by the interviewee. Thus the overall field of enquiry of the Adult Attachment Interview—the nature of early intimate relationships, the impact of rejection, neglect or trauma on developmental processes—made it an appropriate instrument for testing the validity of the integrated model of sadomasochism proposed in Chapter 4.

INSTRUMENT

As explained above, the rating and classification system of the Adult Attachment Interview (Main & Goldwyn, 1985–1994) was originally developed in the Bay Area study of the white upper-class mothers and fathers of infants previously tested in the Ainsworth Strange Situation. Subsequently it has been refined and extended, and increasing evidence of its reliability and validity has been forthcoming, some in prospective studies (e.g., Ward *et al.*, 1990, 1991; Fonagy *et al.*, 1991*b*). An overview is provided by Van Ijzendoorn and Bakermans-Kranenburg (1996).

The interview, lasting between one hour and one-and-a-half hours, probes an adult's representations of early family relationships and their effects on present functioning. It consists of 18 questions regarding relationships with mother, father, siblings and other important figures in childhood. As subjects respond, usually in general, they are encouraged to search for specific episodic memories to support these global impressions, memories to support, for instance, each of five adjectives with which they have described their childhood relationship first with mother, then with father. They are asked what they did when they felt upset during childhood, what happened when they were hurt or ill, whether they were ever threatened or abused by either parent, and why, in their opinion, their parents behaved as they did. Their reactions to any deaths occurring in the family are probed. They are asked whether there have been major changes in relationships since childhood and how they now feel about their parents. The last three questions probe their attitudes and aspirations concerning their own children (real or imagined) and what insights they would hope to pass on to them.

PROCEDURE

After obtaining the subject's permission to audiotape the interview, it was introduced, according to the instructions of Mary Main and colleagues, by a brief explanation of its field of enquiry. The 18 questions and follow-up probes were put to the subject in the prescribed order which had been memorized so that reference to notes should be minimal. Every effort was made during the subject's preliminary description of his family and its circumstances to establish a rapport with him, to gain his confidence and to place him at ease. As recommended, he was given time to think before responding to questions and allowed to establish his own tempo of communication. Apart from accidental interruptions, his flow of thought was only curtailed where he had wandered some distance from the topic of the question. Only where the prescribed wording of a question was inapplicable (e.g., where the subject had no children of his own) was this question reformulated to suit the circumstances (e.g., "If you had a child, how do you think you would respond, in terms of feelings, when you separated from your child?"). Care was taken (though, as usual, execution sometimes fell short of intention) not to suggest responses to the subject, but to show continuous sympathetic interest in what he was saying. After the concluding enquiry as to what he felt he had learnt from his childhood experiences and after making sure he had nothing further to add, the subject was thanked, the tape-recording was stopped and the subject was debriefed. The interview was transcribed verbatim, and the transcript was rated on a series of 9-point scales (see Appendix 2) falling under the headings: scales for experience, scales for states of mind respecting the parents, scales for overall states of mind. The rater then made a final classification of type of attachment, based on the adult subject's current state of mind: Dismissing (Ds), Entangled/Preoccupied (E), or Freely valuing/Secure/Autonomous (F). Besides being placed in one of these three main "organized" categories (organized strategies of response or defence), a subject might also be considered, on the appearance of lapses in his monitoring of discourse or reasoning, to be Unresolved (U) with respect to past bereavement or trauma. Where he presented extreme contradiction in his overall response to attachment issues, dismissing them yet also remaining preoccupied with them, his interview was placed in the Cannot Classify (CC) category.

Rating of Transcripts

All 83 verbatim transcripts were rated by me and, simultaneously, 14 of these were sent to be rated, totally blind, by two other judges who had likewise been trained by Mary Main and Erik Hesse. The rating procedure used is set out in the 163-page Adult Attachment Scoring and Classification Manual, Version 6 of June 1994 (Main & Goldwyn, 1985–1994) and is summarized in Appendix 2. For each of these transcripts—the complete set of 83 judged by me and those randomly extracted to be judged independently by the two other judges—a prescribed 10-page case summary form was completed, giving page and line references to support judgments. The transcripts rated blind in this way were the interviews of 9 index subjects, 3 depressed controls and 2 nondepressed ('neutral') controls. There was two-way agreement (Secure versus Insecure) between the judges in 10 out of 14 cases (71%) and three-way agreement (Ds versus F versus E classification) between the judges in 9 out of 14 cases (64%), i.e., fair to good agreement beyond chance (Cohen, 1960; Fleiss *et al.*, 1969). Agreement at the level of scale scores was also above chance. Besides the ratings carried out by the two trained judges already mentioned, four further transcripts were handed to Mary Main and Erik Hesse themselves.

RESULTS

Two striking results emerging from this investigation require no tabulation. They will therefore be noted briefly at this point and discussed in the next section. (1) As anticipated, index subjects came forward with unmistakable eagerness—48 interviews out of 82 respondents to 2 advertisements. In contrast, it was extremely difficult to obtain control subjects—35 interviews out of 189 respondents to 12,000 questionnaires. Even if this enormous difference in response might be partly due to the differing degree of investment on the part of the two groups in the ostensible research topics of sadomasochism and depression, respectively, the manifest behavior of the sadomasochistic subjects during the interview would still require explanation. In general, they seemed impatient to discuss their deviance, in some cases (e.g., ES8, ES19, ES24) showing physical signs of excitement, such as hand tremors, when supplying details of it. (2) As anticipated, the index group contained far more males than females (43 to 5).

The sex, marital status, age, total score on the Beck Depression Inventory (BDI) and overall classification from the Adult Attachment Interview (AAI), for each subject in both index and control groups, are set out in Table 5.1, mostly in order to facilitate the identification of individual

TABLE 5.1. Sex, marital status, age, total score on the Beck Depression Inventory (BDI) and overall classification from the Adult Attachment Interview (AAI) of (a) 48 index and (b) 35 control subjects (both groups divided into depressed and nondepressed)

Subject	Sex	Marital status	Age	BDI total score	AAI classification
(a) Index Subjects ($n = 48$)					
Depressed ($n = 14$)					
ES7	Male	Unmarried	26	25	E1
ES10	Male	Unmarried	38	17	E1/E2
ES18	Male	Married$^+$	65	22	E3a/E1
ES19	Male	Unmarried	44	18	Ds1
ES20	Male	Unmarried	25	19	E1
ES24	Male	Married	34	21	U/E2
ES27	Male	Unmarried	30	16	CC/E1/E2/Ds2
ES28	Male	Married*	54	25	E1/E2/F4b
ES29	Male	Married*	42	23	E3a,b/E1/U
ES40	Male	Married	77	19	CC/Ds1/E1
ES52	Male	Married*	55	17	Ds3
ES61	Male	Married*	70	39	E1
ES71	Male	Unmarried	64	16	CC/E1/Ds1
ES80	Male	Unmarried	39	17	CC/E3/Ds1/U
Nondepressed ($n = 34$)					
ES1	Male	Unmarried	46	6	CC/Ds2/E2
ES2	Male	Unmarried	63	4	CC/Ds3/E2
ES4	Male	Married	76	11	Ds2
ES8	Male	Married	75	10	E1
ES11	Male	Married$^+$	43	7	E2
ES13	Male	Unmarried	38	6	E1
ES15	Male	Married	53	7	Ds3
ES17	Male	Married	41	7	Ds3
ES21	Male	Unmarried	27	6	Ds3
ES22	Male	Married#	38	7	CC/Ds2/E2
ES23	Male	Married$^+$	35	9	Ds3
ES26	Male	Unmarried	30	2	CC/Ds3/E1
ES30	Male	Unmarried	26	2	E1
ES34	Male	Married	36	12	E1
ES35	Male	Unmarried	33	12	CC/E2/Ds2
ES36	Male	Married*	44	3	CC/Ds2/E2
ES37	Male	Unmarried	34	13	E1
ES39	Male	Married	38	3	E2/E1
ES41	Female	Married*#	53	7	Ds3/F1a
ES42	Female	Unmarried	35	2	CC/E2/Ds1
ES50	Male	Married	47	4	E2/E1
ES51	Male	Married	41	7	E2/U
ES57	Male	Unmarried	30	4	U/Ds3/Ds2
ES58	Female	Married*	36	3	CC/E2/Ds2

(Continued)

TABLE 5.1. (*Continued*)

Subject	Sex	Marital status	Age	BDI total score	AAI classification
ES62	Female	Unmarried	44	4	E3b,a/E1
ES63	Male	Married	42	4	CC/E1/Ds2
ES65	Male	Unmarried	31	10	U/E3/E2
ES66	Male	Married	52	5	Ds1
ES69	Male	Married*	59	2	CC/Ds2/E2
ES74	Male	Unmarried	43	11	E2/E1/F2
ES75	Female	Married*	35	7	Ds3
ES76	Male	Married	44	6	Ds3/Ds2
ES77	Male	Married	43	12	CC/Ds3/E2/U
ES81	Male	Married#	31	5	CC/Ds1/E1
(b) Control Subjects ($n = 35$)					
Depressed (n=20)					
CS121	Male	Married*	60	48	F4b
CS125	Male	Married*#	48	14	CC/E3a/Ds2
CS132	Male	Unmarried	36	28	Ds1/Ds2
CS136	Male	Unmarried	36	24	Ds3/F1a
CS138	Female	Married*	37	33	Ds2/Ds3
CS149	Male	Married+	50	15	F3a
CS157	Male	Married+	45	19	F4b/E1
CS173	Male	Unmarried	37	22	Ds3
CS175	Male	Married	43	27	F4a
CS180	Female	Married*	36	24	E2/F5/U
CS187	Female	Married	44	16	F2/F1a,b
CS190	Female	Unmarried	32	33	U/Ds4/Ds3
CS196	Female	Married#	45	26	E2/F5/U
CS206	Female	Unmarried	51	26	F1a,b
CS226	Male	Unmarried	50	14	Ds3
CS258	Male	Unmarried	47	27	F5/E3b
CS259	Male	Unmarried	38	19	CC/Ds3/E1
CS260	Female	Married+	52	14	U/F4b
CS283	Male	Unmarried	34	21	F2/F5
CS284	Male	Unmarried	33	23	F5/Ds2/U
Nondepressed/Neutral (n=15)					
NS101	Male	Married	47	11	F5/U
NS103	Male	Unmarried	28	4	F4a
NS104	Male	Married	39	1	F5
NS108	Male	Married	38	0	F4a
NS111	Male	Married	62	0	F1a/Ds2/Ds3
NS122	Male	Married	49	1	F2
NS146	Male	Married	63	1	F3a
NS172	Male	Married	65	1	F2/Ds3
NS176	Male	Married	38	3	F2
NS217	Male	Unmarried	37	1	Ds3

(*Continued*)

TABLE 5.1. (*Continued*)

Subject	Sex	Marital status	Age	BDI total score	AAI classification
NS222	Male	Unmarried	24	2	CC/Ds1/E1
NS229	Male	Unmarried	60	0	CC/Ds1/E1
NS269	Male	Married	46	6	E1/F2
NS278	Female	Unmarried	61	0	U/F5/F2
NS285	Female	Married	26	13	F4b/E2/U

'Married' status has been given to subjects who are at present married, or (+) remarried, or (*) who were at one time married, or (#) who have a permanent partner; all others have been classified as 'Unmarried'.

Main AAI categories: Ds = Dismissing, E = Entangled/preoccupied, F = Freely valuing of attachment yet objective, U = Unresolved loss or trauma, CC = Cannot Classify (for subcategories see Appendix 2).

Mean age (range): All 48 index subjects = 43.85 (25–77); 14 depressed = 47.36 (25–77); 34 nondepressed = 42.41 (26–76); All 35 control subjects = 43.91 (24–65); 20 depressed = 42.70 (32–60); 15 nondepressed = 45.53 (24–65);

Mean BDI total score (S.D.): All 48 index subjects = 10.71 (7.90); 14 depressed = 21.00 (6.05); 34 nondepressed = 6.47 (3.30); All 35 control subjects = 14.77 (12.36); 20 depressed = 23.65 (8.23); 15 nondepressed = 2.93 (4.06)

subjects, whilst still, of course, preserving their anonymity, when they are discussed later. The AAI classification is of relevance to the first hypothesis put forward for empirical examination at the beginning of this section, concerning discrepancies between semantic and episodic memories of childhood. Such discrepancies imply increased idealization of parents and the assignment of a Dismissing (Ds) classification. There is in fact, however, no support for this prediction that the idealizing/dismissing style would be characteristic of sadomasochism, since there is a clear predominance of Preoccupied (E) classifications in the sadomasochistic group (18 out of 48 SM subjects received primary E classifications, as compared with only 3 out of 35 control subjects, whereas the difference between the 2 groups was much less with respect to the Ds classification: 11 out of the 48 SM subjects received a primary Ds classification, as compared with 6 out of the 35 controls). Both groups have been subdivided, for purposes of analysis and comparison, according to BDI scores into depressed (total score of 14 or over) and nondepressed (total score of 0 to 13). It can be seen at a glance that all of the 48 index subjects have been classified Insecure on AAI criteria, with the exception of ES28, ES41 and ES74 whose alternative, as distinct from primary, classifications are Secure/Autonomous, though not F3 which exemplifies the Secure category. The control subjects have predominantly Secure classifications—of the 15 nondepressed ('neutral') controls, only 4 (NS217, NS222, NS229, NS269) were given Insecure status as a primary classification; NS278 was classified Unresolved with respect to bereavement. Figure 5.1 summarizes visually how the proportions of primary AAI classifications differ between the index and control groups as a whole.

The means and standard deviations of AAI scale scores for index versus control groups are presented in Table 5.2. It is immediately obvious that the most significant difference between the two groups as a whole

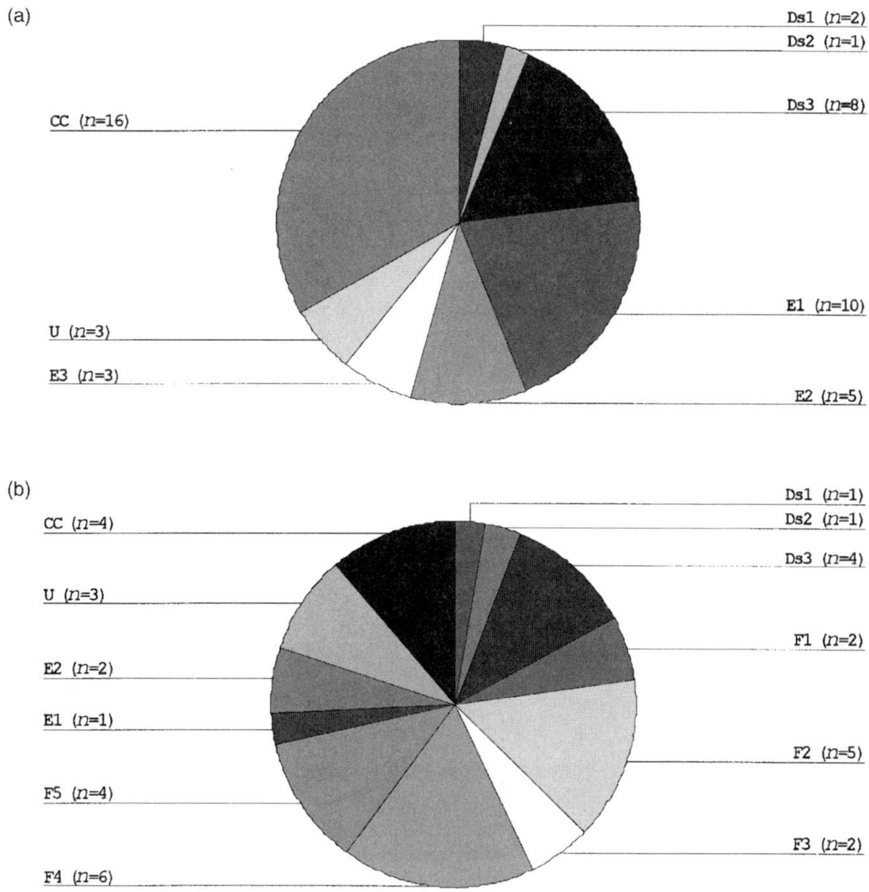

FIGURE 5.1. Proportions of primary AAI classifications in (a) the index group ($n = 48$). It can be seen that no 'Secure' (F) classification was assigned as a primary classification and that 'Cannot Classify' (CC) predominates. (b) the control group ($n = 35$). 'Secure' (F) classifications predominate. Actual numbers of subjects are given in parentheses.

TABLE 5.2. Mean AAI scale scores of index versus control groups

	Index		Control	
	Depressed ($n = 14$)	Nondepressed ($n = 34$)	Depressed ($n = 20$)	Nondepressed ($n = 15$)
Love (M)	2.79 (1.31)	3.09 (1.21)	3.65 (1.56)	4.27 (1.87)
Love (F)	2.57 (1.34)	2.73 (1.19)	3.35 (1.72)	3.93 (1.79)
Reject (M)	3.79 (1.53)	3.32 (1.96)	3.60 (1.79)	3.07 (1.62)
Reject (F)	4.00 (2.22)	4.06 (1.69)	3.40 (1.73)	3.27 (1.62)
Rolerv (M)	4.36 (2.37)	3.12 (2.18)	3.20 (1.82)	2.73 (1.67)
Rolerv (F)	1.71 (1.14)	1.65 (1.15)	1.30 (0.73)	1.07 (0.26)
Achiev (M)	1.36 (0.63)	2.00 (1.58)	1.55 (1.23)	2.00 (1.41)
Achiev (F)	1.57 (1.60)	2.18 (1.58)	1.60 (1.05)	1.80 (1.08)
Neglec (M)	2.29 (1.33)	2.71 (1.66)	2.85 (1.69)	1.80 (1.08)
Neglec (F)	4.07 (1.94)	4.06 (1.91)	3.75 (1.62)	2.93 (1.67)
Ideal (M)	3.36 (1.74)	2.82 (1.47)	2.40 (1.57)	2.73 (2.19)
Ideal (F)	3.14 (1.83)	2.56 (1.60)	2.05 (1.19)	2.87 (1.73)
Anger (M)	2.50 (1.51)	2.71 (1.96)	2.45 (1.57)	2.13 (1.60)
Anger (F)	2.14 (1.61)	2.73 (1.97)	2.25 (1.45)	1.80 (1.42)
Derog (M)	1.64 (0.93)	2.32 (1.74)	2.05 (1.47)	1.60 (0.83)
Derog (F)	2.07 (1.54)	3.00 (2.06)	2.40 (1.60)	1.67 (1.05)
Deroga	1.71 (1.49)	2.71 (1.95)	2.15 (1.35)	1.47 (0.64)
Inabrec	3.71 (2.05)	3.73 (1.85)	3.30 (1.59)	3.20 (1.93)
Metacog	1.14 (0.36)	1.88 (0.81)	2.60 (0.99)	2.27 (1.33)
Passive	5.07 (1.68)	3.41 (1.79)	3.40 (1.39)	3.47 (1.30)
Fearlos	1.14 (0.36)	1.29 (0.68)	1.55 (1.23)	1.20 (0.56)
Unrslos	2.64 (1.55)	2.09 (1.31)	2.45 (1.36)	2.13 (1.41)
Unrstra	2.07 (1.14)	1.94 (1.23)	2.25 (1.37)	1.47 (0.74)
CohereT	3.00 (0.68)	3.29 (0.80)	5.10 (1.33)	5.13 (1.51)
CohereM	2.43 (0.65)	2.85 (0.82)	4.95 (1.50)	5.33 (1.84)

Significant differences between index and control groups as a whole

	t (81df)	p
Loving mother	−2.83	0.0058
Loving father	−2.80	0.0065
Involving/role-reversing father	2.22	0.0290
Metacognitive processes	−3.74	0.0003
Coherence of transcript	−7.98	0.0001
Coherence of mind	−8.78	0.0001

Standard deviations are in parentheses.

Scales for probable experience: Love = Loving, Reject = Rejecting, Rolerv = Involving/Role-reversing, Achiev = Pressure to achieve, Neglec = Neglecting.

M = Mother, F = Father—experience with or state of mind concerning

Scales for states of mind respecting parents: Ideal = Idealizing, Anger = Involving anger, Derog = Derogation.

Scales for overall states of mind: Deroga = Overall derogation of attachment, Inabrec = Insistence on inability to recall, Metacog = Metacognitive processes, Passive = Passivity of thought processes, Fearlos = Fear of loss of child, Unrslos = Unresolved loss through death, Unrstra = Unresolved trauma (including abuse), CohereT = Coherence of Transcript, CohereM = Coherence of Mind.

lies in the area of metacognition and coherence, of direct relevance, therefore, to the second hypothesis adopted for testing at the beginning of this section, concerning understanding of one's own mental processes and those of others. Of course, though generally supportive of hypothesis two, these data lack specificity.

Other significant differences emerged in probable past experience with parents, of relevance to the third hypothesis under examination, concerning possible aetiological factors of sadomasochism. Index subjects had, on average, less loving mothers than controls, less loving fathers than controls, and more involving/role-reversing fathers than controls. Again, these findings are generally supportive, but they fall short of the specific items which are listed in hypothesis three.

Table 5.3, presenting product-moment correlations across all 83 interviews, confirms the finding of previous investigators (Fonagy *et al.*, 1991*b*) that the AAI scales are indeed correlated. The table contains 20 predictable

TABLE 5.3. Pearson product moment correlations of AAI scale scores across all interviews ($n = 83$)

	LoveM	LoveF	RejectM	RejectF	RolervM	RolervF	AchievM	AchievF
LoveF	**0.584**							
RejectM	−**0.654**	−0.217						
RejectF	−0.324	−**0.703**	0.314					
RolervM	−0.034	−0.098	−0.322	−0.168				
RolervF	−0.084	0.034	0.018	−0.107	0.323			
AchievM	0.018	0.043	−0.113	−0.018	0.017	−0.108		
AchievF	0.042	−0.035	−0.056	0.123	−0.067	0.002	**0.560**	
NeglecM	−**0.527**	−0.278	**0.616**	0.342	−0.320	−0.071	−0.063	−0.025
NeglecF	−0.390	−**0.656**	0.201	0.451	0.077	−0.101	0.149	0.041
IdealM	−0.031	−0.308	0.062	0.283	0.034	0.158	−0.031	0.098
IdealF	−0.177	0.082	0.281	−0.050	−0.175	0.126	−0.019	0.030
AngerM	−0.338	−0.125	0.292	0.058	0.189	0.317	−0.031	−0.084
AngerF	−0.175	−0.303	−0.017	0.408	0.116	0.275	−0.083	−0.006
DerogM	−0.294	−0.173	0.146	0.058	0.048	0.110	−0.061	−0.060
DerogF	−0.208	−0.414	−0.008	0.354	0.048	−0.027	−0.024	−0.059
Deroga	−0.233	−0.287	0.113	0.244	−0.135	−0.039	−0.082	−0.011
Inabrec	−0.119	−0.202	0.107	0.113	−0.132	−0.012	0.032	0.167
Metacog	0.197	0.288	−0.087	−0.280	0.155	−0.037	0.070	0.051
Passive	−0.121	−0.086	−0.026	−0.074	0.142	0.050	−0.008	−0.038
Fearlos	−0.112	0.001	0.000	−0.004	0.080	−0.019	0.030	0.027
Unrslos	−0.140	−0.097	0.041	−0.036	0.135	−0.017	0.006	−0.140
Unrstra	−0.308	−0.159	0.303	0.069	0.099	0.084	−0.060	−0.055
CohereT	0.433	0.447	−0.108	−0.267	−0.124	−0.243	−0.005	−0.036
CohereM	**0.506**	**0.501**	−0.140	−0.264	−0.138	−0.243	0.001	−0.015

(*Continued*)

TABLE 5.3. *(Continued)*

	NeglecM	NeglecF	IdealM	IdealF	AngerM	AngerF	DerogM	DerogF
NeglecF	0.333							
IdealM	−0.011	0.125						
IdealF	0.273	−0.060	0.488					
AngerM	0.232	0.172	−0.314	−0.177				
AngerF	0.089	0.142	−0.106	−0.318	**0.556**			
DerogM	0.189	0.136	−0.393	−0.323	0.481	0.425		
DerogF	0.061	0.213	−0.140	**−0.530**	0.284	**0.582**	**0.612**	
Deroga	0.143	0.134	−0.188	−0.340	0.217	0.311	**0.582**	**0.751**
Inabrec	0.059	0.101	**0.502**	0.365	−0.293	−0.298	−0.063	−0.118
Metacog	−0.069	−0.026	−0.241	−0.194	0.173	0.083	0.041	−0.020
Passive	−0.104	0.152	0.055	0.180	−0.106	−0.211	−0.189	−0.210
Fearlos	0.028	0.064	−0.015	0.054	−0.019	0.089	−0.035	−0.060
Unrslos	0.077	0.166	−0.033	−0.087	0.306	0.150	0.017	−0.003
Unrstra	0.358	0.220	−0.115	0.022	0.364	0.218	0.150	0.016
CohereT	−0.075	−0.304	−0.375	−0.255	0.032	−0.037	−0.000	−0.142
CohereM	−0.101	−0.342	−0.344	−0.262	−0.029	−0.085	−0.079	−0.174

	Deroga	Inabrec	Metacog	Passive	Fearlos	Unrslos	Unrstra	CohereT
Inabrec	0.128							
Metacog	−0.155	−0.248						
Passive	−0.251	−0.062	−0.239					
Fearlos	−0.149	−0.091	0.344	0.071				
Unrslos	−0.177	−0.215	0.139	−0.200	0.165			
Unrstra	−0.110	−0.331	0.070	−0.128	0.236	**0.509**		
CohereT	−0.181	−0.349	**0.592**	−0.362	0.050	0.085	0.029	
CohereM	−0.249	−0.348	**0.610**	−0.304	0.071	−0.005	−0.037	**0.943**

Scales for probable experience: Love = Loving, Reject = Rejecting, Rolerv = Involving/Role-reversing, Achiev = Pressure to achieve, Neglec = Neglecting.

M = Mother, F = Father—experience with or state of mind concerning

Scales for states of mind respecting parents: Ideal = Idealizing, Anger = Involving anger, Derog = Derogation.

Scales for overall states of mind: Deroga = Overall derogation of attachment, Inabrec = Insistence on inability to recall, Metacog = Metacognitive processes, Passive = Passivity of thought processes, Fearlos = Fear of loss of child, Unrslos = Unresolved loss through death, Unrstra = Unresolved trauma (including abuse), CohereT = Coherence of Transcript, CohereM = Coherence of Mind.

$r > 0.5$ in bold type.

instances (in bold type) where $r > 0.5$ ($p < 0.001$). The level of association between scales, already sufficient to justify a multivariate approach to their analysis, becomes higher when the index and control groups are examined separately. Further separation of the control group into depressed and nondepressed subjects shows, in the case of the latter ($n = 15$), the strong association between scales which might be expected from normal data, i.e., 67 instances (in bold type) where $r > 0.5$ ($p < 0.05$) (Table 5.4).

TABLE 5.4. Pearson product moment correlations of AAI scale scores across all nondepressed (neutral) controls ($n = 15$)

	LoveM	LoveF	RejectM	RejectF	RolervM	RolervF	AchievM	AchievF
LoveF	**0.752**							
RejectM	**−0.712**	**−0.563**						
RejectF	**−0.731**	**−0.828**	**0.616**					
RolervM	−0.044	−0.054	**−0.547**	−0.051				
RolervF	0.109	0.319	−0.011	−0.386	−0.288			
AchievM	−0.108	−0.141	−0.155	0.124	0.212	−0.196		
AchievF	0.240	0.140	−0.358	−0.130	0.166	−0.204	**0.513**	
NeglecM	**−0.607**	**−0.634**	0.455	**0.642**	−0.032	−0.204	0.047	−0.402
NeglecF	−0.498	**−0.791**	0.345	**0.666**	0.199	−0.321	−0.121	−0.443
IdealM	−0.226	−0.461	−0.115	0.404	0.332	0.034	0.231	−0.024
IdealF	−0.165	−0.188	−0.048	0.192	0.235	0.182	0.117	−0.206
AngerM	−0.491	−0.371	**0.574**	0.426	−0.227	−0.196	−0.221	−0.231
AngerF	−0.488	−0.481	0.438	**0.673**	−0.174	−0.155	0.035	−0.074
DerogM	−0.341	−0.308	0.499	0.351	−0.186	−0.200	−0.183	−0.096
DerogF	−0.353	−0.394	0.476	**0.518**	−0.218	−0.176	0.000	0.000
Deroga	−0.171	0.029	**0.586**	0.078	**−0.544**	0.231	−0.474	−0.165
Inabrec	−0.174	−0.264	−0.209	0.118	0.306	0.114	0.131	0.020
Metacog	0.485	0.307	**−0.569**	−0.431	0.387	−0.263	−0.189	0.237
Passive	−0.290	−0.231	0.221	0.308	0.029	0.326	−0.078	**−0.537**
Fearlos	−0.055	0.228	−0.094	−0.298	0.290	−0.099	−0.090	−0.283
Unrslos	−0.367	−0.308	0.058	0.296	0.047	−0.223	0.000	−0.263
Unrstra	−0.456	**−0.565**	0.327	0.245	0.165	−0.174	0.068	−0.142
CohereT	**0.672**	**0.613**	**−0.500**	**−0.658**	0.129	−0.208	−0.034	0.281
CohereM	**0.658**	**0.571**	−0.486	**−0.606**	0.078	−0.201	−0.027	0.395

	NeglecM	NeglecF	IdealM	IdealF	AngerM	AngerF	DerogM	DerogF
NeglecF	**0.586**							
IdealM	0.489	**0.524**						
IdealF	0.443	0.369	**0.879**					
AngerM	−0.025	0.325	−0.480	**−0.563**				
AngerF	0.158	0.355	−0.133	−0.360	**0.766**			
DerogM	−0.096	0.290	−0.497	**−0.590**	**0.907**	**0.654**		
DerogF	0.000	0.314	−0.354	**−0.540**	**0.840**	**0.863**	**0.907**	
Deroga	0.144	−0.103	**−0.517**	−0.392	0.424	0.266	**0.512**	0.462
Inabrec	0.362	0.270	**0.841**	**0.778**	**−0.587**	−0.425	**−0.615**	**−0.600**
Metacog	−0.455	−0.184	−0.341	−0.479	0.016	−0.271	0.168	−0.034
Passive	0.375	0.476	0.448	**0.570**	0.071	0.247	0.053	0.122
Fearlos	−0.283	−0.138	−0.303	−0.118	0.207	−0.215	0.031	−0.243
Unrslos	0.113	0.308	−0.080	−0.257	**0.595**	**0.513**	0.355	0.323
Unrstra	0.124	0.373	−0.006	−0.115	0.425	0.229	0.325	0.214
CohereT	**−0.684**	**−0.537**	**−0.726**	**−0.707**	0.022	−0.220	0.160	0.030
CohereM	**−0.718**	**−0.598**	**−0.687**	**−0.727**	−0.016	−0.218	0.141	0.025

(Continued)

TABLE 5.4. (*Continued*)

	Deroga	Inabrec	Metacog	Passive	Fearlos	Unrslos	Unrstra	CohereT
Inabrec	**−0.542**							
Metacog	−0.156	−0.160						
Passive	0.063	0.102	**−0.529**					
Fearlos	−0.279	−0.171	0.306	−0.039				
Unrslos	−0.233	−0.063	0.170	0.042	0.416			
Unrstra	−0.040	−0.169	0.010	0.202	0.446	0.346		
CohereT	0.005	**−0.598**	**0.728**	**−0.544**	0.305	−0.076	−0.060	
CohereM	−0.020	**−0.502**	**0.747**	**−0.666**	0.208	−0.101	−0.122	**0.963**

Scales for probable experience: Love = Loving, Reject = Rejecting, Rolerv = Involving/Role-reversing, Achiev = Pressure to achieve, Neglec = Neglecting.

M = Mother, F = Father—experience with or state of mind concerning

Scales for states of mind respecting parents: Ideal = Idealizing, Anger = Involving anger, Derog = Derogation.

Scales for overall states of mind: Deroga = Overall derogation of attachment, Inabrec = Insistence on inability to recall, Metacog = Metacognitive processes, Passive = Passivity of thought processes, Fearlos = Fear of loss of child, Unrslos = Unresolved loss through death, Unrstra = Unresolved trauma (including abuse), CohereT = Coherence of Transcript, CohereM = Coherence of Mind.

$r > 0.5$ in bold type.

The correlation matrix of the depressed control group ($n = 20$) is not shown, but in it a rejecting father appears to be associated with some idealization of mother ($r = 0.520$, $p < 0.02$) and this is in turn associated with derogation of father ($r = 0.561$, $p < 0.01$).

Examining Table 5.4 in more detail, a rejecting mother is negatively associated with metacognition in the neutral (nondepressed) control group ($n = 15$). Her lack of sensitivity to her child's signals is not likely to develop a reflective self function (Fonagy *et al.*, 1991*a*, 1996) in this child. Coherence of transcript is also negatively associated with rejection on the part of either parent. This negative association with coherence is even more pronounced for a neglecting mother. In this neutral control group, the relation between idealization and inability to recall the past, a relation on which the Ds1 (and to a lesser extent the Ds3) classification is based, is particularly marked, leading as might be expected to equally marked negative correlations for coherence of transcript and of mind.

The correlation matrix of the complete index (sadomasochistic) group ($n = 48$) is not shown, but on first scrutinizing it one is struck by the dearth of high correlations—only 14 over 0.5, as compared with 29 for the depressed controls and 67 for the neutral (nondepressed) controls. These 14 associations are moreover to be expected as night may be expected to follow day—for example, it is not surprising that a loving upbringing should be negatively correlated with rejection and neglect, that derogation should apply to both parents and to attachment in general, that passivity of discourse should be negatively associated with coherence of transcript, and the latter in turn should be positively associated with coherence of mind. Why, then, so few meaningful correlations in the matrix of this index group? No formal tests of the significance of the apparent differences between correlations were carried out, but, after all, these scales are indubitably correlated—as already stated, the matrix for all interviewees ($n=83$, Table 5.3) contained 20 correlation coefficients over 0.5. When the complete index group is separated on the basis of a similar criterion to that applied to the complete control group (a critical total BDI score of 14) into 34 nondepressed and 14 depressed sadomasochistic subjects, the picture changes somewhat. More association between AAI scales emerges from the subgroups (20 correlation coefficients over 0.5 in the nondepressed matrix, 32 in the depressed matrix), suggesting that correlations were to some extent cancelling out over the complete index group because of its heterogeneity. The differences between the subgroups were not anticipated, and their analysis at this point and in later chapters, particularly Chapter 8 under the subheading 'A profile of the depressed subgroup of sadomasochists', was therefore exploratory. It was undertaken because, in the course of interviewing these subjects, a picture emerged in which the depressed subgroup stood out as the more quintessentially masochistic. It should be emphasized that the data presented in these exploratory analyses should be viewed with caution and need to be replicated in further studies designed specifically to test differences within the SM group. To return to the present result and the scrutiny of AAI scale scores, however, it is also a possibility that the lack of correlation is partly a reflection of lack of coherence in the individuals comprising this group (mean score for coherence of transcript 3.2, S.E. 0.1, for coherence of mind 2.7, S.E. 0.1, across all 48 sadomasochists). An unusually large number of CC classifications were necessarily allotted to this index group (Table 5.1*a*). 'Cannot Classify' is a rare phenomenon, "a general inability to rally an organized stance" (Hesse, 1996, p. 8) a breakdown in defense strategy at a global level—in short, it betokens an anomaly.

Univariate analyses of variance highlighted certain significant interactions between sadomasochism and depression, with respect to neglect on the part of mother, derogation of father, derogation of attachment in general, metacognition and passivity. These interactions are plotted in Figure 5.2*a*–*e*. The high passivity mean for depressed sadomasochistic subjects (5.07 (S.D. 1.68), Figure 5.2*e*) derives from the predominance of the E1 (passively entangled) AAI classification in this subgroup (Table 5.1*a*). These interactions will, however, be examined in more detail in the next section where possible interpretations of them will be put forward.

Multivariate analysis of variance (MANOVA), performed to test the hypothesis that the index and control groups could be differentiated

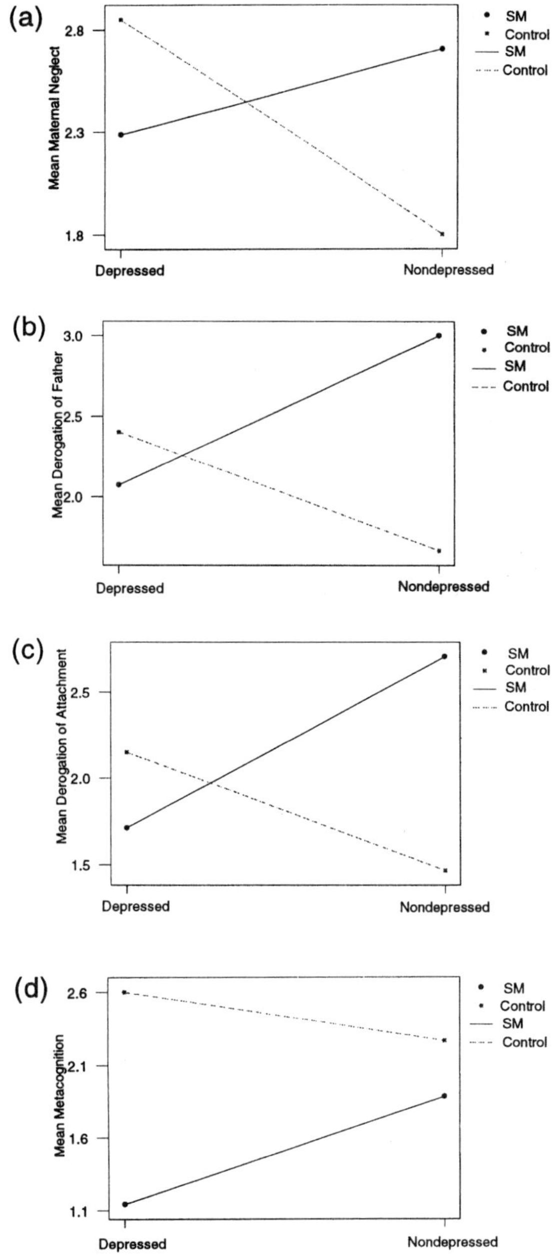

FIGURE 5.2. Interactions significant at the 5% level between sadomasochism and depression as they affect five AAI scales (see means in Table 5.2): (a) Neglecting Mother, (b) Derogation of Father, (c) Derogation of Attachment, (d) Metacognition, (e) Passivity.

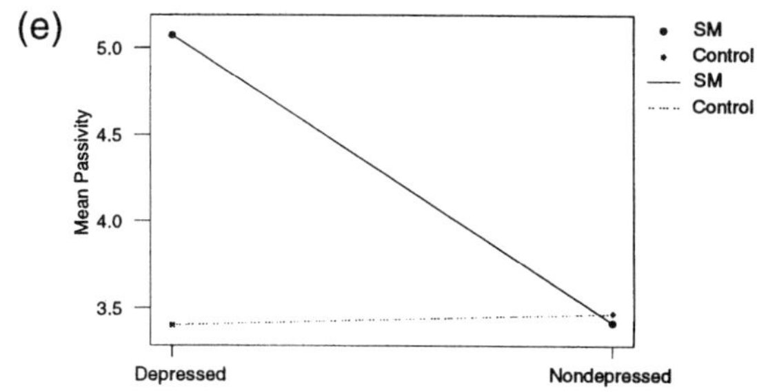

FIGURE 5.2. (*Continued*)

simply on the basis of certain parenting and state of mind scales (loving parents, metacognition and coherence) yielded a highly significant Wilks' lambda (lambda $= 0.502$, approximate $F_{(5,75)} = 14.87$, $p < 0.0001$; Wilks, 1962). These scales were selected for the test because they carried high weightings in a discriminant analysis using all AAI scales and high loadings in a principal component analysis of all the scales, on the first principle component.

In the linear discriminant analysis with all the AAI scales as predictors, a high proportion (0.904) of the 83 interviews were found to have been classified correctly as belonging to the index group or the control group. This result of an objective statistical test may perhaps be regarded as evidence of the consistency with which the interviews were rated. The fact that discrimination between depressed and nondepressed was not quite as good (the proportion found to have been classified correctly into these groupings on the basis of the same predictors was 0.723) may, arguably, point to the self-report nature of the Beck Depression Inventory.

Three control subjects caused some unease as to their group classification. CS125 stated when he was questioned that he sometimes slapped his partner who was submissive in order to give her pleasure. CS175 manifested, at certain points of the interview, some of the characteristics of what Freud described as moral masochism (Freud, 1924*a*, pp. 165–170): "There is a part of me that wants to fail and that, when I'm just on the point of succeeding, I will do something to make sure that I don't *(Mm)* for some reason ... I've done that again and again and again throughout my life and it's not very attractive." NS269 admitted, upon questioning, that he sometimes had sadomasochistic fantasies. I decided not to reclassify these three controls, nor to remove them from the general analysis for four reasons: (a) a control group should be a representative sample of the general population, and sadomasochistic features are certainly observable in the latter; (b) as a result of the preferential recruitment of depressed subjects for purposes of comparison, this control group was already unrepresentative in that it contained a larger proportion of depressed individuals than the population at large, making any further manipulation of its constitution unwise; (c) these three individuals did not meet the DSM-III-R criteria for sadomasochism, criteria met by all of the 48 index subjects; (d) they were correctly assigned to the control group according to the discriminant analysis performed on all 83 subjects, and indeed their assignment to the control rather than the index group was predicted with probabilities of 0.977, 0.999 and 0.662, respectively, in a further discriminant analysis from which their data had been excluded (i.e., treated as test observations). However, these three somewhat anomalous subjects will be mentioned again in the following chapters. As the founder of British genetics, William Bateson (1861–1926), admonished the students of Cambridge University in his inaugural lecture: "Treasure your exceptions! ... Keep them always uncovered and in sight. Exceptions are like the rough brickwork of a growing building which tells that there is more to come and shows where the next construction is to be" (Bateson, 1908).

Since depression might, in principle, be confounding the effect of sadomasochism on coherence, it was treated as a nuisance variable which needed to be statistically controlled by the analysis of covariance, i.e., by regression. To this end, scale scores for metacognition, coherence of transcript and coherence of mind were combined. The mean metacognition/coherence and depression ratings for each group are set out in Table 5.5.

The analysis of covariance summary table is presented as Table 5.6.

The dependent variable is metacognition/coherence, and the covariate or nuisance variable is depression. Group is the independent variable. $F_{(1,80)} = 64.61$ is highly significant ($p < 0.0001$). Controlling for ('partialling out') depression does not therefore undermine the difference between groups.

The possible effect of subjects' marital status, sex and age on this coherence difference between the index and the control groups was also examined by stepwise regression (descriptive use). The order in which

TABLE 5.5. Mean metacognition/coherence and depression scores for index and control groups

	Metacognition/Coherence (3 AAI scales combined)	Depression (BDI total score)	*N*
Index group	7.60 (1.83)	10.71 (7.90)	48
Control group	12.69 (3.83)	14.77 (12.36)	35

Standard deviations are in parentheses.

TABLE 5.6. Analysis of covariance, metacognition/coherence with depression statistically controlled

	DF	SS	MS	*F*	*p*
Reduction in deviance	1	525.31	525.31	64.61	0.0001
BDI total & Group	80	650.34	8.13		
BDI total	81	1175.65			

TABLE 5.7. Correlation of coherence with continuous and discontinuous demographic variables (sex, marital status and age) and with group (index versus control)

	Metacognition/Coherence (3 AAI scales combined)	Sex	Marital status	Age
Sex	−0.227			
Marital status	0.169	−0.059		
Age	0.031	0.071	0.366	
Group	0.666	−0.202	−0.012	0.002

the predictors entered the equation was Group, Marital status, then Sex. The last step was not significant at the 5% level, so Age was not worth entering as a fourth variable. None of these demographic variables effected any appreciable reduction in deviance—Group was the only important predictor of coherence, as was already obvious from the correlations presented in Table 5.7.

Adoption

There were 5 adoptees in the index group. ES4, ES19, ES51 and ES69 stated at the beginning of their interviews that they had been adopted; ES50 recounted a highly implausible story which could only point to his being adopted: "... it was an unusual birth in so far as my mother was very overweight and had always had problems with her periods and she didn't know she was pregnant until, I think, just a few days or a few hours before I was born. *(She didn't know she was expecting a baby?)* No. No. *(Oh goodness!)* It was a very bad winter ... and she'd slipped on some ice and was taken to hospital and I popped out shortly afterwards ... she'd given up the idea of having a family, I think, because of her problems with the periods."

Using the Registrar General's Statistical Review of England and Wales (Office of Population Censuses and Surveys, 1974, pp. 14, 92), the number of adoption orders and the total number of live births were determined for the year of birth of each index subject ($n=48$). Each subject was in this way assigned a probability and these 48 probabilities were summed to give the number (0.88) of adoptees which one might expect to find in a group having this age profile. As stated, 5 adopted cases were observed. The probability of there being 5 or more adoptees in this sadomasochistic group of 48, given the null hypothesis of no special group characteristics, was approximately 0.0019. In other words, such a large incidence of adoption in this group was highly significant and of relevance to hypothesis 3*e*, listed at the beginning of this section, concerning the possible etiological role of early loss of parents in the development of sadomasochism.

Amongst the 35 controls there were 2 adoptees, CS136 and CS284, both depressed (there were no adoptees amongst the nondepressed controls).

TABLE 5.8. Index subjects (14 depressed, 34 nondepressed) listed according to possible causative factors contributing to the development of sadomasochism

	Depressed sadomasochists ($n=14$)	Nondepressed sadomasochists ($n=34$)
(a) *Parental rejection*		
Beating	ES18 ES28 ES29 ES61	ES4 ES11 ES21 ES23 ES37 ES51 ES65 ES69 ES75 ES81
Boarding school	ES52	ES1 ES2 ES15 ES69 ES81
Adoption	ES19	ES4 ES50* ES51 ES69
(b) *Physical illness*		
Injuries	ES7 ES18 ES27	ES62 ES63 ES66
Prolonged pain	ES10 ES24 ES27	ES17 ES21 ES62 ES63* ES65 ES66
Skin problems		ES4 ES15 ES17
Asthma	ES28	ES8 ES13 ES17 ES74 ES77
(c) *Difficulties in sexual development*		
Prudish mother	ES7 ES19 ES61 ES71	ES4 ES8 ES50 ES65
Premature puberty	ES18 ES20 ES24 ES27	ES21 ES30 ES34 ES50 ES51 ES58 ES65 ES74 ES77 ES81
Sexual abuse	ES24	ES51 ES58
Unacknowledged homosexuality	ES20 ES27 ES29 ES40 ES61 ES80	ES8 ES13 ES15 ES66* ES69* ES76*
(d) *Sibling resentment*		
Resented brother	ES20 ES27	ES21 ES36 ES41 ES57 ES58 ES65 ES75 ES76
Resented sister	ES7 ES18 ES19 ES28 ES40 ES52 ES61	ES23 ES26 ES37 ES42 ES63 ES69

Subjects often cited more than one of these factors and are therefore listed more than once. Cases depending on the interviewer's judgment alone are marked with an asterisk.

EARLY LIFE CIRCUMSTANCES POSSIBLY RELEVANT TO THE DEVELOPMENT OF SADOMASOCHISM

Biographical details emerged in the course of the interview which, in the case of many index subjects, seemed relevant to the development of their adult sexuality. In some cases, the subjects themselves volunteered a likely connection. More such information, relevant to the third hypothesis concerning possible etiological factors, formulated at the beginning of this section, was given in a final unstructured discussion with the interviewer of their lives and, indeed, their sexuality in particular. They all, with considerable generosity, permitted the interviewer to make notes of this conversation. The information obtained is summarized in Table 5.8, according to possible causative factors contributing to the development of sadomasochism, and is presented in greater detail, for each index subject, in Appendix 3. (What they themselves wrote in response to the last, open-ended question of the first questionnaire they completed, 'Why do you think you developed SM interests?' is a rather different matter, summarized (Table 8.2) and discussed in Chapter 8.)

DISCUSSION

The alacrity, sometimes already noticeable in the wording of an initial letter, with which index subjects presented themselves for interview did not, on the whole, represent proselytizing, nor was it straightforward exhibitionism. In the case of some older subjects, it was rather a quest for a nonjudgmental listener (they later sent letters of thanks) or even for some explanation of their sexuality. ES52 seemed to want, from somewhere, a short course of treatment which would magically release him from it! In many subjects, there was an underlying uncertainty about personal identity. ES22, in particular, the only quarrelsome one, might almost certainly be classed as a 'borderline' personality (DSM-III-R, pp. 346–347). Precisely the same overall eagerness to cooperate that I encountered with these sadomasochists was noted also by Gosselin and Wilson (1980). I believe Theodor Reik (1939) identified accurately what he termed 'the demonstrative factor' as a characteristic of masochism. Two possible etiological explanations might be put forward tentatively for consideration. (1) The masochist, as just mentioned, often appears to have a weak sense of his own identity, probably because he encountered little 'recognition' (Fonagy *et al.*, 1991*a*; Hegel, 1807; discussed in Chapter 9) as a young child. He thus craves an audience, a mirror, to assure himself that he exists in his own right and has importance. (2) The eagerness to reveal, to display himself on a psychological level is usually paralleled, as can be seen at a glance from subculture magazines, by the urge, conscious or unconscious, to expose himself physically. It reminds one, of course, of an infant's delight in exposing himself and gaining attention.

The other simple and striking finding was also expected (discussed in Chapter 4 and predicted at the beginning of Part II), namely, the preponderance of males in the sadomasochists who came forward: 43 males versus 5 females. Moreover, one of these 5 women, ES41, despite 12 years' active association with the SM 'scene', insisted that her interest lay more in observing than participating, that it was largely an artistic one.

Without exception, the sadomasochistic subjects were classified as primarily Insecure in their attachment to their parents (Table 5.1*a*, Fig. 5.1). The three subjects ES28, ES41 and ES74 received alternative classifications of F4b, F1a and F2, respectively, but these secondary subcategories are not fully Secure/Autonomous. They were awarded in so far as these subjects showed signs of valuing attachment to some extent but they imply reservations (see Appendix 2). The subclassification F4b denotes a difficult childhood that may have included traumatic events such as the death of an attachment figure (the twenty-year-old father of ES28 actually walked out when he was only a few months old) or sexual or physical abuse which still constitute a preoccupation. F1a lies on the border with the Dismissing category and signifies a deliberate reevaluation and redirection of personal life after a childhood lacking warmth if not actually harsh. F2 implies that the individual is somewhat dismissing or restricting of attachment. Is the link between the AAI scales for 'probable childhood experience' and those for 'state of mind' less in evidence in the index group, making the sources of insecurity in this group less clear? Even setting aside the diagnosis offered spontaneously by some subjects themselves (ES58, for instance, said that she had realized quickly that her parents "were not people who could be relied on ... even in an ordinary sense they couldn't be relied on"), one may put forward one possible reason for this wholesale insecurity of attachment in the index group. The mean scores of scales relating to childhood experiences (Table 5.2) suggest that they probably received less than optimal parenting and the majority considered themselves to have been either rejected (e.g., ES4, ES11, ES18, ES69) or stifled (e.g., ES10, ES13, ES39, ES61, ES66, ES71). Often they were neglected at home (e.g., ES11, ES28, ES51, ES81), sometimes sent away to boarding schools (e.g., ES1, ES2, ES15, ES52, ES69, ES81). They were also bullied and maltreated at school (e.g., ES4, ES10, ES17, ES18, ES20, ES23, ES37, ES51, ES62)—another factor predicted at the beginning of this section (additional hypothesis B). The same damaging events also came to light in the control interviews but not to the same extent and more amongst the depressed than the nondepressed controls. Although the mean AAI scale scores (Table 5.2) for rejection and neglect, for instance, are not significantly greater, statistically, for the SM group than the control group, they differ in the same direction and imply that these adverse experiences may have contributed to the greater insecurity of the SM group. Only in the amount of pressure to achieve do the scores point in another direction, albeit the differences again do not achieve statistical significance—the parents of the 'neutral' controls appear, on average, to have applied more pressure whilst those of the depressed controls were more neglectful, though again, the mean level of neglect was not as high as that experienced by the index subjects (Table 5.2). One expectation would be that neglect would cause these index subjects to be depressed at some stage of their childhood and, in fact, several stated explicitly that they were.

However, depression is likely to be, quite generally, only one result of insensitive parenting. The correlation of AAI scale scores shows clearly that for nondepressed control subjects (Table 5.4) rejection on the part of parents is also likely to be associated with damage to metacognitive processes and this damage will almost inevitably be reflected in diminished coherence.

Perhaps it would be wise to pause at this point and establish what is meant in this context by coherence. In her 1991 paper on the subject, Mary Main makes a distinction between two philosophical theories of truth: a *coherence* theory relying upon internal consistency and a *correspondence* theory relying upon plausibility in the wider context of reality (Main, 1991, p. 144). These two concepts are measured by the AAI scales of coherence of transcript and coherence of mind, respectively. Main has, in fact, linked this to Bowlby's working models: coherence of transcript meant that it was possible to construct a single mental model from it. "Coherent subjects seemed to be working with a singular model, whether of favorable or unfavorable experiences and their effects" (Main, 1991, p. 142).

Multiple Models of Attachment

Where the information reaching a child about his parents is severely conflicting—*they* insist they are devoted to his welfare, *he* experiences only harshness and neglect from them—he can either (a) break away from his parents, (b) endorse their version, (c) try to maintain both pictures, oscillating between them, or (d) attempt to integrate them, possibly suffering mental breakdown under their incompatibility (Bowlby, 1973, pp. 362–363). These incompatible representational models are, in fact, created in pairs, each pair comprising a model of his parent and a complementary, confirmatory model of himself. Multiple conflicting images of close family members are likely to relate to discrepancies between memories of actual interactions, stored in episodic memory, and generalized propositions about these people, stored in semantic memory. These discrepancies are precisely what questions 3 and 4 of the Adult Attachment Interview are addressing. The five adjectives selected by the interviewee to describe his early relationships first with his mother then with his father may or may not be supported by actual childhood memories. In the case of the sadomasochistic group, they were often unsupported or contradicted.

This was but one manifestation of the lack of coherence which chiefly distinguished the index from the control group as a whole (see bottom of Tables 5.2 and 5.5). In Mary Main's words: "... these adults were exhibiting (a) multiple models of their histories and attitudes while (b) seemingly intending to present a singular model" (Main, 1991, p. 143). To state their problems using the formulation of Main and Goldwyn (1984), index subjects, more than controls, found it difficult to obtain *access* to information relating to attachment, to maintain *organization* in this information and to prevent it from undergoing *distortion*. The final point made by John Bowlby in delineating this conceptual framework is a critical one: "On the way in which an individual's attachment behavior becomes organized within his personality turns the pattern of affectional bonds he makes during his life" (Bowlby, 1980, p. 41). Both ES35 and ES50 had, for instance, two opposing representational models of women. ES35 wanted to 'worship' a Madonna/whore image (cf. Estela V. Welldon's controversial portrayal of female psychopathology *Mother, Madonna, Whore,* 1988). ES50 carried within him the opposing faces of the teacher in his first nursery class, "a real Tartar of a woman ... feared throughout the land as a very very strict disciplinarian" and of another teacher when he was eight or nine, "just so gorgeous-looking ... she had this lovely Welsh accent ... I always had the feeling I wanted to kiss her ... she was very warm and friendly and interesting". He displayed a marked ambivalence towards his adoptive mother, with whom he lived until her death when he was 41.

The finding that index subjects had significantly less coherence of mind than controls (Tables 5.2 and 5.5) was not unexpected. That they would harbour split and conflicting images of their parents and siblings had been predicted at the beginning of this section (second hypothesis). It was, however, necessary to demonstrate that diminished coherence was characteristic of sadomasochism, that depression was not a confounding variable in this particular result, and neither was it produced by demographic factors such as age, sex or marital status. The issue of depression as a possible nuisance variable was tackled by an analysis of covariance with depression statistically controlled (Table 5.6). Even when depression was 'partialled' out in this way the difference in coherence between index and control subjects remained highly significant. The other concerns were addressed and removed by stepwise regression (descriptive use), though the correlations presented in Table 5.7 already implied that the difference in coherence was genuinely associated with index or control group-membership not with how old subjects were, whether they were male or female, whether they were married or unmarried. It will be recalled that for the purposes of this analysis, the three AAI scales of metacognition, coherence of transcript and coherence of mind were combined. They are, of course, closely related (Table 5.3). It might be said that incoherence arises through a deficit in metacognition. What emerged, in fact, from the interviews of these 48 sadomasochistic subjects, from the accounts they gave of their parents' behavior and their own interpretations of it, was a lack of theory of mind. Their early relationships had afforded most of them little opportunity for the development of an awareness of mental processes motivating behavior. Their low scores for metacognition and coherence were a reflection of this deficit.

Any attempt to interpret the interactions plotted in Figure 5.2*a–e* between sadomasochism and depression as they affect single variables (certain AAI scales) can only be tentative. Univariate analysis of variance revealed that all five of them were significant at the 5% level. In the case of the interactions depicted in Figure 5.2*a–c*, it would appear that accordingly as they were depressed, sadomasochistic subjects suffered rather less neglect from their mothers (or thought they did), were rather less derogatory about their fathers and about attachment in general, whereas the reverse would seem to be true for the control group. It is perhaps hardly surprising that nondepressed ('normal') controls should have less maternal neglect to report and should be less derogating than depressed controls. In the light of the interaction plotted in Figure 5.2*e*, passivity might be an explanation of the contrary behavior of the index group. As already mentioned, a majority (10 out of 14) of the depressed subgroup was passively preoccupied with childhood and attachment issues (assigned an E1 primary or alternative AAI classification, Table 5.1*a*), and they were also older than the other subgroups (mean age 47.36, range 25–77, Table 5.1). The more active sadomasochists were conceivably less depressed in proportion as they externalized their (possibly greater) resentments, for example, frequenting SM clubs. Regarding the interaction appearing in Figure 5.2*d*, it was very noticeable whilst transcribing and rating the interviews of passive and depressed sadomasochists that they were not accustomed to monitoring mental processes—their capacity for metacognition was generally poorer than that exhibited by those who were more angry and less depressed. In contrast, depressed controls were sometimes more realistic and more penetrating in their assessments than 'normal' control subjects, who tended to become more bland the lower their BDI score, a finding which emerged, incidentally, even from my pilot study.

The Adoptees

The unusually large number of adopted subjects in the sado-masochistic group, significant at the 1% level of probability, in a sense provides support for an etiological factor hypothesized at the beginning of this section (hypothesis 3*e*), namely, the early loss of a parent, before assimilation of such a loss was possible. A month before his interview, ES69 went, at the age of 59, to look at his adoptive grandparents' graves, though they were really no relatives of his, and the grandmother had told her daughter at the time of his adoption to "take the bastard back!" However, the need for surrogate blood relatives was equally evident in one of the two adoptees in the control group, CS284, who felt deeply attached to the parents of his adoptive mother.

The disquieting and, at first, surprising element in what these sado-masochistic adoptees related about their upbringing was the damaging treatment they had received from their adoptive parents. One might reasonably expect a couple whose longing for a child has driven them to seek and accept responsibility for someone else's to cherish that infant. It would seem instead that the absence of a genetic relationship was crucial in the life histories I heard. ES4, ES51 and ES69 were frequently and severely beaten. ES69 reflected: "I think they knew my background or they knew my parents and they put it down to inbred badness or whatever—that's what I think. That's what I think." The adoptive mother of ES51 had failed to protect him from sexual abuse by her older male friend and business associate. The sexual development of ES19 and ES50 was inhibited and warped by the prim, puritanical attitude of their adopitive mothers towards sex. Both ES19 and ES69 envied and hated their sisters who had also been adopted.

Claims to Superior Ability

Many index subjects, most notably ES27, ES30, ES50, ES62, ES74, ES77, made claims of outstanding ability at an early age. In the case of ES30 and ES74, it might perhaps be regarded as the spoilt-only-child syndrome: above-average abilities of a precocious nature which then 'drop back'. However, ES35 and ES36 exemplified the pendulum swings in self-assessment from which we all suffer but the masochist, with his *impedimenta* of insecurity and anxiety, probably suffers more acutely than most. These pendulum swings between high and low self-esteem, which make him convinced he is a genius one day and totally inept the next, are, of course, closely linked to his weak sense of personal identity (the conflicting internal working models of himself which complement those of his original caregivers), to his preoccupation with control (each situation must entail either winning or losing, either domination or submission) and probably, on a behavioral or even a physiological level (see the next subsection on somatization), to the scheduling of his sadomasochistic activities.

Authority is not the same as power or control. Authority might be defined as knowledge and experience which permit one to arrive at correct judgments, sound decisions and to speak illuminatingly and with understanding. It is confident in itself. The insecure turn to authoritarian regimes because they are in themselves insecure. It is not surprising that the masochist, who is insecure, should place so much emphasis on power and control, the potentially dangerous substitutes for inner security, for authority.

Somatization

The interview question "what would you do as a child when you were upset?" probes further with respect to childhood illness and injury. As hypothesized at the beginning of this section (additional hypothesis C), this brought to light many instances of prolonged, sometimes excruciating pain in the childhood of index subjects (Table 5.8, Appendix 3). It also revealed their marked tendency to 'somatize', to enact their distress in the 'theatre of the body' (McDougall, 1989). When asked whether his many childhood illnesses meant that he had been in pain a lot, ES27, for instance, replied: "Em—not really, just ill, just a general malaise. I'd get sore throats, you know, and bad like cough, and I had like rheumatism at one point. This was when they realized that like this tonsillitis was really serious—I couldn't move my legs periodically and that was quite painful—but no, I was never in a great deal of enduring pain—it was just—just, you know, 'Damn! I'm ill again!' kind of thing ..."

Physical Characteristics and Behavior

Several index subjects were apparently left-handed—ES30, ES35, ES50, for instance—but probably no more than in the control group or, indeed, the general population.

When, after the interview, the administration of the Beck Depression Inventory and the performance of the 'emotional' Stroop task, discussion finally turned directly to sadomasochism, a few subjects displayed clear physical signs of emotional arousal. ES8, ES19 and ES24, for instance, developed such a marked hand tremor that they had difficulty in writing on the questionnaire forms. The tremor was clearly, in all cases, one of excitement, not one of embarrassment.

Habits of Speech

There was noticeably more stereotypy in the linguistic usage of index subjects than of control subjects. The frequent use of 'basically', 'actually', 'obviously', 'absolutely', for instance on the part of ES34, ES37, ES74, ES76 but also several others amongst the younger men, seemed a form of compensation for vagueness. There was sometimes an entanglement with numbers and with dates, possibly with the same unconscious motivation—to anchor an otherwise vague response—or possibly arising out of something more magical and childlike, akin to the compulsion to count the strokes of a beating (ES15 traced this particular subculture convention to ritualized canings at school). ES26 often introduced percentages without any particular appropriateness. The word 'emotional' held an esoteric, dangerous connotation for him, as it did for several others. The common use of 'tend to' before a verb which could have stood better on its own, without modification, was also characteristic of the index group, possibly reflecting insecurity. The ability to monitor ongoing thought and speech concerning attachment—metacognitive monitoring—is a marker of security it itself, but such metacognition usually takes the form of fresh-sounding remarks. "I tend to find myself doing this …" is more likely to represent a closed or adhesive way of thinking than a genuine monitoring of reaction patterns.

Characteristic of the younger men in the sadomasochistic group (e.g., ES7, ES27, ES30, ES37) was a deep, pervasive dysfluency which only manifested itself incontrovertibly about a half-hour into the transcript. This was a style of language production in short phrases, maybe a hangover from early childhood, and it was usually the vehicle of somewhat banal subject matter, for instance, father-and-son contacts in connection with football! ES76, a little older at 44, brought up on a council estate, had an old-fashioned turn of phrase, presumably derived from his parents: "A little bird told me you were naughty," his father would say when he had been "a rascal"! His parents ultimately lived separately in their council flat.

The accurate verbatim transcription of all these interviews necessitated listening to them, phrase by phrase, many times over. I would like, finally therefore, to record a strong personal impression which formed gradually in the course of transcribing 83 interviews verbatim. I felt in contact with these people. They had come in order to reveal themselves, and for the most part they were striving to be truthful. The contact I sensed was closer than the usual daily exchange of information or of small talk. Of course, there was the unusual event of another human being giving them undivided attention, intent upon understanding what they had to say on a subject of deep interest to them. There may have been another factor at work. From birth onwards, human lives diverge along paths of differing experiences which render communication more and more difficult. In returning to early childhood, we were in a sense reversing this journey into isolation and returning to a point where the paths have only started to diverge.

CHAPTER 6

THE 'EMOTIONAL' STROOP TASK

SUMMARY

A sadomasochistic mind-set in the index group of subjects (n =48) is demonstrated objectively by increased mean response latency to sadomasochistic-content words and by preferential free recall of these words.

INTRODUCTION

The prime virtue of 'emotional' Stroop as a second line of research is that it constitutes an alternative to self-report. Secondly, it is, by definition, a tool for probing the influence of emotion on cognitive processing. Thirdly, it is a promising method for the investigation of an obviously heterogeneous condition, such as masochism, in that word lists can be designed to delineate specific aspects of the phenomenon and test specific hypotheses of its aetiolgy.

But let us go back to the beginning. John Ridley Stroop's (1935) seminal paper has all the clarity and elegant simplicity one would expect of a classic: the name of a color presented in another color increases the response time in naming that other incongruent color. However, even on first reading, one is struck by two facts: (1) strangely enough, he does not test the facilitation ensuing on a presentation of color words in their congruent colors; (2) part of his interpretation is implausible: "... it seems reasonable to conclude that the difference in speed in reading names of colors and in naming colors may be satisfactorily accounted for by the difference in training in the two activities. The word stimulus has been associated with the specific response 'to read', while the color stimulus has been associated with various responses: 'to admire', 'to name', 'to reach for', 'to avoid', etc." (Stroop, 1935, p. 660). Surely a more plausible interpretation is that in reading, the response is given, whereas in naming, the response has to be searched for—an explanation which was already at hand twenty years earlier (Hollingworth, 1915). However, in this, Stroop opted for the explanation of Peterson *et al.* (1925) rather than that of James McKeen Cattell, who pointed out that in reading, "the process has become automatic, whereas in the case of colors and pictures we must by a voluntary effort choose the name" (Cattell, 1886, p. 65). Peterson did, after all, supervise Stroop's dissertation! The implication of their stance, that color is associated with more than one type of response, is, of course, that certain colors should interfere more than others—red, for instance, in suggesting avoidance, might take longer to name than green.

Well over 700 studies of the Stroop effect have appeared since 1935. Jensen & Rohwer (1966) and Dyer (1973) conducted reviews of this literature. Colin M. MacLeod's Herculean effort to encompass it (MacLeod, 1991), with ten pages of references, does not even deal with 'emotional' Stroop since it omits "applied" studies (p. 165). It does, however, discuss the theoretical and, above all, the methodological issues of the basic test and its variants in detail and with admirable thoroughness. Klein (1964) appears to be the first to provide evidence that noncolor words can give rise to interference in color-naming in proportion to their 'attensive' or attention-catching power.

Under the heading 'Variations on the Stroop Procedure', MacLeod (1991) starts by considering different methods of presenting stimuli, and there is surely no better starting point for the consideration of 'emotional' Stroop where mode of presentation would seem to be crucial. The drawbacks of presenting a card of 20, 50 or 100 stimuli to subjects are fairly obvious. (1) Timing of response latencies with a stopwatch is inaccurate by current standards, since it is bound to be distorted by the experimenter's lack of consistency and agility. (2) It invites the development of strategies. For example, one subject, after a swift and even color-naming performance, stated that he had avoided the semantic dimension by focusing on the initial letters of words, easily accomplished by running the eye down the left-hand margin of the list. (3) The effects of repetition of stimuli are likely to be greater since repeated stimuli may remain in the subject's view. (4) To obtain any reliable evidence of a specific hypothesized effect, any reliable differentiation between groups, conditions or concepts, fairly large blocks of stimuli are necessary, running into the confounding variable of fatigue. (5) Most importantly, for emotionally charged stimuli interspersed with others, no measure of interference for the individual stimulus is obtained. The most potentially interesting information is lost. Of course, the advantages, in practical terms, are also considerable, namely, simplicity and mobility. With basic materials, the experimenter can go to the subject. Provided there is an overall consistency of environmental factors, particularly illumination, the test can be conducted almost anywhere.

Transformation of the Stroop test into a card-sorting task, although it lightens the stress on the experimenter and possibly allows him time for subsidiary observations, introduces a confounding variable of such magnitude and intractability—the motor performance of the subject—that it is hardly the same test. The same criticism applies to a 'matching' procedure when it is manual, rather than oral, together with that of loss of economy, since the great asset of Stroop's classic Experiment 2 (1935) is that two dimensions are combined in a single visual stimulus, requiring a single oral response.

MacLeod (1991) reviews several analogues of the classic Stroop, such as the picture-word interference task, but as far as 'emotional' Stroop is concerned, these would seem to hold advantages for child subjects rather than adults, and some, furthermore, introduce the complication of stimulus onset asynchrony (SOA). Auditory or spatial versions would not appear to offer any advantages, for present purposes, over the basic visual presentation using color, with its backing of reliability acquired over the years. The use of two or more verbal stimuli on one and the same trial, one being the target and the other(s) distractor(s), the use of irrelevant 'flankers', could only serve to attenuate still further what is, in all probability, realistically speaking, an already attenuated effect, if not to obscure it altogether.

So let us be realistic and take full note of the necessity of exposing the subject willy-nilly to the semantic dimension. A *sine qua non* of 'emotional' Stroop is that the word must impact on him—otherwise the procedure loses its *raison d'être*. The form of presentation most likely to achieve this is a computer-controlled one—single words in color coming straight at him, foveally, out of a featureless background, one by one, on a VDU, with voice-activated relay equipment providing the measurement of each individual response latency. Sadly, this is also likely to be something of a technological trap, with infuriating malfunctions, "ers", "ums" and mumbles to deplete the data. It also has the disadvantage that the subject must be enticed to the equipment. However, to offset this, there are two potential advantages. First, the overall tempo of the presentation can be regulated, if so desired. Time is, after all, the metric of the dependent variable. The instruction to name colors of listed words, without pausing, as quickly as possible, might well introduce stress of an unwanted, global kind into the equation. Secondly, if the special investigation of certain individual subjects should seem appropriate, word lists could be conveniently reprogrammed.

The selection and ordering of stimuli have given rise to such an abundance of manipulation that only a few personal thoughts are possible in the present context:

(1) The five common colors employed (five, by consensus in the literature) should be clearly distinguishable from one another and so adjusted in hue and intensity as to be equally salient, and they should be equally easy to name. Red, blue, green, brown and purple would seem a satisfactory choice. (Yellow might be too salient against a dark background or lost against a light background. Pink might be too close to red, or equivocal to name.)

(2) Words and their controls should be matched as far as possible for number of letters and number of syllables. Matching for frequency, though obviously important, is a thorny issue and can be disheartening. On the one hand, the rank range of the least frequent words in the corpus analysed by Kucera & Francis (1967), for instance, is 27864–50406; on the other hand, the frequency ranks attributed to some words may well strike one as unrepresentative of general usage. Their corpus, though large, is not the whole of the English (or even American) language, and the valiant endeavor to determine frequencies from their 15 *genres* of text is presumably as accurate as estimating, albeit scrupulously, the number of grains of sand on a beach from the number collected in a child's sand-pail! To make target and control words look and sound as similar as possible might be counterproductive, since if they are, in fact, confused, the result would either be to lose the emotional effect of the target words or to increase, unintentionally, the effect of their repetition. If the confusion itself caused hesitation in color-naming this would be irrelevant and misleading. The only way of even knowing what had actually taken place would appear to be by debriefing the subject—the very self-report which the test is aimed at avoiding.

(3) The ordering of stimuli and of blocks of stimuli has been the subject of almost infinite manipulation, but the undisputed kernel of all these permutations is that the same color or the same word should not be presented immediately next in sequence but separated by several other stimuli. From the point of view of 'emotional' Stroop, concerns of a,b,b,a ordering of conditions, randomization of order, reverse order and all the other ingenious elements of design (which, in subsequent statistical analysis, make the numbers in cells smaller and smaller!) sink, arguably,

to minor importance where it might be precisely an order of concepts, an 'emotional' sequence along the semantic dimension which was of interest. What is the effect of several repetitions of an emotionally charged (hypercathected) word? Is it cumulative or does habituation lessen the interference? This may well depend on the individual.

That different mental processes are involved in 'emotional' Stroop is indicated by a simple fact—the classic color-word Stroop in incongruent colors still invariably gives rise to the longest response latencies. For example, Watts *et al.* (1986, Table 1) report mean color-naming times of spider-phobics, for conflicting color, 'emotional', control (emotional), 'spider' and control (spider) words, respectively, of 99.8, 82.3, 75.0, 92.2 and 73.3 seconds per hundred stimuli. True, their phobic subjects reacted to spiders more than their 'normal' control group (92.2 versus 76.3 seconds), but both groups experienced most difficulty with the classic Stroop test, a different, nonemotional kind of difficulty, one might venture to surmise, that has nothing to do with concept accessibility, construct (Kelly, 1955) or schema, simply the difficulty of processing directly conflicting stimuli. In other words, the difficulty started with input and the active inhibition of one dimension could only be achieved at the expense of attentional resources for processing the other, thus delaying the correct response. Two different but related explanations have been forthcoming for the specificity of 'emotional' Stroop effects: (1) the biassed processing of certain categories of words leads directly to interference; (2) emotional arousal on encountering those words makes the voluntary attentional exclusion of the irrelevant (semantic) dimension increasingly difficult to maintain—it disrupts attentional set.

Watts *et al.* (1986) note that the phobics who averted their gaze most from a real spider showed most retardation on the 'spider' Stroop test, and they explain this in terms of voluntary control of attention: "the same subjects would be expected to be poor both at keeping their gaze directed at a spider in the avoidance test and at excluding spider words from their attention in the Stroop" (p. 105). John A. Bargh (1982) introduces his paper on 'attention and automaticity in the processing of self-relevant information': "Attention serves as a 'gating process', delimiting the range of potential information. This screening of the stimulus field has been found to be an important determinant of the course of information processing" (p. 425). [His several supporting references do not include Freud who pointed to the necessity for a filter, a protective shield, from 1895 onwards (Project, Part I, Sections 5 and 9, Part III, Section 1) and was still doing so in 1920: "These are the sense organs, which consist essentially of apparatus for the reception of certain specific effects of stimulation, but which also include special arrangements for further protection against excessive amounts of stimulation and for excluding unsuitable kinds of stimuli. It is characteristic of them that they deal only with very small quantities of external stimulation and only take in samples of the external world" (*S.E.* 18, p. 28).] Bargh & Pietromonaco (1982) continue to devote a great deal of ingenuity in design to demonstrating that target (social) information can be processed outside of conscious awareness, that is by passive automatic processes. Bargh & Pratto (1986) actually employ the Stroop color-naming paradigm "to test whether one's chronically accessible social constructs constitute such a long-term perceptual readiness" (p. 293). Subjects were paired for four different traits so that the 'accessible constructs' of the one were 'inaccessible' in the other and *vice versa*, and were subsequently given a suprise free-recall test on the stimulus words. "Because automatically processed stimuli are not stored in long-term memory (Fisk & Schneider, 1984), the hypothesized increase in response latencies for the adjectives corresponding to the subjects' chronically accessible constructs should not be related to the subject's ability to recall the stimulus words" (p. 299). The supportive citation is here stretched a little—how, after all, does one prove a negative? Fisk and Schneider (1984), after their two extremely complex recognition experiments on the effect of automatic versus controlled processing on long-term memory, are a little more guarded in reaching their conclusions.

However, returning to the personal, practical concerns lying behind this discussion of 'emotional' Stroop, a free-recall after the test would seem worthwhile in order to ascertain precisely which words, if any, were recalled, regardless of whether they had been consciously perceived—and errors might well be equally interesting! The importance attaching to this issue is likely to depend on the objectives of the experimenter and the nature of his investigation. The empirical studies, just mentioned, take no account of the dynamic concept of the 'preconscious'. Debates on the properties of 'consciousness', like so many areas of controversy in psychology, hinge upon definition.

John Bowlby pointed out that much psychopathology is due to internal working models which have become unserviceable because they are out-of-date or full of inconsistencies and confusions. "It seems likely," he continued, "that revising, extending, and checking models are ill done or done not at all unless a model is subjected from time to time to whatever special benefits accrue from becoming conscious" (Bowlby, 1969, p. 83)—in other words, metacognition.

Masochism is likely to be associated with very early depression and may, in some cases, arise as a defense mechanism against it (Panel, 1984). Many psychiatric studies (e.g., Litman & Swearingen, 1972) have found that adult masochistic patients are depressed. Aaron T. Beck (1967), in considering cognitive patterns in depression, actually delineates 'masochistic' features (pp. 178–182, 339–344). It is therefore essential to identify factors which distinguish masochism from depression. To this end, a control group containing mildly depressed or dysthymic subjects (scoring 14 or more on the Beck Depression Inventory, but with no apparent sexual deviance) was envisaged. The early family relationships of both (masochistic) index subjects and (depressed) control subjects would be probed by semistructured interview (Main *et al.* 1985). 'Emotional' Stroop would, it was reasoned, be a further means of demonstrating consistently emerging differences between the two groups.

It has already been employed with interesting results by Ian Gotlib in two studies concerned with depression (Gotlib & McCann, 1984; Gotlib & Cane, 1987). Hill and Knowles (1991) have made the criticism that his work failed to take account of the fact that depression and anxiety often coexist and may covary, so that his results could reflect a reaction to threat to self-esteem, rather than depression. Not using a Stroop procedure but a 'yes/no' judgment, Greenberg and Alloy (1989) set out to distinguish between depression and anxiety with a different set of potentially self-referent adjectives (p. 212, matched with controls also for 'social desirability'!), both positive and negative. They found their 'depressed' undergraduates "were unique in exhibiting balanced endorsements and processing of positive and negative traits, suggesting that they possessed self-schemata with mixed positive and negative content" (p. 207). 'Anxious' students ascribed more negative anxiety-relevant traits to themselves. The realism of depression is probably a distinguishing feature worth considering versus the fantasy-proneness of masochism. Anxiety is likely to be common to both conditions. Mathews and MacLeod (1985) employed Stroop color-naming of threat cues to demonstrate distinctive domains of anxiety—physical versus social worries. Above all, in seeking to arrive at certain features specific to masochism by using a control group composed partly of mildly depressed individuals, it must be recognized that 'depression' is, like 'masochism', a blanket term, under which are lurking endogenous and exogenous forms. Depression ensuing on neglect, loss, bereavement, frustration, disillusionment, overwork or 'idiopathically' is likely to have a different course in youth than in late middle age.

In so far as masochism, as a psychosexual deviance, is to be defined as the persistent seeking of pain for sexual pleasure, a potential word-source of considerable reliability is at hand in the McGill Pain Questionnaire (Melzack & Wall, 1982), a checklist of adjectives describing pain in its sensory, affective and evaluative aspects. Pearce and Morley (1989), using a Stroop task to investigate its construct validity, found that 16 chronic patients from a Pain Clinic showed more interference than controls with the words drawn from the questionnaire, but no confirmation of their expectation that the response time would be longer for the affective/evaluative descriptors than for the sensory descriptors. The problem which is likely to arise with the use of these 'pain' words in the present context is that they probably also cause interference in the control group. Mildly depressed adults may react to them (a) because they are emotionally or 'mentally' relevant (whilst being 'physically' relevant to the masochistic, or more accurately, sadomasochistic, subjects); (b) because they are simply 'emotive' words. Both groups might be expected, of course, to show increased response latencies for depressed-content words (although a masochist's score on the Beck Depression Inventory might not admit to depression). Possibly the only category of words which could confidently be expected to distinguish between the two groups would be 'fetishistic' (e.g., leather, rubber, fur, whip).

The sheer complexity of language processing has been recognized for over a century—one has only to look back, for instance, to Freud on aphasia (1891, trans. pp. 73–77) or to Isserlin on agrammatism (1922, trans. pp. 324–325) and all the preceding theory they were obliged to address even in their day. In cavalierly entering this domain with the 'emotional' Stroop task, one is also expecting rather a lot of a fairly blunt instrument. A subtle psychological hypothesis, whether priming is used or not, can scarcely be convincingly tested by the naming of colors—probably wiser to limit one's theoretical objectives to the robust. Despite these reservations, it seemed, in principle, that 'emotional' Stroop could be complementary to self-report in the form of a questionnaire (the Beck Depression Inventory) and an interview (the Adult Attachment Interview). It could be a means of combining dynamic and cognitive concepts in an economic, confirmatory and possibly even heuristic way. It seemed probable that the internal working models (Bowlby, 1969, 1973, 1980) of, for instance, mother and self, elaborated by sadomasochistic subjects would be different from those of controls. Their power for interference might well differ between the two groups. To test this important hypothesis, it seemed essential to include the words 'mother', 'father', 'brother' and 'sister' in the word presentation.

Instrument

A computer-driven 'emotional' Stroop task has already been employed with some success in several studies concerned with depression. Gotlib and McCann (1984) reported longer response latencies to depressed-content words (versus neutral and manic words) in depressed students, but no such differential response in nondepressed students, thus supporting Beck's cognitive model of depression. Gotlib and Cane (1987) replicated this finding with clinically depressed inpatients, using the same words. These had originally been rated as self-descriptive by psychiatric patients and tested in previous studies. Professor Ian H. Gotlib kindly sent me his word lists for use in this study. The 50 'Depressed-content' words, the 50 'Neutral-content' words and the 20 'Manic-content' words used in this presentation are thus his, and of established reliability and validity. The 20 'manic' words were used at the beginning and end of the presentation, and afterwards excluded from analysis. The first ten (short) words enabled the subject to become familiar with the task whilst being confronted with decidedly more pleasant words than those which were to follow. The last ten (long) words were encountered when the subject was fatigued and were designed to provide an upbeat conclusion—a matter of some concern since many of the subjects were depressed to start with. The 50 'Sadomasochistic-content' words were taken partly from the McGill Pain Questionnaire (Melzack & Wall, 1988) but some fetishistic words (e.g., 'leather', 'rubber') and the words 'mother', 'father', 'brother', 'sister' were added. The latter were thought likely to be more emotionally 'fraught' for the majority of index subjects than for the majority of controls.

Procedure

Identical instructions for the Stroop task were given to all subjects whilst seating them at a distance of approximately 50 cm (18 inches) from the VDU and adjusting the microphone. After the initial enquiry: "You're not color-blind, are you?" the Spiel proceeded: "Well, would you name some colors for me? (Indicating squares of color on the screen) Red, green, blue, purple, brown. When we press the button, a word will appear in the centre of the screen and all you have to do is to say as quickly as possible, but there's nothing competitive about it, which of these five colors it is written in. This will bring the next word up onto the screen. There will be 170 words in all, so it will take about 3 minutes. If you could sit with your mouth almost touching the microphone and say loud and clear, without any 'ers' or 'ums' or chatting, (very decisively articulated) 'red', 'green', 'blue', 'purple' or 'brown'... Ready? Off we go! Name the color!" As the presentation commenced, the tape recorder, moved after the interview to beside the computer, was also restarted. Any mistake or malfunction was thus identified and corrected afterwards by comparing the printout of the subject's response times with the audiotape of his voice.

A 3-minute free recall of the words just viewed was timed with a stopwatch. The blank sheet of paper on which the subject had jotted any words he thought he had seen on the screen was then used also for debriefing notes.

Materials and Equipment

One hundred and fifty words were used in the final analysis, after the 10 'happy' words which had introduced the presentation and the 10 which had concluded it, had been excluded. These 150 words are listed in Table 6.1.

The 'happy' words introducing the task were free, brave, high, glad, great, alert, sunny, happy, merry, jolly. Those concluding it on a cheerful note were confident, assertive, optimistic, fortunate, efficient, productive, enthusiastic, accelerated, outstanding, wonderful. These were generously supplied to me, as were the 'depressed-content' and 'neutral-content' words, by Professor Ian H. Gotlib. He describes their provenance as follows (Gotlib & McCann, 1984, p. 429): "One hundred of these words were drawn from a list developed by Myers (1980), who obtained ratings of the degree of self-description of each of 400 adjectives from psychiatric patients diagnosed as either depressed or manic. The 50 adjectives rated both by the depressed patients as most self-descriptive and by the manic patients as least self-descriptive were selected as the depressed-content words; similarly, the 50 adjectives rated both by the depressed patients as least descriptive and by the manic patients as most descriptive were chosen as the manic-content words. Finally, 50 neutral-content words were chosen from the list presented by Thorndike and Lorge (1944), and were matched with the depression- and manic-content words with respect to frequency of occurrence in English. None of the neutral-content words were contained in the list of 400 self-descriptive adjectives used by Myers."

As already stated, the 50 'sadomasochistic-content' words were predominantly from the McGill Pain Questionnaire (Melzack & Wall, 1982, revised edition, 1988, pp. 39–40), with the addition of well-known fetishistic words from the subculture. The validity of these 50 crucial words is discussed later.

The entire presentation was the same for all subjects. It ran from short to long words, no color following itself immediately, no category following itself immediately, but otherwise in random order.

Each of these 170 words was presented as a single stimulus in the middle of a dark grey background. A Dell 310 (IBM-compatible PC) was programmed by Mr Simon Zielinski, MSc, computer-technician in the Department of Psychology, University College London, who also connected a Revox microphone to a voice key (Campden Instruments Ltd), through a connection box to the computer input port. A push button started

TABLE 6.1. Words used for analysis according to category (depressed, sadomasochistic, neutral) and color (red, green, blue, purple, brown)

	Word Type		
Color	Depressed	Masochistic	Neutral
Red	Low	Sore	Hat
	Glum	Pain	Fork
	Empty	Bully	Table
	Doomed	Tight	Stereo
	Tearful	Searing	Teapot
	Defeated	Leather	Cabinet
	Hopeless	Betrayal	Picture
	Inferior	Scalding	Suitcase
	Worthless	Harnessed	Television
	Insignificant	Submissive	Intermission
Green	Inept	Spite	Pen
	Weary	Power	Plane
	Guilty	Rubber	Kettle
	Morbid	Mother	Rocket
	Unloved	Nagging	Antenna
	Diseased	Piercing	Freezer
	Suicidal	Dominant	Mattress
	Deficient	Agonizing	Apparatus
	Miserable	Matriarch	Typewriter
	Pessimistic	Persecutor	Electricity
Blue	Sad	Win	Car
	Dull	Hang	Tree
	Dismal	Sister	Basket
	Failure	Father	Bottle
	Useless	Torment	Tractor
	Lifeless	Potency	Trailer
	Sluggish	Stabbing	Textbook
	Depressed	Deprived	Telephone
	Inadequate	Torturing	Motorcycle
	Downhearted	Invincible	Thermometer
Purple	Shy	Fur	Tap
	Weak	Chain	Couch
	Flabby	Tattoo	Windoe
	Dreary	Despot	Machine
	Downcast	Victory	Furnace
	Helpless	Vicious	Armchair
	Unwanted	Brother	Magazine
	Sorrowful	Gruelling	Saxophone
	Discouraged	Humilated	Supermarket
	Disappointed	Retribution	Refrigerator

(Continued)

TABLE 6.1. (*Continued*)

Color	Word Type		
	Depressed	Masochistic	Neutral
Brown	Awful	Whip	Paint
	Bleak	Grudge	Plant
	Tired	Beaten	Spoon
	Gloomy	Gagged	Carton
	Crushed	Revenge	Bicycle
	Lonesome	Champion	Cracker
	Pathetic	Punished	Football
	Apathetic	Grievance	Catalogue
	Desparing	Compulsion	Blackboard
	Incompetent	Subjugation	Subdivision

the presentation which was in double-size modified EGA character set (all 7 mm tall × 5 mm wide capitals). The time interval between the subject's response (his voice into the microphone, causing the disappearance of the stimulus) and the appearance of the next stimulus was set at 1000 ms (exactly one second). The crucial measurement, the response latency, the time the subject took to name the color, was, of course, recorded by the computer for each word in milliseconds.

Statistical Analysis

To obtain a measure of the overall impact of, specifically, the sadomasochistic-content words on the index group, thus obtaining a measure of sadomasochistic mind-set, an SM quotient was calculated for each index subject. This SM quotient was the ratio of the subject's mean response time for SM-category words to his overall mean response time (since each subject obviously had his own overall tempo of response). The measure could then be used to investigate further the AAI classifications already assigned and reported in Chapter 5.

RESULTS

The mean response times (with their standard errors) of index and control groups, subdivided according to depressed or nondepressed status, are set out in Table 6.2 according to word category (depressed-content, sadomasochistic-content, neutral-content). These mean response latencies are also given in Appendix 4 for each individual subject.

TABLE 6.2. 'Emotional' Stroop task: Mean response times (with standard errors) in naming the colors in which three categories of words (depressed-content, sadomasochistic-content, neutral-content) were presented to index vs control subjects (depressed vs nondepressed)

	Depressed-content words ($n = 50$)	Sadomasochistic-content words ($n = 50$)	Neutral-content words ($n = 50$)
(a) *Mean response times (milliseconds) in naming colors*			
Index group ($n = 48$)	809.8 (29.6)	843.6 (32.0)	811.5 (25.8)
Depressed ($n = 14$)	811.8 (74.0)	830.7 (77.0)	805.9 (63.2)
Nondepressed ($n = 34$)	809.0 (29.5)	848.9 (33.0)	813.8 (26.3)
Control group ($n = 35$)	750.2 (21.2)	754.1 (21.3)	746.2 (17.4)
Depressed ($n = 20$)	710.5 (20.3)	720.2 (24.0)	710.9 (17.2)
Nondepressed ($n = 15$)	803.1 (38.1)	799.2 (35.8)	793.2 (30.1)

(b) *Mean number of corrections and percentage of the 150-word presentation of these corrections constitute*

	Errors/malfunctions per subject	%
Index group ($n = 48$)	6.20	4.1
Depressed ($n = 14$)	6.43	4.3
Nondepressed ($n = 34$)	6.12	4.1
Control group ($n = 35$)	6.17	4.1
Depressed ($n = 20$)	5.30	3.5
Nondepressed ($n = 15$)	7.33	4.9
All subjects ($n = 83$)	6.19	4.1

These mean reaction times are presented in Appendix 4 for each individual subject. For completeness, corrections necessitated by subjects' errors and equipment malfunction are also shown as part (b) of the table.

Table 6.2 shows clearly an increased mean response time on the part of the index group of subjects ($n = 48$) to sadomasochistic-content words as compared with depressed-content words and neutral-content words. This differential is even more marked in the case of the nondepressed subgroup of sadomasochistic subjects ($n = 34$). It is true that the control group ($n = 35$) also had a marginally greater mean response time (not statistically significant) for these 'SM' words but nothing comparable to the index group and, in any case, deriving from the depressed subgroup of controls ($n = 20$) and thus directly suggesting the overlap, not unexpected, between depression and sadomasochism, which emerges also from Tables 6.3 and 6.6 and which will be addressed in the Discussion.

When examined in several models of mixed factorial analysis of variance, 'word-category' as a 'within subjects' (repeated measures) factor was, therefore, significant as a main effect ($F_{(2,162)} = 7.39$, $p < 0.001$, in the simplest 'group × word-category' model). The interaction between 'group' and 'word-category' was also significant ($F_{(2,162)} = 3.68$, $p < 0.05$, again in this simplest model).

Errors and Equipment Malfunction

After checking each subject's computer printout against his voice on audiotape, a small number of errors and occasional equipment malfunction were identified. The most common occurrence requiring correction was the need to repeat, for instance, "green" because it had been pronounced too softly to trigger the next word. It became obvious that one subject, ES66, was partially color-blind, but, since he was perfectly consistent in his color *mis*naming ("green" meant brown, "yellow" meant green, "blue" meant purple and "purple" meant blue!) his performance was not excluded from the analysis. As can be seen from part (b) of Table 6.2, these errors and malfunctions were not numerous, never exceeding 4.9% of the presentation, on average. They were corrected for each performance in which they occurred, in three stages: first they were extracted and denoted as missing values, then a contingency table of response times (5 colors × 3 word-categories) was generated, and finally they were replaced in each case by a neutral value calculated from this table according to the following formula for filling in missing data (Iles, 1993, p. 73): add the mean of the row to the mean of the column, and subtract the overall mean for that subject.

Analysis by Response Latency to Individual Words

When the mean response time of the entire index group of subjects ($n = 48$) to each word in the 150-word presentation was computed and then rank-ordered (in descending order) according to length in milliseconds of response latency (i.e., presumed interference or impact of the semantic dimension), a striking picture emerged. The 'top eight words' are presented in Table 6.3. It can be seen immediately that these are all

TABLE 6.3. Result of rank-ordering (in descending order) the mean response latencies (milliseconds) across all 48 index subjects in naming the color of each word in the 150-word presentation—'top eight words'

Word	Category	Color	Mean response time (ms)
(a) *Index group* ($n = 48$)[1]			
Submissive	SM	Red	1000.08
Humiliated	SM	Purple	994.98
Whip	SM	Brown	988.44
Matriarch	SM	Green	978.77
Subjugation	SM	Brown	977.35
Rubber	SM	Green	937.85
Retribution	SM	Purple	937.65
Harnessed	SM	Red	924.12
(b) *Control group* ($n = 35$)[2]			
Brother	SM	Purple	902.86
Humiliated	SM	Purple	896.06
Magazine	Neutral	Purple	894.89
Pathetic	Depressed	Brown	857.57
Downcast	Depressed	Purple	855.43
Refrigerator	Neutral	Purple	855.14
Sluggish	Depressed	Blue	843.71
Discouraged	Depressed	Purple	840.74

[1] Probability of 8 or more SM words coming to the top of the 150-word list by chance is 0.0001
[2] For completeness, the 'top eight words', ascertained by a similar computation across all 35 control subjects, are presented as part (b) of this table. No trend comparable to that displayed in part (a) emerges from this list (see text for discussion)

sadomasochistic-category words, whereas the colors in which they were presented show no trend. The probability of 8 or more SM words, out of a balanced then randomized presentation of 150 words, coming to the top, given the null hypothesis of all arrangements being equally likely, is

$$\text{Binomial}[142,42]/\text{Binomial}[150,50] = 46483/455169819 = 0.0001.$$

This is an important result for several reasons: (a) it contains no element of subjectivity—the computer simply recorded the time which elapsed before each subject named the color in which each of these words was presented, and in using the statistical package MINITAB to rank-order the mean values, I had no idea which words would come to the top of the list; (b) it validates the inclusion of these words in the presentation as words of sadomasochistic content; (c) it validates the concept of 'emotional' Stroop itself; (d) it points, through the actual words (submissive, humiliated, whip, matriarch, subjugation, rubber, retribution, harnessed), to certain, possibly subliminal, concerns of sadomasochism and even to a possible etiology. This will, of course, be considered further in the Discussion section. For completeness, a list of the 'top eight words', similarly computed across the entire group of control subjects ($n = 35$), is presented as part (b) of Table 6.3. Words of all three categories figure in this control list, and three different colors are represented. If purple seems somewhat overrepresented, this only strengthens the demonstration of the impact of the semantic dimension on the index group in part (a). When debriefed after the task and the 3-minute free recall which immediately followed it, many subjects, irrespective of group, said they found purple the most difficult color to name.

Table 6.4 represents an attempt to assess the average emotional impact of the four words 'mother', father', 'brother', 'sister', on the complete group of sadomasochists ($n = 48$) and the complete group of controls ($n = 35$). The same method of rank-ordering the 150 words of the presentation in descending order of response time (in milliseconds) enabled a rank to be assigned to each of these four words. In the event they did not, on average, impact as much as expected on the sadomasochists: 'brother', 'mother', 'father' and 'sister' ranked only 43rd, 59th, 77th and 122nd, respectively, in the degree of interference to which they gave rise. By contrast, the controls were, on average, more affected by these same words, with ranks of 1, 39, 71 and 86, respectively. 'Brother', with a mean response time of 902.86 milliseconds, appears to have had genuine overall impact for these controls.

The sex of a child is likely to lead to differences in relating to either parent. Since there were so few female subjects in this study, it was only feasible to look at equal subgroups of males. These depressed and nondepressed subgroups could each only consist of 13 individuals since there were only 13 males available in two of them (the depressed and nondepressed controls). For the other two, the 13 most depressed and the 13 least depressed sadomasochists were used. The results produced by this painstaking subdivision of the main groups enjoin caution on account of the smaller number of subjects involved, but it might be noted that 'mother' appears to have had less average impact on the 13 least depressed sadomasochists than on the 13 most depressed, slipping to a rank of 72 (mean response latency 811.46 ms) from a rank of 16 (mean response latency 848.15 ms). 'Sister' would seem to have generated little interference in any group.

The Importance of Color as an Effect

'Color' was unlikely to contribute findings of interest to this study, but, since it was potentially a confounding variable, considerable time and attention was given to the examination of its influence. As a 'within

TABLE 6.4. An attempt to assess, by the rank-ordering (in descending order) of mean response latencies (milliseconds), the impact of the words 'mother', 'father', 'brother', 'sister' in the Stroop presentation, firstly on the complete index and control groups, secondly on subdivisions of both groups into depressed and nondepressed, each of the four subgroups consisting of 13 male subjects

	Rank (in 150 words)	Word	Color	Mean response time (ms)
All index subjects				
($n = 48$)	43	Brother	Purple	851.96
	59	Mother	Green	831.65
	77	Father	Blue	815.60
	122	Sister	Blue	769.37
Depressed males				
($n = 13$)	16	Mother	Green	848.15
	27	Brother	Purple	815.00
	69	Father	Blue	769.85
	75	Sister	Blue	765.54
Nondepressed males				
($n = 13$)	59	Father	Blue	840.38
	62	Brother	Purple	836.23
	72	Mother	Green	811.46
	129	Sister	Blue	736.31
All control subjects				
($n = 35$)	1	Brother	Purple	902.86
	39	Mother	Green	782.34
	71	Father	Blue	747.40
	86	Sister	Blue	736.40
Depressed males				
($n = 13$)	12	Brother	Purple	826.08
	41	Father	Blue	754.77
	43	Mother	Green	747.00
	105	Sister	Blue	688.69
Nondepressed males				
($n = 13$)	11	Brother	Purple	888.08
	62	Father	Blue	790.15
	66	Mother	Green	783.54
	72	Sister	Blue	775.54

In order to exclude a sex difference and to have equal numbers, the subgroups had necessarily to consist of 13 males since, for both the control subgroups, only 13 males were available.

subjects' (repeated measures) factor, like 'word-category', 'color' was tested in the same mixed factorial (split-plot) models of analysis of variance and, like 'word-category' found to have a significant main effect ($F_{(4,324)} = 10.94$, $p < 0.001$, in the simplest 'group × color' model). Unlike 'word-category', however, the interaction between 'group' and 'color' was not significant ($F_{(4,324)} = 1.25$, $p = 0.290$, in this simple model).

From the mean response times depicted in Figure 6.1, it is evident that the response latency for purple was, on average, the largest, across all subjects, both index and control. The five colors had, in fact, been carefully adjusted in intensity so as to be equally salient. However, as mentioned above, each subject was subsequently asked (a) which color, if any, he had found most salient and (b) which color, if any, he found most difficult to name. Not all subjects expressed a clear opinion in response to these questions—some wavered, some placed their own interpretation on the questions, whilst others stated they had experienced no difference between the colors. Of those who did express an opinion, irrespective of group (index or control) and irrespective of depressed or nondepressed status, blue, green, red and purple, in that order, were found to be most salient by 49.3%, 29.3%, 17.3% and 4% (37, 22, 13 and 4 subjects out of 75), respectively—brown was not found to be salient by anyone. Purple was found to be the most difficult color to name by 75% (48 out of 64) of subjects giving a clear response to question (b), again irrespective of group or depressed status. (Since purple has been depicted as a depressive color, it might have been of some interest to have found a significant interaction between color and depression, but there was none.) Several reasons were volunteered by subjects to explain why they thought 'purple' might have been slightly more difficult to name: for example, they thought of it as 'magenta' or 'mauve' or 'maroon', or "it had two syllables". Again, these difficulties were not experienced by any group specifically, but they are likely to account for the somewhat increased mean response time in naming this color, and indeed for the statistical significance of color as a main effect. In the words of St Matthew (chapter 5, verse 45): "... he maketh his sun to rise on the evil and on the good, and sendeth rain on the just and on the unjust."

The Relation of AAI Classifications to Stroop Results

As 'Cannot Classify' implies, the CC classification represents the absence of one 'organized' working model of attachment. It is important in assessing the index group of subjects on two counts: (a) there are 16 CC out of 48 primary classifications (33%) in this group, as compared with 4 out of 35 (11%) in the control group (Table 5.1, Figure 5.1); (b) as shown in Table 6.5, the CC classification, together with the E (Preoccupied) classification, is associated with the highest mean SM quotient, an average of the quotient calculated for each index subject by the formula:

$$\frac{\text{mean response time for SM category words}}{\text{overall mean response time}}$$

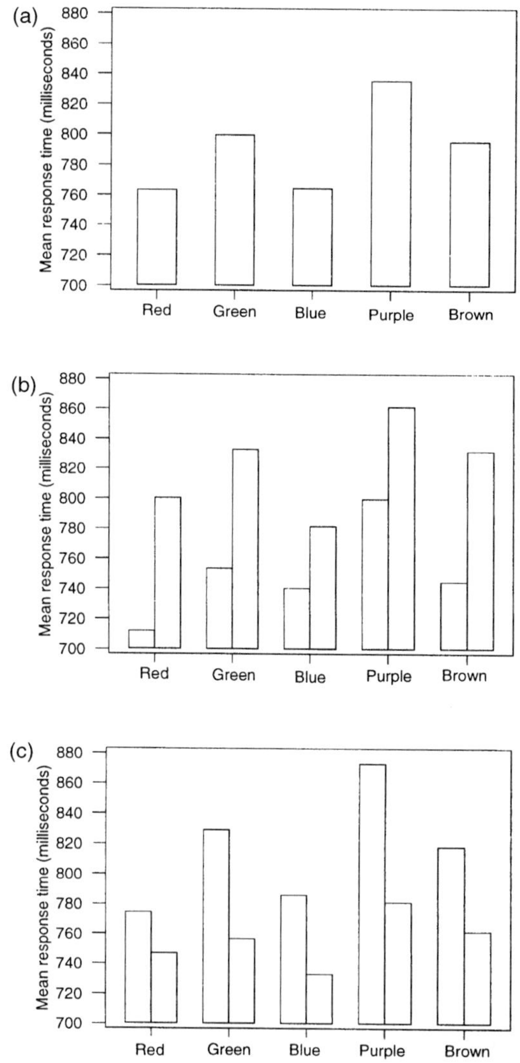

FIGURE 6.1. Mean response times (milliseconds) for the 5 colours of the 'emotional' Stroop presentation: (a) all subjects ($n = 83$), (b) control (left) ($n = 35$) vs index (right) ($n = 48$), (c) nondepressed (left) ($n = 49$) vs depressed (right) ($n = 34$). In each case the vertical axis displays 700–880 ms. The increased response latency for purple is clearly across all subjects, irrespective of group.

TABLE 6.5. A comparison of the mean SM quotient (a measure of sadomasochistic mind-set derived from performance of the 'emotional' Stroop task) obtained for the complete index group ($n = 48$) with those obtained when the group is divided according to AAI classification*

	Mean SM quotient
All index subjects ($n = 48$)	843.6/821.7 = 1.027
Ds classifications† ($n = 21$)	807.1/793.5 = 1.017
E classifications† ($n = 27$)	872.0/843.6 = 1.034
CC classifications ($n = 16$)	870.8/841.6 = 1.035

The SM quotient is the mean response time for SM words divided by the overall mean response time.

It is apparent that the Preoccupied/entangled (E) attachment model has a greater association with sadomasochistic mental processing than the Dismissive (Ds) internal model, but 'Cannot Classify' (CC), signifying a conflicted model, is equally closely associated with the sadomasochistic mind-set, in fact its association is even very slightly greater.

* For details of Adult Attachment Interview classifications and how they are derived see Appendix 2.

† Assigned either as first classification or assigned, as required by protocol, as best-fitting classification following CC or U.

It is therefore apparent, on the basis of these Stroop results, which are totally objective—the computer recorded the milliseconds which elapsed before the subject's voice, naming the color, reached the microphone—that the CC classification is equally as representative of sadomasochistic mental processing as either of the two Insecure classifications, Ds or E, which signify 'organized' or 'patterned' internal models. Of these two, however, the E category emerges as the more representative, both in terms of the frequency with which it was awarded (to 27 index subjects vs 21 index subjects classified Ds) and in terms of mind-set (SM quotient of 1.034 vs 1.017). The first hypothesis put forward at the beginning of Part II, that sadomasochists, whether depressed or nondepressed, would provide general descriptions of childhood relationships which were either upsupported or contradicted by episodic memories, where these memories were forthcoming at all, implied the more frequent assignment of a dismissive (Ds1 or Ds3) classification. In the event, this expectation was, therefore, not confirmed. The Secure (F) classification is simply not associated with the sadomasochistic group (Table 5.1*a*, Figure 5.1*a*). It should, of course, be emphasized that this analysis has only been made long after AAI classifications were assigned.

THREE CONTROL SUBJECTS UNDER SPECIAL OBSERVATION

The three control subjects, mentioned in the previous chapter, whose classification as controls was retained only after considerable reflection because certain pointers to sadomasochism came to light during discussion with them, namely, CS125, CS175 and NS269, all had increased mean response times for sadomasochistic-content words: 835.18 ms (overall mean 807.59 ms), 962.98 ms (overall mean 915.75 ms) and 1033.24 ms (overall mean 1023.74 ms), respectively.

FREE RECALL

Reporting the results of 3 minutes' free recall (timed precisely with a stopwatch) on the part of all 83 subjects was a problem of some complexity. The most meaningful method of tabulation, permitting any existing tendencies to be inferred, was to count the number of words correctly remembered by each subject (i.e., words that had in fact been presented to him on screen) and express the proportion for each category as a percentage of all category-words ($n = 150$) recalled by this subject.

Table 6.6(a) gives the mean percentage (with standard error) of words freely recalled in each of the three categories (depressed-content, sadomasochistic-content, neutral-content) by the index and control groups, subdivided according to depressed or nondepressed status. (Included as Table 6.6(b), for completeness, is any recall of the 20 'happy' words, which were removed from the main analysis presented in Table 6.2(a), and any erroneous 'recall' of words not seen at all on the screen. Part (b) of the table is also according to group and is simply in the form of a mean number of 'other words' recalled by each subject.)

The mean percentage of 'SM' words freely recalled by the index group as a whole ($n = 48$) is strikingly greater than the mean percentage of 'depressed' or 'neutral' words recalled by this group. As can be seen from Table 6.7, the mean difference between 'SM' and 'depressed' recall is 55.73%, over 3.3 times its standard error (4.38), making this difference significant at the 0.001 level. The mean difference between 'SM' and 'neutral' recall is 49.83%, not quite as large but still more than 3.3 times its standard error (4.96), making this difference also significant at the 0.001 level. The same level of significance attached to these differences when the index

TABLE 6.6. Free recall of words presented in the 'emotional' Stroop task according to word category (depressed-content, sadomasochistic-content, neutral-content) and group of subjects (index vs control, depressed vs nondepressed)

	Depressed-content words ($n = 50$)	Sadomasochistic-content words ($n = 50$)	Neutral-content words ($n = 50$)
(a) Mean percentage (S.E.) of words recalled			
Index group ($n = 48$)	12.79 (2.19)	68.52 (2.84)	18.69 (2.57)
Depressed ($n = 14$)	15.11 (4.07)	69.96 (4.60)	14.93 (4.21)
Nondepressed ($n = 34$)	11.84 (2.62)	67.93 (3.58)	20.23 (3.19)
Control group ($n = 35$)	31.83 (3.90)	41.44 (3.85)	26.73 (3.05)
Depressed ($n = 20$)	34.55 (5.23)	39.40 (5.53)	26.05 (4.13)
Nondepressed ($n = 15$)	28.20 (5.93)	44.17 (5.27)	27.63 (4.65)

(b) Mean number of other words recalled by each subject

	'Happy' words ($n = 20$)	Wrong words (total 123)
Index group ($n = 48$)	0.45	1.60
Depressed ($n = 14$)	0.39	2.00
Nondepressed ($n = 34$)	0.47	1.44
Control group ($n = 35$)	0.51	1.31
Depressed ($n = 20$)	0.40	0.90
Nondepressed ($n = 15$)	0.67	1.87

Words which were not quite accurately recalled were scored 0.5 rather than 1. Included as part (b) of the table, for completeness, is the free recall of any of the 'happy' words with which the presentation began and ended and also the erroneous 'recall' of words not presented at all.

group was subdivided into depressed subjects ($n = 14$) and nondepressed subjects ($n = 34$). Turning to the control group, the picture is very different. The control group as a whole ($n = 35$) also remembered more 'SM' words—they are, after all, unusual and emotive words—but with nothing like the same differential. Only the mean difference between 'SM' and 'neutral' recall (14.71%, S.E. 5.75, and 16.53%, S.E. 7.98, for all 35 control subjects and 15 nondepressed control subjects, respectively) achieved

TABLE 6.7. Mean differences (standard errors) between index and control groups (depressed and nondepressed) in free recall of three word categories (depressed-content, sadomasochistic-content, neutral-content) measured as percentages

	Mean difference (standard error)	
	SM—Depressed	SM—Neutral
Index group ($n = 48$)	55.73 (4.38)***	49.83 (4.96)***
Depressed ($n = 14$)	54.86 (7.60)***	55.04 (7.82)***
Nondpressed ($n = 34$)	56.09 (5.40)***	47.69 (6.25)***
Control group ($n = 35$)	9.61 (7.13)	14.71 (5.75)*
Depressed ($n = 20$)	4.85 (9.93)	13.35 (8.25)
Nondepressed ($n = 15$)	16.0 (10.20)	16.53 (7.98)*

* $p < 0.05$, *** $p < 0.001$.

significance, and since these means were just greater than twice their standard errors, significance was only barely achieved at the 0.05 level. What is important to note about the free recall of this control group, containing a majority ($n = 20$) of depressed subjects, is the overlap which emerges from both Table 6.6 and Table 6.7 between depression and sadomasochism, an overlap which was always expected and which will receive further consideration in the Discussion.

Words which were not quite accurately recalled (e.g., "harness" instead of "harnessed", "punish(ment)" instead of "punished", "torture (d)" instead of "torturing") were scored as a half rather than one.

Occasionally words were recalled because of previous discussion. ES58 listed "thermometer" because the ineptitude of a child-minder with a thermometer had been described in the course of the preceding Adult Attachment Interview. ES8 wrote down "bottle" because he had a rubber hot-water bottle in mind as a fetish object.

Although excluded from the main analysis of the Stroop results, the 'happy' words with which the presentation began and ended (20 in all) were, of course, occasionally remembered. "Assertive", then "confident" were the most frequently recalled of these deliberately positive words on the part of index subjects. It appeared likely that the particular impact of these two words related to their association with control, a preoccupation of sadomasochism.

However interesting a complete account of all the words listed by every subject in the 3-minute free recall might be—and interesting reading they were!—such a tabulation is, of course, impossible. To give some flavour of this, however, and at the same time provide a first glimpse of the 14 women subjects, who have remained shadowy figures until now, a complete listing is presented in Table 6.8 of the actual words written down by the following small groups: (a) the female subjects ($n = 14$), (b) the adopted subjects ($n = 7$), (c) the male controls under special scrutiny ($n = 3$). In each of these groups the main differences emerging from the free recall are, of course, individual personality differences and unquantifiable. The words listed are best left to speak for themselves, but a brief mention will be made in the Discussion section which follows of any tendencies distinguishing groups.

The words which subjects thought they had seen on screen were often interesting and informative in general but again, of course, impossible to tabulate satisfactorily. As can be seen from Table 6.6, the depressed index

TABLE 6.8. Actual words freely recalled from the Stroop presentation, including those 'recalled' erroneously or not quite correctly, in the order in which they were listed by (a) the female subjects, (b) the adopted subjects, (c) the 3 controls under special scrutiny

Subject	Actual words listed during 3 minutes free recall
(a) *Female subjects* ($n = 14$)[1]	
ES41	Intermission+ Help! Tattoo* Piercing* Pain* Patriarchal! Brother* Body!
ES42	Disappointed^ Thermometer+ Refrigerator+ Tortured~* Harness~* Whip* Glad> Pain* Hang* Tattoo* Dominant* Bondage! Happy> Sad^ Jolly> Contented! Television+ Rubber* Piercing*
ES58	Thermometer+ Harness~* Discriminate! Pain* Confident> Matriarch*
ES62	Leather* Subjugation* Unwanted^ Refrigerator+ Dominant* Mother* Father* Whip* Restraint!
ES75	Assertive> Efficient> Submissive* Dominant* Leather* Unloved^ Inferior^ Grievance* Harnessed* Tattoo* Subjugate~* Teapot+
CS138	Brother* Sister* Bottle+ Fahter* Cabinet+ Sad^ Telephone+ Armchair+ (Blue) Bicycle+
CS180	Sluggish^ Mother* Telephone+ Crushed^ Defeated^ Guilty^ Saxophone+ Tired^
CS187	Mother* Brother* Gloomy^ Sad^ Father* Subjugation*

(*Continued*)

TABLE 6.8. (*Continued*)

Subject	Actual words listed during 3 minutes free recall
CS190	Enthusiastic> Supermarket+ Anger! Despair~^ Worthless^ Unloved^ Fear! Football+
CS196	Television+ Sad^ Worthy! Sore*
CS206	Assertive> Depressed^ Supermarket+ Basket+ Mother* Submissive* Teapot+
CS260	Supermarket+ Sorrowful^ Humiliated* Win*
NS278	Stabbing* Sorrowful^ Catalogue+ Suicide~^ Lonely~^ Armchair+
NS285	Depressed^ Suicidal^ Accelerated> Submissive* Signal! Accident!
(b) *Adopted subjects* ($n = 7$, all male)	
ES4	Electricity+
ES19	Assertive> Kettle+ Subjugate~* Hopeless^ Failure^ Power* Worthless^ Easy! Help! Punish~* Strain! Enforce! Defeat~^ Pressure! Dedication! Destroy! Life! Fridge~+ Pain* Teapot+
ES50	Bicycle+ Leather* Rubber* Worthless^ Humiliated* Submissive* Whip* Typewriter+ Lonely~^
ES51	Assertive> Pain* Television+ Whip* Confident> Chain* Teapot+ Leather* Rubber* Suicidal^ Mattress+ Mother* Hopeless^
ES69	Dominant* Submissive* Whip* Failure^ Fridge~+ Inevitable! Mother* Kettle+ Sister* Work! Travel! Suitcase+
CS136	Mother* Father* Whip* Refrigerator+ Decadent! Struggle! Resistant! Loneliness~^
CS284	Matriarch* Depression~^ Mother* Brother* Subdivision+ Sluggish^ Suicidal^
(c) *Control subjects under special scrutiny* ($n = 3$, all male)	
CS125	Sister* Adequate! Angry! Mother* Teapot+
CS175	Thermometer+ Regrigerator+ Submissive* Incompetent^ Matriarch* Father* Assertive> Failure^ Tractor+ Persecute~* Torture~* Depressed^ Ball! Prison! Trapped! (Submissive*) (Persecute~*) Aggressive!
NS269	Wonderful> Outstanding> Humiliated* Subdivided~+ Alert> Whip* Dominant* Tree+

[1] The names 'red', 'green', 'blue', 'purple', 'brown', actually appeared on screen beneath blocks of their respective colors before the word presentation started. Where recalled, these names have not been scored and are here simply placed in parentheses.

ES numbers denote sadomasochistic subjects, CS numbers denote controls with depression scores of 14 or more, NS numbers denote 'neutral' controls with depression scores of less than 14.

^ Depressed-content, * sadomasochistic-content, + neutral-content, ~ almost correct (slight modification of the word presented), > 'happy' (positive words at the beginning and end of the presentation), ! wrong (erroneously 'recalled'). Where the same word has been listed a second time, it has been placed in parentheses.

subjects were the most cavalier with respect to erroneous 'recall', then the 'neutral' controls (on average 2 and 1.87 words wrongly remembered per subject, respectively). NS146 managed to get 11 wrong and only 2 right, but this level of inventiveness, which included listing "reward" twice although he had not seen it on screen, is perhaps understandable in a journalist, the most fluent of all interviewees to boot! The depressed controls were the most accurate group (only 0.90, less than one mistake per subject on average).

Words were sometimes repeated in a revealing manner. For instance, ES61 wrote down "punish" 3 times in a list which contained 10 items in all, most of them *not* appearing in the presentation on screen: "punish, intimidate, hate, cane, mother, school, punish, discipline, strict, punish". The word which had actually appeared on the screen was "punished". This subject had scrawled "punish" somewhat illegibly in the top left corner of the sheet of paper supplied to him and had been requested to print any words he thought he recalled in capitals for legibility, whereupon he obligingly wrote it again in capitals, alongside, and continued his list beneath it in capitals, so he did in fact write the word 4 times (though only 3 times spontaneously) and when asked which word had had most impact, replied as no great surprise: "punish"!

DISCUSSION

As anticipated, the sadomasochistic group of 48 subjects as a whole experienced most semantic interference from SM-content as compared with depressed-content and neutral-content words. The mean response latency for this word-category was even greater, compared with the other two categories, in the nondepressed subgroup. To preempt much future discussion, one might advance the interpretation, albeit tentatively at this stage, that these more active practitioners (Figure 5.2*e*) had 'converted' depression to sadomasochism more succcessfully than those who remained depressed.

The controls were also affected marginally more by 'SM' words than by 'depressed' or 'neutral' words but, as can be seen from Table 6.2*a*, the difference derived from the depressed subgroup of controls who were in the majority (20 versus 15). It points to the overlap between depression and sadomasochism, explicitly recognized by Aaron Beck (Beck, 1967, Chapter 13, Appendix, pp. 339–344) and, indeed, almost certainly evident to any reasonably percipient person who has had real contact with depressed and with sadomasochistic individuals. As Freud observed in *Mourning and Melancholia*, the depressed person "reproaches himself, vilifies himself and expects to be cast out and punished. He abases himself before everyone" (Freud, 1917, p. 246). It might almost be a sadomasochistic ritual except that the roles of 'dominant' and 'submissive' have not been cast concretely in the external, physical world but are being played out within the psyche of the depressed person by the sadistic 'critical agency' and a part of the 'ego' (the sadomasochist is, of course, also playing both roles himself in fantasy). Freud's characterization continues with a further observation which might apply as much to the sadomasochist as to the depressive whom he is describing: instead of feelings of shame, "One might emphasize the presence in him of an almost opposite trait of insistent communicativeness which finds satisfaction in self-exposure" (p. 247). This overlap between sadomasochism and depression emerges equally in the results of free recall reported in Table 6.6.

The evidence presented in Table 6.3 for a mind-set specific to the sadomasochistic group is compelling. The 'top eight words', across the complete index group of 48 subjects, when the 150-word-presentation was rank-ordered by mean response time, were all sadomasochistic: "submissive, humiliated, whip, matriarch, subjugation, rubber, retribution, harnessed". Together they seem to depict an inner world, an unsubtle world, similar to that in the comics or science fiction which many of these subjects cited as their preferred reading in childhood and a formative influence. They even suggest a gloom-laden scenario: the submissive is the protagonist who is first humiliated then whipped by the dominatrix-mother into subjugation, in clammy rubber—a staging of retribution with the trappings of bondage. The word 'retribution' is quintessentially sadomasochistic in that it connotes punishment, revenge and inevitability. 'Whip' and 'harnessed', besides their concrete and symbolic loading, are probably also mnemic cues for many of these index subjects, activating memories not only of adulthood but also of childhood.

In considering the results presented in Table 6.4, it must be remembered that the four words, 'mother', 'father', 'brother', 'sister', had been heard and spoken many times by each subject during interview only a matter of minutes previously. They were, that is, either highly primed or, quite to the contrary, their emotional charge was possibly already released. Nevertheless, it would appear that the 13 males in the depressed subgroup of sadomasochists were considerably more affected overall by the word 'mother' than the 13 least depressed sadomasochists. It might plausibly be inferred that the former had remained more emotionally entangled with their mothers than the latter. The overall effect of the word 'matriarch' is, however, both more striking in terms of its impact and more informative in terms of a sadomasochistic mind-set. 'Brother' appears to have had real semantic impact for the control group as a whole. 'Sister' was apparently of least significance for all groups.

An Examination of Possible Sources of Systematic Error

It seemed essential to include the words 'mother', 'father', 'brother', 'sister' in the Stroop presentation. They were, after all, only 4 in 150 words but they might cast light on subjects' representational models of these attachment figures (Bowlby, 1969). After reflection, but arguably still ill-advisedly, I decided to place the four words in the sadomasochistic word category, with the following 'rationale': (1) Although they were likely to be words of universal emotive content, they were likely to be more emotionally charged for the sadomasochistic subjects than the controls. (2) They should therefore be made SM words by analogy with 'leather' and 'rubber', which were also intrinsically innocent of such connotations but which indubitably carried a special fetishistic significance for sadomasochists and were also likely to cause more semantic interference for them than for controls. (3) It is, to take this argument to its logical conclusion, impossible to find any word which is totally neutral for everyone. (4) The four words in question (like a hair in one's soup!) are not, in fact, likely to be neutral for anyone, nor are they likely to have a depressed content for the majority of people, nor can they have any statistical viability on their own, disrupting the balanced design of the 150-word presentation. (5) Most persuasively, *if* the result of placing 'mother', 'father', 'brother' and 'sister' in the SM word category *were* to increase the index group's mean response time for this category, it could only validate the expectation that these words would disturb them.

As can be seen from Table 6.4, what actually resulted was that these words had higher ranks, on average, for controls than for sadomasochists, thus slightly inflating the SM-word-category mean for controls, eroding the difference between the groups of subjects in a conservative direction (Table 6.2*a*).

Like the longer average time to name 'purple' than the other four colors (Figure 6.1), this effect was across the board and therefore did not lead to any seriously wrong conclusion.

Table 6.5 presents the first of three measures of the degree of a subject's sadomasochistic orientation (the other two measures, SM sum 1 and SM sum 2, based on questionnaire data are introduced in Chapter 8). What I have called SM quotient, namely the ratio, calculated for each index subject, of his mean response time for SM words to his overall mean response time, might be regarded as a measure of sadomasochistic mind-set since it derives from a preconscious level of mental processing. It is, of course, greater than 'one' for the large majority (37 out of 48) of sadomasochistic subjects—another justification for using the term 'mind-set'. It has been used in Table 6.5 to relate Stroop results to Adult Attachment Interview classifications. The finding concerning the importance of the CC classification, both from the point of view of frequency and from the point of view of individual internal working model, confirms the hypothesis, put forward at the end of Chapter 4 and reiterated at the beginning of Part II, that sadomasochistic subjects would have failed to achieve an integration of painful experiences, that they would have a split and conflicting image, rather than a whole image, of the people who had inflicted these experiences. In short, many would have evolved no unified defence strategy. As already stated in reporting the results of Table 6.5, the hypothesis of marked discrepancy between global characterization of early relationships and episodic memories relating to them, where available at all, with its implied prediction of more frequent dismissive (Ds1 or Ds3) categorization, was not confirmed. In the event, the entangled/preoccupied (E) classification proved more characteristic of the sadomasochistic group, particularly of its more depressed members.

In proceeding to the analysis of the data provided by free recall (Tables 6.6 and 6.7), one becomes even more aware of a mind-set in the case of the index group of subjects. Their lists of words, noted down in the allotted 3 minutes, were not edifying reading. The objection may immediately be made: "What could you expect from the gruesome assortment of words you presented them with and were now requiring them, without warning, to recall?!" Agreed. But the overall impression created by the words recalled by index subjects was different from that received when analysing the lists written by control subjects, even though the latter also contained SM words. The most striking feature of the sadomasochists' word lists was sameness, and this emanated largely from the recurrence of fetishistic words. As stated towards the end of the Introduction, it was anticipated that these words, such as 'leather', 'rubber', 'whip', might ultimately be the most useful in distinguishing between the two groups of subjects. This expectation was confirmed. Seeing it rise off the written page does, however, bring home the limiting effect of this mind-set. Further, it draws one's attention to the limitation imposed on an individual's functioning by fetishism in general: emotional reaction determined by and restricted to a concrete object, mental processing dependent upon and limited by the physical. In his extreme, but also extremely thought-provoking, semiautobiographical study *The Facts of Life*, R.D. Laing may throw some light, albeit a bizarre light, when he records the perinatal feelings of a forty-year-old stockbroker: "From time to time very intensely, at other times always, but less so, he feels exposed, naked, raw, flayed (stripped of vernix caseosa), helpless, at the mercy of others, no strength. It feels to him as if he were a newborn baby. He has devised a procedure that mitigates his torment. He covers himself, or has his wife cover him, in leather (restoration of fetal or newborn skin, feeling as yet unborn). Covered in leather he feels as though he is mummified and has oil poured between his skin and leather, affording him one of the most pleasant and consoling 'feelings'—sensations—he knows" (Laing, 1976, p. 57).

Turning now to the words freely recalled or erroneously 'recalled' by the 14 women subjects (Table 6.8*a*), one finds in the lists produced by the index women (with ES numbers) a higher incidence of fetishistic words, as predicted, and of words relating to actual SM practice. In the words listed by the depressed women controls (with CS numbers), there is more a suggestion of sadness, even though SM words are also present. There is, as recognized several times already, an undeniable overlap between depression and sadomasochism. In devising the Stroop presentation, several words could have been placed in either category. What then, it may eventually be asked, constitutes the real difference in flavour between depressed-content and sadomasochistic-content words? It is not difficult to distinguish the latter—in essence they convey a certain relish of the negative. At the 1982 meeting of the American Psychoanalytic Association, Arnold Cooper expressed it thus: "Depression always refers to a *painful* affective state... On the other hand, masochism refers to a capacity for pleasure in unpleasure or pain" (Panel, 1984, p. 609). As to the other two women controls (with NS numbers), it may be relevant to their free recall to reveal that they both struck me during interview as having a fine sense for the dramatic! The 61-year-old NS278, who was unmarried and who had had two abortions, had an increased mean response time for depressed-content words (Appendix 4). NS285, who was 26 years old and married, had an increased mean response time for SM words. During her interview, she said that she thought her father, a collector of Nazi memorabilia, was probably sadistic. Thumbnail sketches of all fourteen of these women subjects are given in Chapter 7 where they are reported at somewhat greater length.

With respect to the 7 adopted subjects (Table 6.8*b*), a similar tendency to recall fetishistic words is discernable in 3 of the 5 sadomasochistic subjects. It is perhaps also worth noting that both ES19 and ES51 began their lists with 'assertive', whilst ES69 began his with 'dominant'. It almost always emerged on questioning that the first word written down was the word which had most impact on the subject. 'Assertive' was, of course, one of the 20 positive words not used in the main statistical analysis, but it would be very likely to have a similar connotation to 'dominant' for these subjects, a connotation referring, as already suggested, to control. As to the two depressed control subjects, CS136, who placed 'mother' first on his list, during interview said of his adoptive mother that 'the blanket of her love was choking'; CS284, writing 'matriarch' first, 'depression' second, and 'mother' third, explained during interview that his adoptive mother was suffering from depression throughout his childhood so that he felt partly responsible for his adoptive sisters and brother.

The 3 control subjects who have been kept under scrutiny after doubts arose about their suitability as controls all remembered words in the SM category (Table 6.8*c*), but their lists have little else in common. CS125, who recalled 'sister' first, actually had a twin sister. His mother, who had tried to dress them alike, had been denigrated during his interview as stupid and fickle. CS175 wrote the words 'submissive' and 'persecute' twice. NS269 recalled 'humiliated', 'whip' and 'dominant'. One might infer that the latter two subjects had possible sadomasochistic tendencies, but that would already be a considerable assumption based on very slender evidence. The sadomasochistic tendencies of these three control subjects, if they existed, were slow in manifesting, for CS125 was 48 years old, CS175 was 43 and NS269 was 46.

In conclusion, I submit that the 'emotional' Stroop task has provided evidence for a sadomasochistic mind-set, thus confirming my own observations on rigidity, made before undertaking this empirical investigation and set out in Chapter 4. Here both response latency (Table 6.2) and free recall (Table 6.6) are strongly oriented towards sadomasochism in the index group. The Stroop procedure may be a blunt instrument, but it is not self-report—it is computer-driven and free from subjective decisions. The most robust evidence for a sadomasochistic mind-set is probably that presented in Table 6.3: over 48 self-declared sadomasochists, the eight words with most impact, causing the most interference on the preconscious, semantic level, were all clearly sadomasochistic. Since we are speaking of a sadomasochistic mind-set, let us be quite clear as to its nature. Typical of the mind-set we are dealing with would be the words freely recalled by ES15, a 53-year-old married subject with a depression score of 7: "dominant, rubber, mistress, leather, whip, unloved, submissive, chain, mattress" ('mistress' would almost certainly mean 'dominatrix' rather than 'lover' for this subject). Equally typical would be the words listed by ES52, divorced, 55 years old, with a depression score of 17: "torturing, matriarch, leather, magazine, chained, supermarket, whip, dominant, humiliated". Both men were intelligent and well-educated.

CHAPTER 7

THE BECK DEPRESSION INVENTORY

SUMMARY

An attempt is made to examine the difference and the overlap between sadomasochism and depression. In particular, the female sadomasochists (n =5) are compared with the female controls (n =9).

INTRODUCTION

There have been various approaches to the complex phenomenon of depression—psychodynamic, existential, physiological and cognitive. Abraham (1911, 1916, 1924) postulated an increased orality: the depressive's sexual development is, predominantly, fixated at the oral stage and he, characteristically, wishes to eat up or incorporate his love object. This view may now seem to come from a bygone age, but it still finds some support in the frequent association of depression with the eating disorders (anorexia, bulimia) and the habit of compensatory eating. Freud (1917) considered depression as retroflected hostility. In denigrating himself, the 'melancholic' is really aiming his accusations against the lost love object he has introjected. Rado (1928) saw the depressive as narcissistic and needing to manipulate significant persons in his environment. Depression is a drama of self-vilification, played out on the psychic plane, designed to win back love by rechannelling aggressive impulses against the ego. Melanie Klein (1934) viewed adult depression as a reactivation of an early infantile depression, usually in the first year of life and associated with weaning.

When the angry child, helpless in his frustration, does not meet with sufficient maternal love, he will be predisposed to return to the depressive position, to feelings of loss and lack of self-esteem. Helene Deutsch (1937) considered that childhood bereavement could lead either to mourning or, more pathologically, to a defensive absence of affect. Later compulsive self-reliance and episodes of depression were the result of this disconnection of feeling from the childhood event. This delineation seemed worth pursuing in the case of the 7 adoptees in the present study. They had all virtually suffered a type of early bereavement in that their blood parents had gone out of their lives in infancy. Would they in fact, as Deutsch (1937) describes, display an absence of affect and a compulsive self-reliance?

In the existential approach of Hubert Tellenbach (1961), the depressive is dominated by strict orderliness, conscientiousness, a need to do right by those close to him. His hypersensitivity to guilt results in his life being consumed by simultaneous strivings to reach his own aspirations and standards of orderliness and to fulfil his obligations, so that he is precariously balanced between the two and is haunted by the fear of falling short on one or the other.

Kraines (1965) attempted a physiological explanation: stimuli from the cerebral cortex excite the somatovisceral system via the hypothalamus, and the stimulation in the form of feedback passes via the reticular system to be elaborated in the thalamus and the limbic system. The impulses terminate in the cerebral cortex, thus completing a complex 'emotional circuit', producing a sensory experience of depressed mood. Pathological hypothalamic function is primarily responsible for manic-depressive illness, and psychological symptoms are secondary defenses against this alarming physiological condition of the diencephalon. Much printer's ink has, of course, flowed under the bridge since Kraines' 1965 account. Duman *et al.* (1997) offer an interesting overview of current physiological theories of depression. These authors suggest that depletion of the monoamines, serotonin and norepinephrine, is unlikely to be the only factor involved in depression since, even though synaptic levels of these monoamines are increased rapidly by antidepressant treatment with the tricyclics and monoamine oxidase inhibitors, the time required for their therapeutic action is several weeks. They conclude, therefore, that additional factors must contribute both to antidepressant responses and to the onset of depression. For instance, the activated cyclic adenosine 3′,5′-monophosphate (cAMP) system leads to the regulation of specific target genes, including the increased expression of brain-derived neurotrophic factor (BDNF) in certain populations of neurons in the hippocampus and cerebral cortex. Recent studies demonstrate that chronic stress decreases the expression of BDNF in the hippocampus. Siuciak *et al.* (1997) found, in fact, that centrally administered BDNF had an antidepressant effect in two animal models of depression—learned helplessness (Seligman & Beagley, 1975) in rats preexposed to inescapable electric shock, and the forced swim test in 16 inches of water, so that rats can neither touch the bottom nor escape from the plastic container. Midbrain infusion of BDNF restored normal escape behavior in the first case and reduced the time by 70% that the rats remained immobile, neither swimming not trying to escape, in the second case. There is mounting evidence (Duman *et al.* 1997, pp. 603–604) that chronic psychosocial stress and long-term elevation of glucocorticoid levels can cause atrophy and even death of vulnerable hippocampal neurons (particularly CA3 pyramidal neurons), creating a diathesis for depression.

Aaron Beck (1967) agreed with Grinker *et al.* (1961) that a wide spectrum of pathological phenomena must be addressed in any account of depression: affective (feelings of sadness, loneliness, emptiness, hopelessness, boredom), motivational (cries for help, escapism, paralysis of the will, suicidal thoughts), physical (motor retardation, fatigue, loss of appetite, sleep disturbance, loss of libido), and cognitive (pessimism, negative concept of the self, negative interpretation of experiences). In seeking a summary formulation, Beck arrived at a primary triad in depression: a negative view of the self, of the world and of the future. He concluded that both etiology and treatment should be approached largely from a cognitive point of view. Cognitions (arbitrary inferences, wrong attributions, gloomy generalizations) and the affects they evoke set up a vicious circle, or rather, a downward spiral: "The more negatively the patient thinks, the worse he feels; the worse he feels, the more negatively he thinks" (Beck, 1967, p. 289).

There are, however, two other observations recorded by Beck which made his work particularly relevant to the present investigation of masochism, controlling for depression. First, he identified a pervasive "masochistic" attitude in his depressed patients, manifesting as a need to suffer and an enduring cognitive distortion in evaluating, always with a negative bias, their worth, adequacy, social acceptability or achievements. Their feelings were frequently of humiliation, deprivation, frustration and social isolation. In collaboration with Marvin Hurvich, he examined the manifest content of his patients' dreams (Beck, 1967, chapter 13) and found these same unpleasant themes occurring with greater frequency in depressives than in nondepressives. This led to the development of a dichotomous scoring system for "masochistic" dreams (Beck, 1967, Appendix, pp. 339–344): manifest content presenting the dreamer as less fortunate or attractive than he was in reality (for instance, as ugly, sick or defective) or as thwarted, rejected or deprived was scored "+", otherwise "0".

Secondly, and potentially of equal relevance, Beck (1967, chapter 14) examined the histories of adult depressives for the incidence of childhood bereavement and found that this was 27%, as contrasted with 12% in the case of nondepressives. He concluded, like Deutsch (1937), that "a drastic experience such as the loss of a parent in childhood may be determinant in the later development of severe depression" (p. 225).

The potential relevance of this finding lay in the possibility it suggested of testing such a hypothesis in the course of investigating early family relationships and, specifically, in terms of the attachment theory of John Bowlby (1969, 1973, 1980, 1988). The third volume of Bowlby's *magnum opus, Attachment and Loss*, is, in fact, subtitled "Sadness and Depression" (1980) and in it he comments that Beck formulates a cognitive theory of depressive disorders "cast in the same mould as the theory of cognitive biases proposed here. Both formulations postulate that depressive-prone individuals possess cognitive schemas having certain unusual but characteristic features which result in their construing events in their lives in the idiosyncratic ways they do" (p. 249).

Subjects

The basic composition of all groups of respondents to the Beck Depression Inventory is set out in Table 7.1.

TABLE 7.1. Basic Composition of all Groups of Respondents to the Beck Depression Inventory

		Males		Females		Males + Females	
	Total *N*	CS	NS	CS	NS	CS	NS
All respondents (other than index subjects)	189	36 (19%)	78 (41%)	28 (15%)	47 (25%)	64 (34%)	125 (66%)
Potential controls (not attending for interview)	154	23 (15%)	65 (42%)	21 (14%)	45 (29%)	44 (29%)	110 (71%)
All control subjects	35	13 (37%)	13 (37%)	7 (20%)	2 (6%)	20 (57%)	15 (43%)
	N	Males		Females			
All index subjects	48	43 (90%)		5 (10%)			
Index subjects scoring 14 or more	14	14 (100%)		0 (0%)			
Index subjects scoring less than 14	34	29 (85%)		5 (15%)			

'Control subjects' ($n = 35$) are those respondents who subsequently attended for personal interview and who have been studied for purposes of comparison with the sadomasochistic index group of subjects.
CS = those scoring 14 or more; NS = ('neutral') those scoring less than 14.
Actual numbers of respondents with percentages in parentheses.
All index subjects received an 'ES' ('experimental') number, irrespective of their BDI scores.

All completed questionnaires received from potential control subjects were recorded on computer as a benchmark ($n = 189$). Those with total scores of 14 or more ($n = 64$) were given CS ('depressed') numbers and those with total scores of 13 or less ($n = 125$) were given NS ('non-depressed' or 'neutral') numbers. Of those who did not come for interview ($n = 154$), 44 had BDI total scores of 14 or more, 110 had total scores of 13 or less. One questionnaire (CS281) was obviously facetious so its exaggeratedly depressed input was neutralized by substituting mean values of the 'depressed' group for all its responses. Another (NS215) was returned with a critical comment but otherwise uncompleted and was similarly dealt with by supplying mean values of the 'nondepressed' group. All the other questionnaires appeared genuine, but many were returned without a self-addressed envelope, presumably signalling that no further involvement was desired.

INSTRUMENT

The reliability (internal consistency and stability) and validity (content, concurrent, discriminant and construct validity) of the Beck Depression Inventory (BDI) have been established over the three decades of its use. There have been many reviews of its psychometric properties (e.g., Beck & Lester, 1973; Beck *et al.* 1988; Mental Measurements Yearbook, 1992).

Two subscales are referred to in the manual accompanying the questionnaire: the cognitive/affective subscale and the somatic/performance subscale. The first 13 items, comprising the former, refer to sadness, pessimism, sense of failure, dissatisfaction, guilt, expectation of punishment, self-dislike, self-accusations, suicidal ideas, crying, irritability, social withdrawal and indecisiveness. The 8 items of the second subscale relate to body image change, work retardation, insomnia, tiredness, anorexia, weight loss, hypochondriasis and loss of libido. These 21 symptoms and attitudes (13 items in the shorter form of the Inventory) were arrived at by systematic clinical observation. Each is depicted in sentences ranging from 0 to 3 in intensity (no complaint to severe complaint).

PROCEDURE

As stated at the beginning of Part II, all control subjects were, in fact, recruited through the questionnaire on 'Morale' (actually the Beck Depression Inventory) which they returned from one of the two selected newspapers, *New Statesman & Society* or *The Spectator*. They had been requested to ring the number of the relevant statement in each group and post the questionnaire together with a stamped, self-addressed envelope.

The following procedure was used for the index subjects who were all presented with the questionnaire immediately debriefing on the interview was concluded. Following Beck's own instructions (Beck, 1967, p. 336) for administration of the Depression Inventory, subjects were handed a copy and asked to choose one statement out of each group (read aloud by the experimenter) which best reflected their present mental or physical state (the accompanying manual produced in 1987 instructs "during the past week"). If the subject responded with a number, confirmation of the statement against that number was sought, at least until it was clear that the subject had understood the numbering system. Where the subject indicated that two statements would apply, the higher value was recorded; where the subject hovered between two statements, either the value of the one he/she felt closer to or the lower value was recorded. No suggestions were made which might influence choice and, on conclusion, the subject was asked how he/she had found the questionnaire. The total score for each subject was determined by simply summing the values (0, 1, 2 or 3) recorded as his/her responses to the 21 items of the questionnaire, the higher numbers being endorsements of more negative statements.

Statistical Procedure

The nondepression/depression cutoff point between 13 and 14 was not adopted arbitrarily. The pilot study conducted before this investigation used a small sample of only 14 subjects and could therefore hardly be considered representative of the general population, but nevertheless, the mean BDI total score of those 7 'nondepressed' and 7 'depressed' subjects was 13.79 (S.D. 8.64) and the median total score was 14.0. Beck himself (1967, p. 203) placed a dividing line between 'nondepressed' and 'depressed' around 13.

There is, however, something slightly preposterous, not to put too fine a point on it, crazy, about the notion that a person scoring 13 is not depressed but one scoring 14 has become depressed. To make amends therefore, albeit belatedly, for the impropriety of dichotomizing a continuous variable (the statistical dangers of this practice are elegantly demonstrated by Maxwell & Delaney (1993)), I propose to treat depression, represented by Beck total scores, as a continuum for much of this chapter.

RESULTS

Although depression was found by Beck and many others to be more prevalent in women than in men, it can be seen from Table 7.1 that only

75 out of the 189 completed questionnaires were returned by women. A 40% female presence was, however, more than might have been expected when *New Statesman & Society* and *The Spectator* had been deliberately chosen to reach as many male readers as possible, and it was more than enough for purposes of comparing depressed with sadomasochistic women. The comparison is made later in this section under the heading 'The women', and discussed in the following section under the same heading. It has, in fact been made the occasion for taking a special look at the women in this study.

The mean and median total scores of different groups of respondents to the Beck Depression Inventory are set out in Table 7.2. It is noticeable that those index subjects who scored under 14 (the erstwhile 'nondepressed' group) not only had a low mean score (6.47) but a low standard deviation (3.30). The control subjects scoring under 14 had a lower mean total score (2.93) but a higher standard deviation (4.06) although they

TABLE 7.2. Mean and Median total Scores of Different Groups of Respondents to the Beck Depression Inventory

		BDI total scores		
	N	Mean	S.D.	Median
All respondents (other than index subjects)	189	10.85	9.14	9
All female respondents (other than index subjects)	75	11.80	9.28	10
Potential controls (not attending for interview)	154	9.96	8.02	8
Female respondents (not attending for interview)	66	10.61	8.48	8.5
All control subjects	35	14.77	12.36	14
Control subjects scoring 14 or more	20	23.65	8.23	23.5
Control subjects scoring less than 14	15	2.93	4.06	1
All female controls	9	20.56	10.75	24
All index subjects	48	10.71	7.90	7
Index subjects scoring 14 or more	14	21.00	6.05	19
Index subjects scoring less than 14	34	6.47	3.30	6
All female index subjects	5	4.60	2.30	4

'Control subjects' ($n = 35$) are those respondents who subsequently attended for personal interview and who have been studied for purposes of comparison with the sadomasochistic index group of subjects.

were less than half as many in number (15 as compared with 34 subjects); this presumably reflected greater heterogeneity. It will be noted that the complete group of 35 control subjects had a mean total score of 14.77 (S.D. 12.36) and a median of precisely 14, the cutoff point selected to designate depression. Thus, although the control group was so constituted as to enable meaningful comparisons between depressed and sadomasochistic subjects, the low total scores of the randomly obtained 'neutral' controls at the other end of the distribution counterbalanced to create a reasonable spectrum and avoid excessive 'skewness'.

As can be seen from Table 7.2 and seen at a glance from Figure 7.1, the level and prevalence of depression over the complete group of sadomasochists ($n = 48$) were not appreciably different from the level and prevalence in what might be regarded as a fair sample of the general population, namely, those postal respondents who did not subsequently come for an interview ($n = 154$). In both cases, 29% of individuals scored 14 or more on the Beck Depression Inventory. The median scores of both groups were very similar: 7 for the sadomasochists, 8 for the population sample.

The sadomasochists would thus appear, at least superficially and as they themselves reported, no different from anyone else in their susceptibility to become depressed. What was different was the way in which their depression manifested, their symptomatology, and this is illustrated in Figure 7.2. Here it can be seen that the profiles, constructed from response to the 21 groups of statements of the Beck Depression Inventory, show certain differences between the population sample ($n = 154$) and the sadomasochistic group ($n = 48$). Specifically, the sadomasochists have higher mean scores for a sense of failure (0.69, S.E. 0.12, as compared with 0.47, S.E. 0.06 in the population sample), for expectation of punishment (0.73, S.E. 0.16, as compared with 0.37, S.E. 0.05), for self-accusations (0.88, S.E. 0.10, as compared with 0.66, S.E. 0.06), for body image change (0.77, S.E. 0.12, as compared with 0.54, S.E. 0.06). Even more informative is the fact that sadomasochistic depression does not manifest to the same extent in loss of libido, i.e., the mean score of the index group for this symptom was considerably less than that of the population sample (0.35, S.E. 0.08, as compared with 0.57, S.E. 0.07). These differences from the 'normal' picture of depression will receive further attention in the Discussion section of this chapter, where one similarity will also be considered: the mean score for somatic preoccupation, in other words, hypochondriasis, was 0.44 in both the sadomasochistic group and the population sample (S.E. 0.09 and 0.05, respectively). It perhaps gives a clue to the nature of the undeniable overlap between sadomasochism and depression.

Since loss of libido is obviously of prime relevance to a sexual deviation such as sadomasochism, its association with the total depression

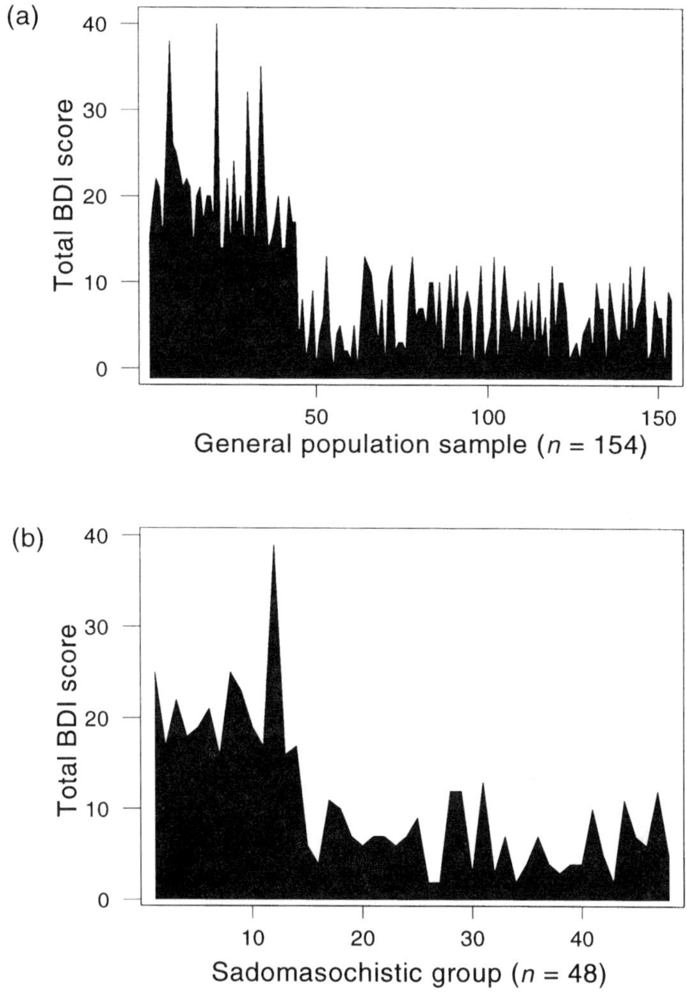

FIGURE 7.1. Plots depicting level of depression measured by the Beck Depression Inventroy (a) in the 154 respondents from the general population who did not subsequently attend for interview, (b) in the complete group of 48 sadomasochists. In both cases total BDI scores have been plotted from left to right along the horizontal axis in ascending order of the identification numbers allotted to individuals, but with those scoring 14 or more grouped on the left. It can be seen that there is no marked difference in level or prevalence of depression between the two plots.

score is scrutinized, overall, in Table 7.3. Quite strikingly, the sadomasochistic group as a whole ($n = 48$) is alone in showing no association between depression and loss of libido ($r = 0.092$) and, even more strikingly, for the subgroup of sadomasochists scoring 14 or more, depression

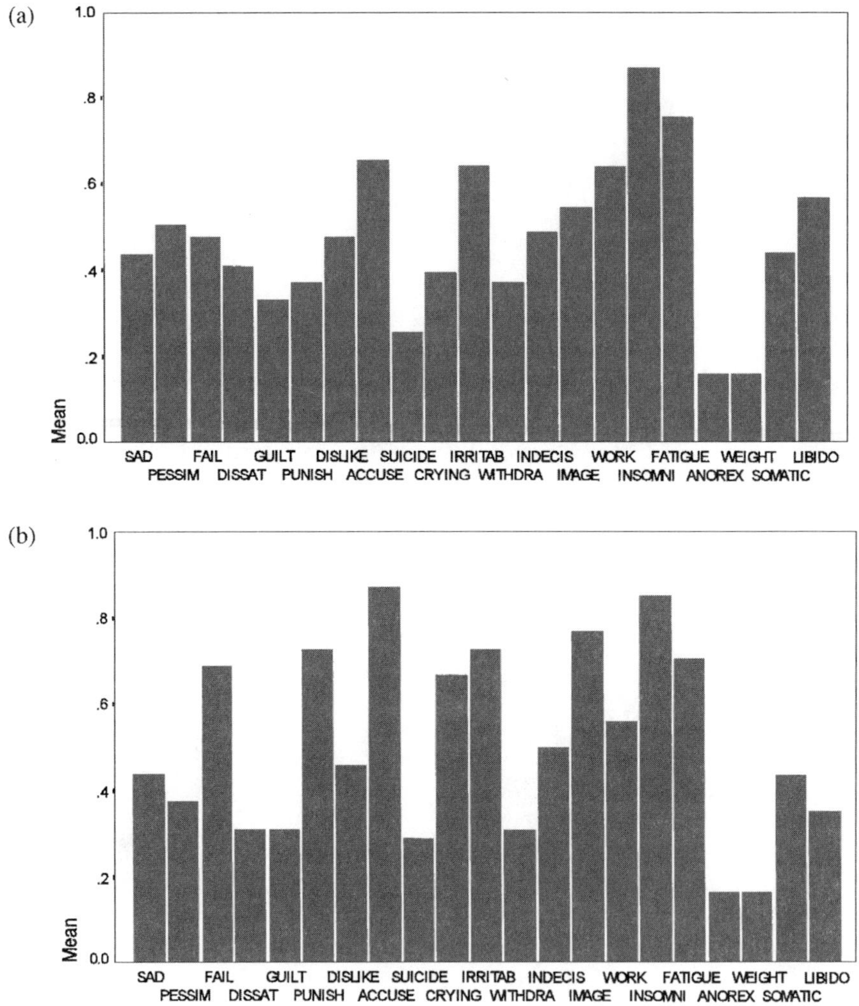

FIGURE 7.2. Differing BDI profiles of (a) the 154 respondents from the general population who did not subsequently attend for interview, (b) the complete group of 48 sadmoschists. Mean scores are shown for 21 symptoms of depression, measured from 0 (not depressed) to 3 (very depressed): sadness, pessimism, sense of failure, dissatisfaction, guilt, expectation of punishment, self-dislike, self-accusations, suicidal ideas, crying, irritability, social withdrawal, indecisiveness, body image change, work retardation, insomnia, fatigability, anorexia, weight loss, somatic preoccupation, loss of libido.

is negatively correlated with loss of libido ($r = -0.248$). The highest correlation ($r = 0.561, p < 0.001$, 2-tailed) emerges in the case of the interviewed subjects who formed the control group ($n = 35$). This is not connected with the preponderance of depressed individuals in this group since the

TABLE 7.3. Pearson Product-Moment Correlations Between 'Loss of Libido' and Total Scores for Different Groups of Respondents to the Beck Depression Inventory

	N	*r*
All respondents (other than index subjects)	189	0.378***
All female respondents (other than index subjects)	75	0.324**
Potential controls (not attending for interview)	154	0.301**
Female respondents (not attending for interview)	66	0.316*
All control subjects	35	0.561***
Control subjects scoring 14 or more	20	0.299
Control subjects scoring less than 14	15	0.307
All female controls	9	0.264
All index subjects	48	0.092
Index subjects scoring 14 or more	14	−0.248
Index subjects scoring less than 14	34	0.220
All female index subjects	5	0.267

'Control subjects' (n = 35) are those respondents who subsequently attended for personal interview and who have been studied for purposes of comparison with the sadomasochistic index group of subjects
$*p<0.05$, $**p<0.01$, $***p<0.001$, 2-tailed.

association between depression and loss of libido is slightly stronger ($r = 0.307$ versus $r = 0.299$) in those controls scoring less than 14 ($n = 15$) than in those scoring 14 or more ($n = 20$). The larger groupings of postal respondents showed similar significant correlations between depression and loss of libido.

When the sadomasochistic group ($n = 48$) and the control group ($n = 35$) were submitted to a linear discriminant function analysis, using depression (BDI total score) and metacognition/coherence (combined AAI scale scores for metacognitive processes, coherence of interview transcript and overall coherence of mind) as predictors, 70 out of the 83 subjects were assigned to their correct group (proportion correct: 0.843). When the linear discriminant analysis was repeated with three groups, i.e., the sadomasochistic group and the control group divided into CS-numbered subjects (the 20 subjects scoring high for depression) and NS-numbered subjects (the 15 'neutral' subjects scoring low for depression), the separation

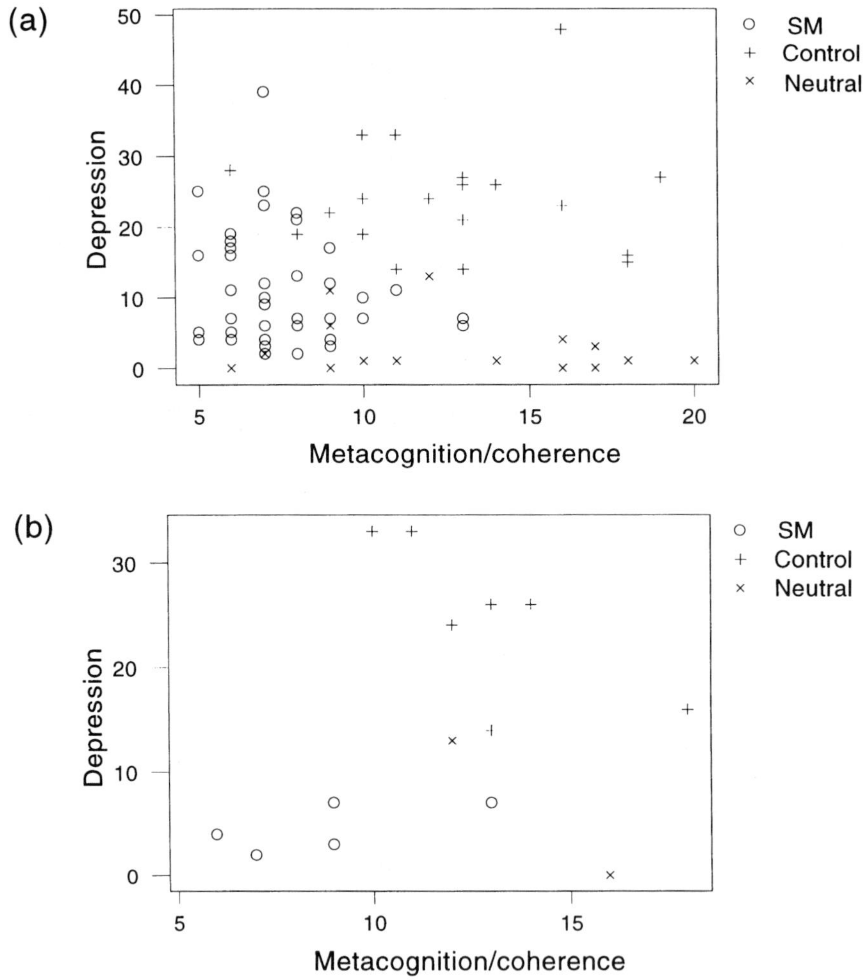

FIGURE 7.3. Discrimination between sadomasochistic (ES-numbered), control (CS-numbered) and neutral (NS-numbered) groups of subjects by means of depression (BDI total socre) and metacognition/coherence (combined AAI scales for metacognitive monitoring, coherence of transcript, coherence of mind), achieved (a) for the complete sample of 83 subjects who came for interview, (b) for the 14 female subjects in that sample. In the case of the women, the separation of the groups is extremely clear.

was even better: 72 of the 83 subjects were assigned to their correct group (proportion correct: 0.867). Figure 7.3*a* displays the striking separation of groups produced when these two variables (depression and metacognition/coherence) are plotted against each other. An attempt will be made in the Discussion section to examine the curious relations between depression, coherence and sadomasochism.

The Women

According to DSM-III-R: "In almost all studies of Major Depression in adults in industrialized countries, the disorder is estimated to be twice as common in females as in males" (p. 229). More relevant to this study is dysthymia: "Among adults the disorder is apparently more common in females" (p. 231). This is confirmed in several ways (relating both to prevalence and to degree of depression) by the sample from the general population of postal respondents to the Beck Depression Inventory ($n = 189$). Of the 75 women who returned questionnaires, 28 (37%) scored 14 or more; of the 114 men, only 36 (32%) scored 14 or more (Table 7.1). These 75 women had a mean score of 11.80 (S.D. 9.28) and a median of 10 (Table 7.2); the 114 men had a mean score of 10.23 (S.D. 9.03) and a median of 7.5. Of the 35 respondents who finally agreed to come for an interview, 9 were women. Their mean score was 20.56 (S.D. 10.75), and their median score, at 24, was the highest of those listed in Table 7.2; the 26 male controls who agreed to be interviewed had a mean score of 12.77 (S.D. 12.44) and a median score of 12.5.

Against this background of female depression, the 5 sadomasochistic women I interviewed stood out, therefore, as rather strikingly *non*depressed, according to their own projection, with a mean BDI score of 4.60 (S.D. 2.30) and a median score of only 4. Like the female controls, however, they had much to relate from their childhoods which might reasonably have led to depression. A thumbnail sketch of all 14 female subjects is given in the Discussion section of this chapter.

For these 14 women, the correlation between depression (BDI total score) and metacognition/coherence (combined AAI scale scores for metacognitive monitoring, coherence of transcript and coherence of mind) was 0.417. When plotted against each other, these variables produced (Figure 7.3*b*) an even clearer separation of the index and control groups in the case of the female subjects alone than was achieved with the complete groups of men and women (Figure 7.3*a*). In fact, the proportion correctly assigned to their group in a linear discriminant analysis using depression and metacognition/coherence as predictors was 0.929 (13 out of 14 subjects). If, besides the 5 sadomasochistic women, only the 7 female controls with high scores for depression, i.e., those with CS numbers, were used, excluding the 2 'neutral' controls with low BDI scores and NS numbers, then the proportion correctly assigned was 1.0 (all 12 women were correctly assigned either to the sadomasochistic or to the control group).

TABLE 7.4. AAI Classifications, BDI Total Scores, Age, Sex and Marital Status of the 7 Adoptees (5 Sadomasochists, 2 Controls)

Subject	AAI classification	BDI total score	Age	Sex	Marital status
ES4	Ds2	11	76	Male	Married
ES19	Ds1	18	44	Male	Unmarried
ES50	E2/E1	4	47	Male	Married
ES51	E2/U	7	41	Male	Married
ES69	CC/Ds2/E2	2	59	Male	Married*
CS136	Ds3/F1a	24	36	Male	Unmarried
CS284	F5/Ds2/U	23	33	Male	Unmarried

ES numbers signify sadomasochistic subjects; CS numbers signify controls.
'Married' status was given to subjects who are at present married, or remarried, or (*) who were at one time married, or who have a permanent partner; all others were classified as 'Unmarried'.
Main AAI categories: Ds = Dismissing, E = Entangled/preoccupied, F = Freely valuing of attachment yet objective, U = Unresolved loss or trauma, CC = Cannot Classify (for subcategories see Appendix 2).
It can be seen that Ds (Dismissing) was the classification most frequently assigned to these adopted subjects, irrespective of whether they belonged to the sadomasochistic or the control group.

The Adoptees

If Helene Deutsch (1937) was right in her observation that early bereavement could sometimes act pathologically to produce an absence of affect and, later, a compulsive self-reliance with episodes of depression, then this might well be confirmed by the 7 adoptees who had all been virtually bereaved in infancy. Table 7.4 sets out the same information as was given in Table 5.1 of Chapter 5, but it facilitates scrutiny of these particular subjects and of their AAI classifications in particular. It can be seen that these adopted subjects were, indeed, placed most frequently in the Dismissing (Ds) category whether they belonged to the index group or the control group. ES19 was classified Ds1 'dismissing of attachment' (see Appendix 2), CS136 was classified Ds3, 'restricted in feeling', and yet more confirmatory, ES4, ES69 and CS284 received either a primary or a secondary classification of Ds2, 'devaluing of attachment'. This classification is rarely assigned and connotes precisely a compulsive self-reliance. The two index subjects who were not dismissive (Ds) were angrily entangled (E2) with attachment figures.

DISCUSSION

The factor of depression points both forward and backward in this analysis of several strands of data. Looking back, one is reminded by

Tables 5.5 and 5.6 of Chapter 5 that depression can, in fact, be treated as a potential nuisance variable and statistically 'partialled out', leaving the sadomasochistic group ($n = 48$) still with significantly less coherence and ability to 'mentalize' (i.e., with significantly less theory of mind) than the control group ($n = 35$). Looking forward, one realizes that the Beck Depression Inventory, the only questionnaire presented to a wide spectrum of individuals (Table 7.1), must be kept in view, somewhat like a backdrop, when considering the questionnaires, presented specifically to the sadomasochistic group of subjects, in Chapter 8. Attempts to clarify historical, attitudinal and behavioral differences within that group (Tables 8.2, 8.4, 8.5, Figure 8.3) are in fact made from the basis of BDI scores. Meanwhile, in the present chapter, Table 7.1 is a timely reminder that there are women as well as men in this study and, although far fewer attended for interview, these women repay some belated attention. This they receive in special subsections, the one above reporting results and the one below discussing these results, both headed in 'politically correct' style 'The women'!

As can be seen from Table 7.2, the mean total BDI score of the 34 sadomasochists at the lower end of the index distribution (mean = 6.47, S.D. 3.30) was considerably less than the benchmark mean total (mean = 10.85, S.D. 9.14) of all 189 postal respondents from which the control group was formed. These sadomasochists were, thus, markedly less depressed, according to their own reporting, than the nearest approximation to the general population. The mean score quoted by Aaron T. Beck himself for the 115 patients with no depression in his sample of 409 routine outpatient and inpatient admissions was 10.9 with a standard deviation of 8.1 (Beck, 1967, p. 196), an almost identical value to that of the 'general population' in this study. What is, however, also of interest in the result mentioned above is that the *standard deviation* of these 34 low-scoring sadomasochists is so small (3.30) by comparison with most other groups of respondents. (It may be remembered that another distinguishing characteristic of this group emerged in Chapter 5: they showed less correlation between Adult Attachment Interview scales than controls, and this was interpreted as a possible indication of their lesser coherence.) One may thus reasonably infer that, with respect to their morale, they are similar individuals who may justifiably be treated as a subgroup. Such was indeed my personal impression: they struck me as generally more open and confident in manner than those sadomasochists who were more depressed. However, this behavioral difference within the index group is not necessarily attributable solely to depression. All other groupings in Table 7.2 contain more variance as indicated by their standard deviations (the 5 sadomasochistic women were part of the low-scoring group at present under consideration), so there remains a behavioral difference to be explained. It will be addressed in Chapter 8.

Figures 7.1 and 7.2 endeavor to make the point that sadomasochists are, according to their own reports, no more and no less likely to feel depressed than 'the man in the street' (29% of the sadomasochists ($n = 48$) and 29% of the postal respondents to the questionnaire ($n = 154$) scored 14 or more and their median total scores were 7 and 8, respectively), but they are likely to manifest depression in a different manner. Certain symptoms, of those 21 pinpointed by Beck, are more in evidence and, after the picture painted so laboriously from the literature in Chapter 2, they can hardly come as a surprise: a sense of failure, expectation of punishment, self-accusations and anxiety over change for the worse in physical appearance. In the light of the earliest experiences of these people, such symptoms are even less surprising. They mostly encountered, as revealed by their interviews, a cruel and baffling world in which, more often than not, threatening, unreliable or unpredictable caregivers did little to dispel the ominous atmosphere, to help them make sense of feelings and behavior as emanating from intentional beings. I submit that they frequently experienced depression before they were old enough to recognize it and they adopted the defense of sexualizing the pain, often masturbating, helpless in the face of an intolerable situation. Hence the overriding need to control or to be controlled (discussed at some length in Part III) and hence the anomaly depicted in Figure 7.2 of depression with less than 'normal' loss of libido.

That the two profiles (Figure 7.2*a*,*b*) display virtually the same mean score for somatic preoccupation in the form of ever-increasing concern over aches and pains, may point to the overlap, the common ground of sadomasochism and depression, which is in fact the use of the body as a theatre (McDougall, 1989). What they both share are the psychological and physiological mechanisms of somatization but, with the erotization of pain, masochism has gone further and probably started much earlier.

The result of chief interest in Table 7.3 carries the argument for making a distinction between the sadomasochistic subjects according to their depression scores a stage further: the high-scoring sadomasochists ($n = 14$) are the *only* group for whom, as a whole, depression is *negatively* associated with loss of libido. This is an important consideration when sadomasochism is a sexual deviance. An attempt will therefore be made in Chapter 8, when reporting the questionnaire data gathered specifically from the sadomasochistic group, to build up a profile, statistically, of this 'depressed' subgroup who, unlike all other subjects, tend to remain more interested in sex, the more depressed they are. The significant interaction, depicted in Figure 5.2*e* of Chapter 5, between sadomasochism and depression with respect to passivity, suggested that characterization of this subgroup was worth pursuing. They present a different picture from the more active sadomasochists, who tend apparently to be less depressed, and with smaller group variance, than the average man in the street.

To sum up, the same inference may be drawn from Table 7.3 as from Figure 7.2, namely, that sadomasochists are anomalous in not losing their interest in sex when they are depressed. The interpretation, already advanced, of sadomasochism as first a somatization of psychological pain and then a defensive erotization of this pain, has, of course, found support in the past (Panel, 1984; Glenn, 1984*a*,*b*). Clearly, once pain, whether psychological, physical or both, has become associated with sexual pleasure, the painful array of symptoms which constitute depression only become grist for the mill and one has masochism proper, defiantly retaining its libido.

Childhood Depression

In the opinion expressed by ES36, his parents' rows depressed him. The stress over several years "was precipitating depressions that I didn't have a word for". This points to a consideration which is more important, the younger the child. A child before the age of three simply has not developed the mental apparatus with which to recognize and work over his own feelings, yet his feelings are never more intense. Where parenting has been insensitive, he has had no assistance with this developmental task. As Mary Main points out: "The secure child may also have more epistemic 'space' in which to review her actions, situations, or thinking processes because her thinking processes are not compartmentalized ... defensive and/or self-deceiving processes are compartmentalizing processes" (Main, 1991, p. 146). The defenses which are likely to be adopted as time goes on are those which come to light in the Adult Attachment Interview as idealization, dismissal, derogation, suppression of memory.

If Freud was right, and he almost certainly was, in supposing that the painfulness of mourning lay in the necessarily piecemeal detachment from the lost person, where each memory and expectation must be brought up over time and detached from an object which no longer exists in reality (Freud, 1895*b*, p. 162; 1917, pp. 244–245), then a very young child simply does not yet possess the mental capacity for this. How much less could an infant, abandoned by his natural parents and adopted by others only to be unloved or smothered, ever work through any healing process of mourning to arrive at a reconciled frame of mind?

Certainly many of my depressed interviewees, sadomasochists and controls alike, considered they had been forsaken and ill-treated as children.

Many index subjects had been stifled and bored. The point I am emphasizing here is that there would often be no conscious awareness of the factors contributing to their sad mood, or even that they were feeling sad—just a heavy greyness where nothing mattered. To escape from this world drained of color, from this paralysis, into autoerotic activity, later into bizarre fantasy, would not be surprising. It has, in fact, been filmed in institutions for the handicapped in Greece and Romania.

THE WOMEN

The fact that here there were in all, from the general population, only 75 female as compared with 114 male respondents to the Beck Depression Inventory is, of course, a reflection of the predominantly male readership of *New Statesman & Society* and *The Spectator*. These journals had, it will be recalled, been selected as vehicles on that account, but one can't have it all ways—although there are apparently more sadomasochistic males, there are really more depressed females (Beck, 1967, p. 205) in the general population.

The five women who were self-declared sadomasochists and who came, without inhibition, for interview were all assertive and intelligent but otherwise were completely individual in personality and physical appearance. ES41 was short in height, somewhat pretentious, even snobbish, and guarded. ES42, who was ebullient and impulsive, declared that as she grew up she thought as a boy and picked up male attitudes to sex. ES58 was beautiful and announced that she was a 'professional', highly remunerated by male sadomasochists for her services, as well as a practitioner by choice and bisexual. ES62, a lesbian and a vegetarian, could not tolerate computers so had to have the microphone hand-held whilst performing the Stroop task. ES75, who styled herself 'a love slave', was extremely plump and quick-witted. Also aware of social status, she filled in questionnaires with unusual swiftness and seemed impatient to move on, to get on with things!

The nine female control subjects were apparently glad to have a sympathetic listener. CS138, a vegetarian, felt that she was highly sexed and was in one-to-one therapy with a woman. CS180, who was also a vegetarian and had also had counselling, felt that her sex-drive was low and that she had a strong masculine side; she had been bulimic and had herself sterilized when she was 29. CS187 seemed to have high standards, to be realistic and honest with herself, but caring for privacy and independence. CS90 started to cry when she spoke of sexual abuse from her grandfather and continued to weep through a long portion of her interview, saying that she had always wanted to be a boy. CS196 had also been sexually abused and battered as a child; this left her afraid of most men and with little current interest in sex. CS206, who looked older than her 51 years, made an honest, straightforward impression but tended to be overconscientious in her work and overscrupulous in her consideration for others. CS260 was a charming, inconsistent woman with a good sense of humour but a tendency to idealize. NS278 was a volatile person with a gift for painting vivid pictures but what might be called a severe superego. NS285 had a childish voice and manner but seemed to become more mature as her interview progressed, even manipulative. The childhood events which emerged from the interviews of the majority of the female controls with high BDI scores could thus quite feasibly have created a predisposition to depression.

Turning again now to the female sadomasochists, who were, according to self-report, uniformly low-scorers for depression, ES42 lost her mother before she was two, and her father remarried when she was four-and-a-half: "I remember the van come up and her get out ... That's when she first came. That's burnt into my mind, that sight—here is the new mother coming!" A half-sister and a half-brother were born: "It was always my fault and I got sent to my room, I got punished ... And so I had a feeling of injustice—it's always—always my fault, and it's not fair, it's not fair—just absolute burning anger and resentment for years." Of her childhood ES58 said: "I think I just wandered around a lot on my own. I remember most of my childhood wandering around a lot on my own." Of her parents she said: "I think I also realized quite quickly that they were not people who could be relied on—even in a—even in an ordinary sense they couldn't be relied on." It might reasonably be asked: why were ES42 and ES58, who were both classified by the AAI system as preoccupied with their unhappy childhoods, not depressed? The index subjects at the upper end of the BDI distribution had a preponderance of 'E' (entangled/preoccupied) classifications—why were they depressed? The mental entanglement of ES42 and ES58 is, however, angry (E2) and therein may lie their defense—their persisting resentment is expressed actively and at length. The classification amongst the more depressed index subjects is primarily E1, passively entangled.

For these 14 women, the association between depression and metacognition/coherence (Pearson's $r = 0.417$) is clear from Figure 7.3*b*. The groups can be separated on the basis of these two variables. Using them as predictors in a linear discriminant analysis, 13 out of the 14 women were assigned to the correct group. If only the 7 women with high scores for depression and CS numbers were used as controls, dropping the 2 'neutral' controls with low scores and NS numbers from the linear analysis, then discrimination between groups was complete—all 12 women were correctly assigned to their groups. However, as everyone knows (or at least piously proclaims!), correlation does not necessarily imply causality. In Chapter 5 (Tables 5.5, 5.6), it was demonstrated that the difference in coherence between the sadomasochistic group, women and men ($n = 48$), and the control group, women and men ($n = 35$), remained significant, even when depression had been statistically controlled ('partialled out'). Furthermore, the 'depressed' control subjects were, on average, slightly better at metacognitive monitoring than the 'nondepressed' (Table 5.2, Figure 5.2*d*).

The idea that depression might bring about a *reduction* in coherence is not, on the face of it, implausible but, in the light of the present results from adult subjects, it is evidently not true. The more depressed adult control subjects in this study have, on average, a *greater* metacognitive faculty than those who are less depressed (Figure 7.3*a*). It is, however, totally implausible that depression with its accompanying mental incapacitation has brought this about. Let us get the horse back in position before the cart! If the control subjects are currently more coherent than the sadomasochists, it is not because they are more depressed but probably because the sadomasochists have long been less coherent. There must have been, and there must be still, another factor at work.

A sadomasochist's reaction to a harsh childhood is likely to have been in some important way different from that of an adult depressive. The Beck Depression Inventory and the Adult Attachment Interview seemed, from the start, appropriate instruments for probing this difference. Having employed the questionnaire, one appreciates that, with great economy of time and effort, it does, in fact, cover all the quintessential features of adult depression. For this context, it has two drawbacks: (a) it throws no light on childhood depression; (b) many respondents are self-deceptive. Offsetting these drawbacks, however, for the study of masochism, several items it contains have, as anticipated, proved to have discriminant potential—sense of failure, expectation of punishment, self-accusations, anxiety concerning body image change, and in the other direction, (little or no) loss of libido (Figure 7.2). I was already alerted by the results of the pilot study on depression, conducted in preparation for the present investigation, that one of the most important factors measured by the Adult Attachment Interview was coherence. Most of the depressed subjects in that pilot study, somewhat counterintuitively, scored high on coherence. With the larger numbers of the present study, the result is confirmed. How is one to explain it? Could these depressed people simply be more accurate in their perceptions of reality? The theory of 'the depressive as realist', subscribed to by Golin *et al.* (1977, 1979), Lewinsohn *et al.* (1980), Alloy & Abramson (1988) and others, links up with the 'appearance-reality distinction'

(Flavell *et al.* 1983) which Mary Main and colleagues are addressing with the interview scale of 'metacognitive monitoring'. The final link in this argument is that reality is sometimes depressing.

To be quite sure of making my train of thought plain, I will express it in a crass overstatement. The sadomasochists almost certainly were depressed also, but they fled to The Land of Masturbation Fantasy where witches and ogres could be made to yield pleasure as well as pain. One of the prices paid for this attempt to superimpose incompatible representations was coherence of mind.

The Adoptees

As evidenced in Table 7.4, these 7 adopted subjects did indeed provide support for the picture painted by Helene Deutsch (1937) of the pathological defences which may be called into play by early bereavement. Deutsch sometimes observed an absence of affect and later an exaggerated self-reliance, interspersed with periods of depression. In her view, this was the result of never mourning the childhood loss. As mentioned in the Introduction to this chapter, Aaron Beck also found a significant association between childhood bereavement and adult depression (Beck, 1967, chapter 14). Early bereavement, before assimilation of such a loss was possible and which was therefore never mourned, was, in fact, one of the possible aetiological factors of masochism I hypothesized at the beginning of this section. The fact, of itself, that five of these adoptees are sadomasochists and the other two are depressed would seem to support this hypothesis. What is worth noting is that the two depressed subjects, CS136 and CS284, received 'F' (valuing attachment) as well as 'Ds' (dismissing) classifications, and these were, of course, awarded long before this analysis was undertaken. Although CS284 said during his interview that he always felt like a cuckoo in somebody else's nest, and albeit F1a and F5 are at the borders of the 'F' category and not, as is F3, representative of it, these 'F' classifications nevertheless imply that these two men had not dismissed attachment issues completely. They were both, in fact, involved with public service, CS136 with the care of homeless people, alcoholics and those with mental health problems, CS284 with the representation of union members before tribunals. Both had been in therapy and both had made efforts to trace their natural mothers.

The sadomasochistic adoptees were angrily preoccupied (E2) where they were not dismissive. They had, of course, very different personalities one from another. ES4, for instance, was extremely unforthcoming throughout his interview, whereas ES69 had a fine, almost biblical, feeling for language. From the start of his interview, he expressed his hurt and resentment at being "dumped" (in his case, quite literally) by his natural mother. He did not, however, acknowledge any element of revenge in his SM activities: "everything and anything I do that is in the field of sadomasochism is consensual." This declaration was unprompted. It would seem to lend some support to the characteristic self-deception I mentioned in Chapter 4 under the heading 'hypocrisy'.

A Personal Theory Concerning Character Traits Tending to Lead to Depression

There are many different roads to depression, as there are to masochism. I believe Hubert Tellenbach's existential approach to depression, summarized in the Introduction to this chapter, is a persuasive one, often borne out in day-to-day experience. In my own control group, several depressed subjects appeared to be conscientious, scrupulous people who, as a result of these very qualities, arrived at a conflict of personal aspiration and commitment to others. One depressed female control subject in this investigation, CS206, even seemed to epitomize the qualities Tellenbach observed in many of his Heidelberg patients (Tellenbach, 1961). She was, as already described, a highly principled woman who perhaps took too much account of other people's feelings for her own good. She told me that she did not share her own problems much with other people, rather shut herself away when not putting in unpaid overtime. The strain of overwork is exacerbated for people like her when they are even interrupted, impeded, beleaguered in the struggle to perform tasks which are tiresome to them. The whole day is burdensome and joyless—all they ask is to be permitted to get on, not with their pleasures, but with their duties without obstruction.

I have made the somewhat related observation that a desire for privacy and a commitment to personal goals conspire to lead to loneliness, and thence sometimes to depression. To reveal feelings not only assuages them, it frequently evokes a warm response in others (witness the extraordinary public response to the death of Diana, Princess of Wales, probably due less to her good works than to her undoubted courage in revealing her feelings), but the habit of privacy usually springs from past betrayals of trust, mostly though not always, of course, in childhood. The achievement of personal goals often requires solitude. Other people make demands of attention and time which militate against completion of the undertakings on which one wishes to concentrate. But then the sacrifice of personal contact for the pursuit of an aspiration can suddenly seem sterile, particularly when it ends in fatigue rather than satisfaction. And then unfortunately, a clutching at company, be it human or animal, is seldom met with the hoped-for response.

Bereavement in adulthood, particularly where the person lost constituted the last remaining source of human warmth and emotional security, can precipitate depression at an even more basic level—that of identity. The stark insight which comes as you stand alone on the precipice and look into the void is that you *are* the various roles you fulfil and the experiences, not only your own, engraved in memory, but those adopted from others. Insofar as you have identified with another, the 'ego' is depleted in bereavement, and depression ensues.

I believe we become depressed when there are too many unacceptable insights present just beneath consciousness, when we have looked too hard at the human condition. We have shed illusions about our conspecifics and we carry the awareness that we have lost or are going to lose those nearest to us, even as we are going to die soon ourselves. This is eating of the tree of knowledge—simply knowing, having these things present in the mind, is enough to banish us from Eden. This is what the South African poet and naturalist Eugène Marais referred to as 'the pain of consciousness', pointing out with remarkable penetration that each person has his own form of intoxicating poison with which he tries to escape from this pain. As a morphine addict and almost certainly also a masochist, Marais was in a position to know. As we get older, life consists less of travelling hopefully and more of damage limitation, a struggle against the second law of thermodynamics. Little involuntary movements parallel the little uninvited thoughts which invade our minds. Arthur Miller once responded to an interviewer's question: "Well, most things *end* badly, don't they?" This is the meeting place of exogenous and endogenous depression. Life's sorrows can be dismissed to a limited extent and when that limit is reached, depression ensues—Winston Churchill's black dog emerges and lurks growling in the shadows. In other words, the etiology of depression is quantitative. One of Freud's major contributions was his economic model of mental processes—their seeming vagaries are quantitative. In this case, the dismissive defense against suffering is an effective one whilst it lasts, but when the last straw is laid, the retaining wall starts to crumble, and the sad misshapen creatures spring out startlingly from the past. Cognitive techniques of healthier habits of thought (Beck, 1967, pp. 318–330) can perhaps stave off a major depressive episode. Frequently, however, the theatre of the mind, because it can no longer tolerate being ignored, becomes the theatre of the body (McDougall, 1985, 1989)—somatization sets in and becomes ever more insistent. From middle age onwards, the physiological processes of involution are likely to add an endogenous element to exogenous depression, but meanwhile, mercifully, psychological defenses will probably keep unwelcome perceptions at bay, for nothing whatever follows from pessimism—"nothing will come of nothing," as King Lear rightly observed, though not otherwise notable for his judgment. Meanwhile, optimism, even resting partly on illusion, is more adaptive. The higher species are optimistic because they have to be in order to survive. If you are a wildebeest, it does not pay to think the lion is going to get *you*!

CHAPTER 8

QUESTIONNAIRES CONCERNING CHRONICITY, PRACTICE AND MOTIVATION OF SADOMASOCHISM

SUMMARY

Information gathered by 4 questionnaires is used to demonstrate attitudinal and behavioral differences within the sadomasochistic group (n = 48). As probably the most quintessential of masochism, a profile of the largely passive, depressed subgroup of males (n = 14) is pieced together statistically.

INTRODUCTION

Although the main thrust of this investigation was to throw light on the etiology of sadomasochism and although its main interest was a psychological one, it was, of course, indispensable to gain information on the actual behavior of the index group, and what motivated it. Discussion is revealing, but the most systematic and economic means of gathering such information remains the questionnaire. Dr Glenn Wilson and Dr Chris Gosselin of the Institute of Psychiatry (the old Maudsley Hospital, London) were extremely helpful when I was planning this area of the study. I had profitable conversations with both of them, and they both kindly agreed that I might adapt two of their well-tested questionnaires to my own purposes.

After the Adult Attachment Interview, the Beck Depression Inventory and the 'emotional' Stroop task had been concluded, therefore, two questionnaires were completed by all index subjects ($n = 48$), their responses to a third questionnaire were noted down by the interviewer ($n = 48$), a fourth questionnaire was handed or later posted to 20 of the index group who appeared most articulate and this questionnaire was completed, sometimes copiously, in all but 5 cases ($n = 15$). The exact wording of these four questionnaires is given in Appendix 5.

INSTRUMENTS

Each questionnaire was typewritten on a single sheet of paper.

(1) The first questionnaire was adapted from that appearing in Table 4 of Gosselin *et al.* (1991). It sought information on how often SM activities were included in the subject's sex life, whether he undertook a dominant or a submissive role, how easily the role could be switched, whether sexual orientation was heterosexual, bisexual or homosexual, how long he had been involved in the SM 'scene', whether the concern was for his own or his partner's enjoyment, what form that enjoyment took, how satisfactory he considered his sex life. The subject was asked to underline the most appropriate response to these questions (forced choice between two, three or four alternatives). Lastly, he was asked why he thought he had developed SM interests (an open-ended response).

(2) The second questionnaire was adapted from the Wilson Sex Fantasy Questionnaire (Wilson, 1988, pp. 46–48). It was very much shorter and was, in fact, headed 'Fantasy Questionnaire'. The activities probed were the four which were expected to be most widely representative of the index group, and they were listed first in passive then in active mode: being forced to do something, forcing someone else to do something, being whipped or spanked, whipping or spanking someone else, being hurt, inflicting pain on a partner, being tied up (bondage), tying someone else up. The subject was requested to evaluate on a scale of 0 to 3 the frequency with which he engaged in these activities, first in fantasy, then in reality. He was asked to state which of the listed activities he found most exciting, first in fantasy, then in reality. Finally, he was requested to describe briefly any favorite fantasy which had not been included in the list.

(3) The third questionnaire was headed 'Informal Questions,' and it was devised in part to obtain more detailed information as to chronicity, in part to check consistency with some of the

responses already made in the preceding questionnaires. Subjects were asked when they first became aware of their SM interests, what had first occasioned that awareness, how they had felt about it at the time, which activities they currently prefer, how often they engage in them, when precisely they last enacted one of these rituals, what they felt they gained from it, what their physical sensations were during one of these practices.

(4) The fourth questionnaire, 'Requesting your Opinion', was an attempt to obtain, from some of the more articulate members of the index group, explanations of issues which are perennially baffling: what constitutes the difference between an SM relationship and any other relationship, to what extent the subject's sexuality is focussed in the genitals, what attitude he takes to the subject of cruelty, whether there was an element of revenge involved and, if so, what the offense was which was inciting revenge, to what extent 'love' was associated with 'tenderness', with 'teasing', with 'pain', with 'betrayal', whether the subject had ever witnessed sexual intercourse as a child and interpreted it as aggression. Finally, comment is invited on an opaque definition of 'a generalized masochism', given by James Rusbridger before his death—masochistic pleasure is said to occur with the suppression of a strong reaction to an offensive situation in which there is also a sexual stimulus. (The precise quotation is given in the Discussion section and in Appendix 5. What is thereby being sought is, in fact, the subject's own explanation of the puzzle of masochism.)

Procedure

The answers to the first two questionnaires were written by the subject after the Adult Attachment Interview, the Beck Depression Inventory, the 'emotional' Stroop task and the free recall of words in the Stroop presentation had been concluded. The answers to the third questionnaire were mostly written down by the interviewer as the subject gave his response to each question. The fourth questionnaire was either handed to the subject or posted to the subject for his completion after due reflection. It was returned by post.

Statistical Analysis

It was established after relating AAI classifications to Stroop results (Chapter 6, Table 6.5) that the two classifications most closely associated with the sadomasochistic mind-set were the CC (Cannot Classify) and

E (Preoccupied or Entangled) classifications. This was determined after calculating an SM quotient, the ratio of each index subject's mean response time for the SM words in the Stroop presentation to his overall mean response time. The mean SM quotient obtained for the complete index group was then compared with the mean SM quotients obtained when the group was divided according to main AAI classifications.

The present chapter deals with external, day-to-day behavior and internal thought behavior (fantasies, attitudes) rather than unconscious or preconscious mental processing of stimuli. Another major difference is that it is based on the subjects' self-report, not an objective, computer-driven procedure. Nevertheless, mind-set is likely to be reflected in behavior, so two further measures of the influence of sadomasochism were devised:

(1) SM sum 1 derives from questions 1, 5 and 8 of Questionnaire 1 (see Appendix 5), probing how frequent, over how many years, how satisfactory SM involvement has been. The sum of scores on these responses would seem a fair measure of each subject's commitment to the sadomasochistic 'scene'.
(2) SM sum 2 derives from questions 1–8 of Questionnaire 2 (see Appendix 5). The frequencies with which the four main themes (forcing, whipping, hurting, bondage) are engaged in, both actively and passively, both in fantasy and in reality, would similarly, when scored and summed, seem to reflect fairly the degree of each subject's involvement in sadomasochistic practice.

These 3 measures (SM quotient, SM sum 1, SM sum 2) were together used to demonstrate a difference in extent of SM commitment between depressed and nondepressed index subjects. A further analysis of this difference was then undertaken by calculating separately, from the scores of Questionnaire 2, a Masochistic Sum, a Sadistic Sum, a Fantasy Sum and a Reality Sum. The correlation matrix, into which AAI passivity scale scores and BDI total scores were also introduced, would perhaps help to build a profile of the depressed index group in particular.

RESULTS

QUESTIONNAIRE 1

Details of sexual orientation, chronicity, practice and motivation of the sadomasochistic group ($n = 48$) are presented in Table 8.1. The numerical findings, summarizing the responses to all the forced-choice questions 1–8

TABLE 8.1. Details of Chronicity, Practice and Motivation of the Sadomasochistic Group ($n = 48$)

		Number of subjects	Percentage of index group
(1) Sex life in general involves SM activities	(a) Only sometimes	19	39.6
	(b) Fairly often	14	29.2
	(c) Nearly always	15	31.3
(2) In SM activities prefer to be	(a) Mostly or totally dominant	21	43.8
	(b) Mostly or totally submissive	27	56.3
(3) Can switch dominant submissive roles	(a) Very easily	14	29.2
	(b) Fairly easily	15	31.3
	(c) With difficulty or not at all	19	39.6
(4) Sexual orientation	(a) Totally or largely heterosexual	42	87.5
	(b) Totally or largely bisexual	5	10.4
	(c) Totally or largely homosexual	1	2.1
(5) In the SM 'scene'	(a) Less than 3 years	6	12.5
	(b) Three to six years	2	4.2
	(c) More than 6 years	40	83.3
(6) Take on SM role	(a) Mostly for own enjoyment	22	45.8
	(b) Equally for own and partner's enjoyment	24	50.0
	(c) Mostly for partner's enjoyment	2	4.2
(7) Type of enjoyment got out of SM	(a) A sexual turn-on	31	64.6
	(b) A mental 'high'	11	22.9
	(c) A sense of power	2	4.2
	(d) A thrill from partner's enjoyment	4	8.3
(8) Overall, sex life rated	(a) Very satisfactory	16	33.3
	(b) Moderately satisfactory	20	41.7
	(c) Not satisfactory	12	25.0

Section numbers on the left refer to the questions put in the first questionnaire (see Appendix 5).

of the first questionnaire, are set out so as to parallel the wording of the questionnaire (see Appendix 5). Responses to the last open-ended question, 'Why do you think you developed SM interests?' are dealt with separately in Table 8.2.

TABLE 8.2. Explanations Given by Index Subjects ($n = 48$) for their Development of SM Interests

	Depressed sadomasochists ($n = 14$)	Nondepressed sadomasochists ($n = 34$)
(a) Began with a fetish (rubber, leather, PVC)	ES7 ES27 ES40	ES8 ES39 ES63 ES76
(b) Adverse conditions in childhood		
(i) Mother to blame	ES20 ES28 ES61 ES80	ES21 ES37 ES50 ES63 ES74
(ii) Father to blame	ES28 ES52	ES21 ES23 ES37 ES63 ES74
(iii) School to blame	ES20 ES61	ES23 ES66 ES81
(iv) Inability to make friends	ES29	
(c) Precocious sexual development	ES18	
(d) Predisposition		
(i) Inherited	ES52	ES1 ES2 ES17 ES22 ES34 ES36 ES75
(ii) Observed behaviour (of father)	ES71	
(e) Specific experience or spectacle causing excitement	ES10	ES77
(f) Guilt requiring either punishment or coercion		ES15 ES50
(g) Escape from responsibility		ES50 ES51 ES62
(h) Shyness with opposite sex		ES26 ES50
(i) Reading SM literature	ES19	ES4
(j) Violent television or films		ES30 ES35
(k) SM clothing an art form		ES13 ES41
(l) SM as therapy		ES42 ES65
(m) Birth under certain astrological sign	ES20	
(n) No explanation	ES24	ES11 ES57 ES58 ES69

In response to the last, unnumbered question on Questionnaire 1, 'Why do you think you developed SM interests?' subjects occasionally volunteered more than one explanation and are therefore listed more than once. Some subjects felt unable to offer any explanation.

Fifteen subjects (31.3%) reported that their sex life nearly always involved SM activities (Table 8.1) and, as expected, more subjects preferred to adopt a submissive rather than a dominant role (56.3% vs 43.8%).

As to ability to 'switch' roles, 14 subjects reported that they could do so very easily, 15 fairly easily, and 19 with difficulty or not at all. The marked differences in these respects which emerged between the depressed and the nondepressed subgroups are discussed in the next section under the heading 'A profile of the depressed subgroup of sadomasochists'. The depressed subjects were more rigidly entrenched in a masochistic role, with a proportion of 11 : 3 submissive to dominant, and 8 out of 14 of the subjects in this subgroup unable to switch roles or finding any attempt to do so difficult.

Despite a strong impression of latent homosexuality in several cases, only one subject stated he was homosexual. As to the orientation of the other 47 subjects, 5 reported it as bisexual, the remaining 42 as heterosexual. ES69 was distinctly homophobic.

A large majority (40 out of 48 subjects) had been involved in the SM 'scene' for over 6 years. As to their reported motivation, 22 out of 48 performed mostly for their own enjoyment, 24 equally for their own and their partner's, only 2 performed mostly for their partner's enjoyment. The majority (31 out of 48 subjects) did so for a sexual 'turn-on', but there is, again on this point, a difference between the subgroups. Of the 14 depressed subjects, 12 apparently engaged in SM activity for a sexual 'turn-on', one subject (ES20) for a mental 'high', and the one remaining subject (ES10) for power. In the case of the 34 nondepressed subjects, although the majority (19 subjects) also engaged in SM ritual for a sexual 'turn-on', nevertheless 10 subjects did so because they obtained a mental 'high'.

Not surprisingly, 7 out of 14 (50%) depressed index subjects stated that they found their sex life unsatisfactory, as contrasted with 5 out of 34 (14.7%) nondepressed subjects. This suggested that the difference between the two subgroups was probably worth pursuing by means of the measure of SM commitment already outlined under 'Statistical analysis' at the end of the previous section. Designated SM sum 1, it was obtained for each subject simply by adding his scores on questions 1, 5 and 8 (see Table 8.1, Appendix 5), deemed a fair reflection of the extent of his SM involvement. The frequency of sadomasochistic practice and the length of time of the involvement were both scored 1, 2 or 3; degree of sexual satisfaction was scored 2, 1 or 0. This measure was applied in combination with another derived from Questionnaire 2 and designated SM sum 2. The results are therefore reported in Table 8.4 of the following subsection.

The explanations volunteered by all 48 index subjects in reply to the final question, 'Why do you think you developed SM interests?' are summarized in Table 8.2 and expanded in the Discussion section.

Individual subjects are listed against the causes they cited, and it can be seen at a glance (Table 8.2) that an inherited predisposition was a popular explanation with the nondepressed subgroup.

QUESTIONNAIRE 2

The results of questions 1–8, probing the frequency of involvement in four main themes (forcing, whipping, hurting, bondage) in both active and passive mode, in both fantasy and reality, are set out in Table 8.3, so

TABLE 8.3. Frequency of the Most Common SM Fantasies and Enactments as Reported by all 48 Index Subjects

	Never		Rarely		Sometimes		Often	
	F	R	F	R	F	R	F	R
Being forced	7	11	7	14	14	16	20	7
to do something	(14.6)	(22.9)	(14.6)	(29.2)	(29.2)	(33.3)	(41.7)	(14.6)
Forcing someone	14	20	12	14	13	8	9	6
to do something	(29.2)	(41.7)	(25.0)	(29.2)	(27.1)	(16.7)	(18.8)	(12.5)
Being whipped	7	6	11	11	8	18	22	13
or spanked	(14.6)	(12.5)	(22.9)	(22.9)	(16.7)	(37.5)	(45.9)	(27.1)
Whipping or	15	15	11	11	8	9	14	13
spanking someone	(31.3)	(31.3)	(22.9)	(22.9)	(16.7)	(18.8)	(29.2)	(27.1)
Being hurt	17	14	10	17	7	9	14	8
by a partner	(35.4)	(29.2)	(20.8)	(35.4)	(14.6)	(18.8)	(29.2)	(16.7)
Hurting	25	24	10	13	4	4	9	7
a partner	(52.1)	(50.0)	(20.8)	(27.1)	(8.3)	(8.3)	(18.8)	(14.6)
Being tied up	10	11	7	12	10	15	21	10
	(20.8)	(22.9)	(14.6)	(25.0)	(20.8)	(31.3)	(43.8)	(20.8)
Tying someone up	20	19	9	9	8	13	11	7
	(41.7)	(39.6)	(18.8)	(18.8)	(16.7)	(27.1)	(22.9)	(14.6)

Prevalence of these themes, assessed by adding subjects' scores on each

	Passive mode	*Active mode*	*Overall*
Forcing	162	113	275
Whipping	179	137	316
Hurting	125	87	212
Bondage	162	114	276

Use of these themes in passive (masochistic) mode can be seen to be significantly more prevalent than their use in active (sadistic) mode ($t_{46} = 2.80$, $p < 0.01$)

Employment of all four themes in fantasy = 581
Enactment of all four themes in reality = 498

Numbers given are actual numbers of subjects making the report, with percentages beneath in parentheses. F = Fantasy, R = Reality.

Their employment in fantasy can be seen to be significantly more prevalent than their enactment in reality ($t_{46} = 2.20$, $p < 0.05$).

as to parallel the layout of the questionnaire (see Appendix 5). Across the whole group of 48 index subjects, the order of prevalence of these themes was 'whipping', 'bondage', 'forcing' and 'hurting' (sums of scores: 316, 276, 275, 212, respectively). The differential between 'bondage' and 'forcing' is negligible here, but it becomes quite distinct when one moves from the frequency with which these themes are invoked to their respective excitement potentials (Figures 8.1 and 8.2).

As anticipated, the passive, or masochistic, mode of employing these themes emerged as significantly more prevalent than the active, or sadistic, mode ($t_{46} = 2.80$, $p < 0.01$). Unsurprisingly also, their employment in fantasy was significantly greater than their enactment in reality ($t_{46} = 2.20$, $p < 0.05$).

As already mentioned in the previous subsection, a third measure of SM commitment (the first two measures were SM quotient, derived from Stroop results, and SM sum 1, derived from Questionnaire 1) was calculated for each subject by simply adding all his scores in response to these 8 questions. The frequency with which he fantasized or enacted the four themes in both active and passive mode (scored 0 = never, 1 = rarely, 2 = sometimes, 3 = often), appearing to reflect fairly the extent of his SM involvement, was designated SM sum 2. All these measures were applied together in Table 8.4, with the aim of exploring further the difference in SM commitment between the depressed and the nondepressed index subjects. Although SM sum 1 was, in fact, the only one to achieve statistical significance ($t_{46} = 2.15$, $p = 0.037$), it can be seen that all three measures are in the same direction, showing the nondepressed group as apparently more committed to sadomasochism than the depressed group (SM quotient = 1.03 vs 1.01, SM sum 1 = 6.03 vs 4.93, SM sum 2 = 23.32 vs 20.43). One interpretation would be that the sadomasochism of the nondepressed subjects is more overt, but to be secure in this interpretation it would naturally be desirable to repeat the tests with larger numbers of subjects, when all three measures might show statistically significant differences between the subgroups.

This result, recalling the interaction which came to light in Chapter 5 between sadomasochism and depression with respect to passivity (Figure 5.2*e*), suggested that it might be possible to arrive at a profile of the depressed sadomasochists in particular. Table 8.5 presents mean scores and Pearson product-moment correlations which are relevant to this endeavour. Probably the most revealing and germane to the differentiation of the two subgroups are the Fantasy Sum, the Reality Sum, the Masochistic Sum and the Sadistic Sum. They were calculated by adding, respectively, as their designations imply, the scores in the left-hand 'fantasy' column, the right-hand 'reality' column, the scores of the masochistic themes (questions 1, 3,

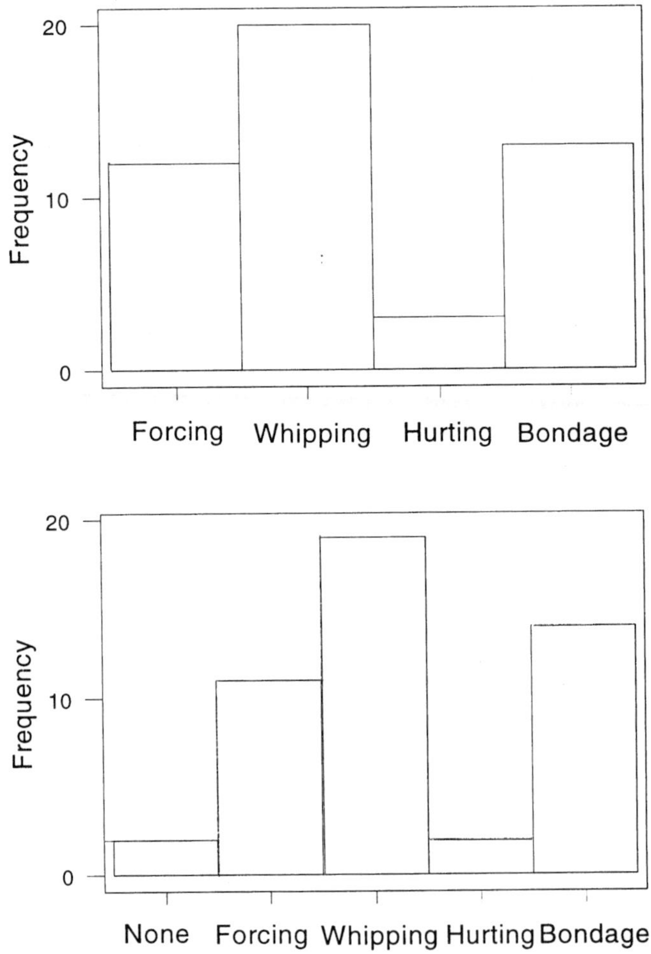

FIGURE 8.1. The SM theme (irrespective of whether in active or passive mode) found to be the most exciting of those listed in Table 8.3, in fantasy (above), in reality (below), as reported by all 48 index subjects. In each case the vertical axis shows the number of subjects. The order of preference is clearly Whipping, Bondage, Forcing, Hurting, both in fantasy and in reality. Two subjects, ES71 and ES76, claimed that they had enacted none of these themes in reality, only fantasized.

5, 7), and those of the sadistic themes (questions 2, 4, 6, 8) of Questionnaire 2 (see Appendix 5). The depressed group in which we are interested appears to be more sadistic than masochistic when fantasizing ($r = 0.740$, $p < 0.01$, as compared with $r = 0.326$, n.s., both 2–tailed) and also more given to fantasy than enactment in reality (mean Fantasy

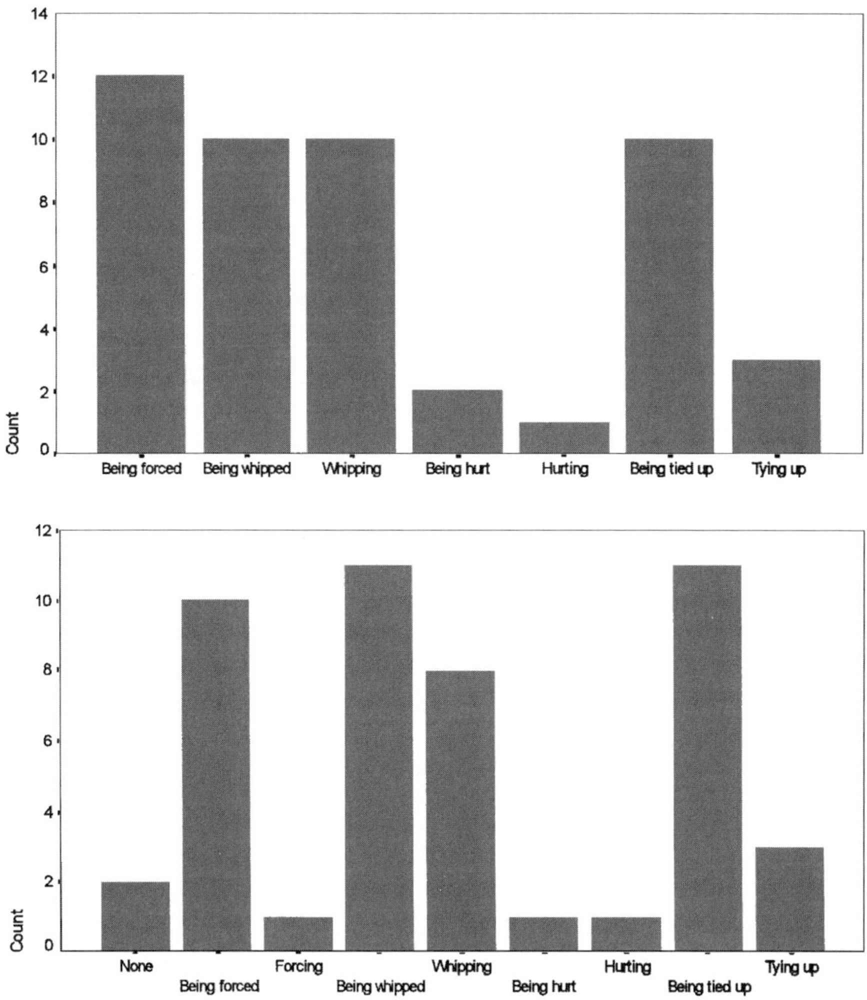

FIGURE 8.2. The SM theme (active and passive modes now separated) found to be the most exciting of those listed in Table 8.3, in fantasy (above), in reality (below), as reported by all 48 index subjects. In each case the vertical axis shows the number of subjects. No subject reported 'Forcing' as most exciting fantasy. Two subjects, ES71 and ES76, claimed that they had enacted none of these themes in reality, only fantasized.

Sum = 12.21, S.E. 0.90, mean Reality Sum = 8.21, S.E. 1.17). In their actualizations in reality, they are, of course, apparently more masochistic than sadistic ($r = 0.665$, $p < 0.01$, as compared with $r = 0.494$, n.s., both 2-tailed). These associations are reversed in the case of the nondepressed

Table 8.4. A difference in the extent of sadomasochistic commitment between depressed index subjects and nondepressed index subjects, as indicated by three measures: mean SM quotient, mean SM sum 1, mean SM sum 2

SM quotient (derived from Stroop results*)	$= \dfrac{\text{mean response time for SM words}}{\text{overall mean response time}}$
SM sum 1 (derived from Questionnaire 1⁺)	= question 1 score + question 5 score + question 8 score = how often (score 1, 2 or 3) + how long (score 1, 2, or 3) + how satisfactory (score 2, 1 or 0)
SM sum 2 (derived from Questionnaire 2⁺)	= sum of all scores on questions 1–8 = sum of frequencies of forcing, whipping, hurting, bondage fantasies or enactments in reality (scored 0 = never, 1 = rarely, 2 = sometimes, 3 = often)
Depressed sadomasochists ($n = 14$)	SM quotient = 1.01 SM sum 1 = 4.93 SM sum 2 = 20.43
Nondepressed sadomasochists ($n = 34$)	SM quotient = 1.03 SM sum 1 = 6.03 SM sum 2 = 23.32

SM sum 1 was the only measure to show a statistically significant difference between the subgroups ($t_{46} = 2.15$, $p = 0.037$), but this may be a function of sample size. With present numbers, the nondepressed group appears to have more sadomasochistic involvement on all three measures than the depressed group, and in future work with larger numbers, these mean differences might all be reasonably expected to become statistically significant.
*See Appendix 4.
⁺See Appendix 5.

group: they are slightly more masochistic than sadistic in their fantasies ($r = 0.632$, $p < 0.001$, as compared with $r = 0.607$, $p < 0.001$, both 2-tailed) but enactment in reality does not lag as far behind fantasy as it does in the case of the other subgroup (mean Fantasy Sum = 12.06, S.E. 0.97, mean Reality Sum 11.27, S.E. 0.92). In their activities in reality, they are, it appears, more sadistic than masochistic ($r = 0.710$, $p < 0.001$, as compared with $r = 0.479$, $p < 0.01$, both 2-tailed). These correlations are not independent, since they are based on the same subjects within either subgroup (14 depressed, 34 nondepressed, respectively), so it was necessary to take this lack of independence into account when testing their statistical significance. Williams (1959) devised a more stringent test of the difference between two nonindependent correlations than the traditional solution proposed by Hotelling (1931) and this test was later endorsed by Steiger (1980).

TABLE 8.5. An attempt to differentiate the depressed and nondepressed subgroups of sadomasochists by means of 6 variables: Masochistic Sum, Sadistic Sum, Fantasy Sum, Reality Sum, Passivity (AAI scale), Depression (BDI total score), presented as (a) means (standard errors in parenthesis), (b) Pearson product-moment correlations

	All subjects ($n = 48$)		Depressed subjects ($n = 14$)		Nondepressed subjects ($n = 34$)	
(a)						
Masochistic Sum	13.08	(0.82)	13.71	(1.44)	12.82	(1.01)
Sadistic Sum	9.40	(0.99)	6.71	(1.58)	10.50	(1.20)
Fantasy Sum	12.10	(0.73)	12.21	(0.90)	12.06	(0.97)
Reality Sum	10.38	(0.75)	8.21	(1.17)	11.27	(0.92)
Passivity (AAI scale)	3.90	(0.28)	5.07	(0.45)	3.41	(0.31)
Depression (BDI total)	10.71	(1.14)	21.00	(1.62)	6.47	(0.57)

(b)	Mas.Sum	Sad.Sum	Fantasy	Reality	Passivity
(i) *All index subjects* ($n = 48$)					
Sad.Sum	−0.044				
Fantasy	0.569	0.600			
Reality	0.481	0.686	0.441		
Passivity	0.183	−0.384	−0.052	−0.255	
Depression	0.195	−0.203	0.112	−0.162	0.371
(ii) *Depressed subjects* ($n = 14$)					
Sad.Sum	−0.234				
Fantasy	0.326	0.740**			
Reality	0.665**	0.494	0.634**		
Passivity	0.205	−0.291	0.011	−0.148	
Depression	0.610*	−0.125	0.182	0.443	0.219
(iii) *Nondepressed subjects* ($n = 34$)					
Sad.Sum	0.036				
Fantasy	0.632***	0.607***			
Reality	0.479**	0.710***	0.433**		
Passivity	0.157	−0.328	−0.080	−0.173	
Depression	0.039	0.114	0.226	−0.047	−0.029

Masochistic Sum, Sadistic Sum, Fantasy Sum, Reality Sum calculated, for each subject, by adding, respectively, his scores on masochistic themes (questions 1, 3, 5, 7), scores on sadistic themes (questions 2, 4, 6, 8), scores in the left-hand 'fantasy' column, scores in the right-hand 'reality' column of Questionnaire 2 (see Appendix 5).
*$p < 0.05$, **$p < 0.01$, ***$p < 0.001$.

Williams' formula, which is also recommended by Howell (1987, p. 243), was therefore applied to the values from Table 8.5 just reported above. They did not, in fact, reach statistical significance but, again, this might be because of the relatively small numbers involved. To demonstrate conclusively that these are real differences would require the tests to be repeated on larger groups of subjects. Meanwhile, the behavioral differences which may be inferred from these (albeit at this point nonsignificant) statistical differences are examined in the Discussion section, under the subheading 'A profile of the depressed subgroup of sadomasochists'.

Response to the question on Questionnaire 2 concerning the most exciting of the themes listed above it, (a) in fantasy, (b) in reality, is depicted visually in Figures 8.1 and 8.2. Figure 8.1 shows clearly that whipping, bondage and forcing, in descending order, are the preferred themes both in fantasy and in reality. Only three subjects admitted excitement from the infliction of pain: ES20 found it exciting to be hurt in fantasy, ES52 in both fantasy and reality; only ES58, a female subject, found it exciting to hurt someone else, both in fantasy and in reality. There were two subjects, ES71 and ES76, who stated that they had enacted none of these themes in reality, only fantasized. (On the other hand, ES69 was adamant that he only carried rituals out in reality, never fantasized, however, with not unusual sadomasochistic inconsistency, when he came to this question he found whipping someone exciting in fantasy as well as in reality!) Figure 8.2 separates the response to this question into active/dominant versus passive/submissive mode. It can be seen that no subject found most excitement in the fantasy of forcing someone to do something and only one (ES4) in the reality. Tying someone up is markedly less rewarding, it appears, than being tied up: 3 votes vs 10 in fantasy, 3 vs 11 in reality!

The final question on Questionnaire 2 which enquires whether a favorite fantasy has been omitted and, if so, invites the subject to describe it briefly, is dealt with in the next section where responses are noted and simultaneously discussed.

QUESTIONNAIRE 3

Figure 8.3 presents the approximate age at which SM interests were first noticed, as reported by all 48 index subjects. The depressed subjects are shown on the left, the nondepressed on the right, with each subgroup arranged in ascending order of 'ES' numbers. The mean age at which such interests were first noticed, according to the reports of the index group as a whole ($n = 48$), was 13.56 years. When the subgroups are plotted separately (below), the age reported by the depressed subgroup ($n = 14$) is, on average, two years younger than that reported, on average, by the nondepressed subgroup ($n = 34$) (12.07 and 14.18 years, respectively). Since this picture is slightly distorted by the presence of outliers, it is worth noting that the median age at which SM interests were noticed was 13, 12.5 and 13 years, for the whole index group, the depressed subgroup and the

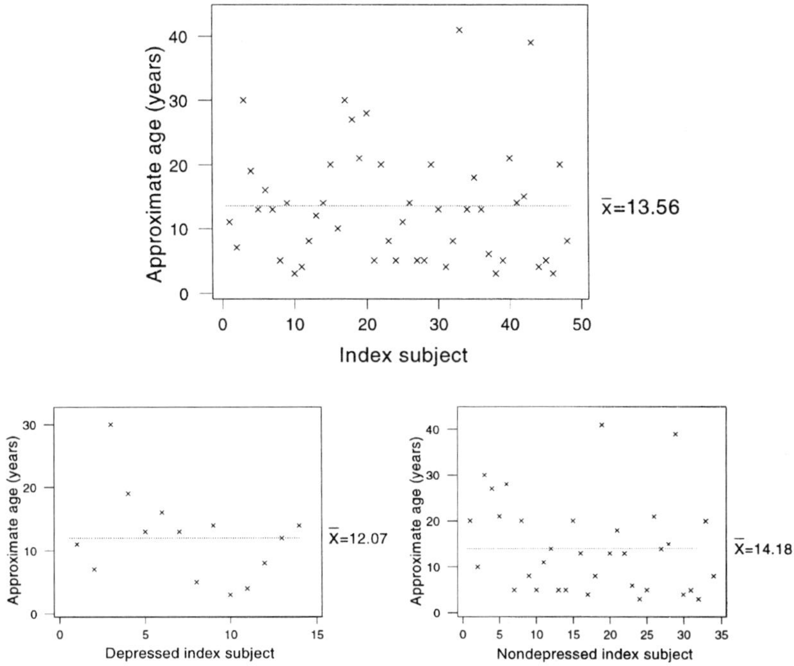

FIGURE 8.3. The approximate age (in years) at which SM interests were noticed, as reported by all 48 index subjects. Depressed subjects ($n = 14$) on the left, nondepressed subjects ($n = 34$) on the right, each subgroup arranged in ascending order of 'ES' numbers; both subgroups combined (above), subgroups separated (below). The age at which depressed subjects reported noticing their SM interests was, on average, two years earlier than that reported, on average, by nondepressed subjects, both having a mean around the age of puberty but several reports of SM interest long before the usual age of puberty.

nondepressed subgroup, respectively. Both subgroups have, therefore, a mean and a median around the age of puberty but it will be noticed that there are many reports of interest in sadomasochism long before the usual age of puberty. Precocious sexual development is, I would suggest, one of the hallmarks of sadomasochism. Overall, there were 22 reports of awareness of SM proclivities before the age of 12 years—6 out of 14 in the depressed subgroup, 16 out of 34 in the nondepressed. If one includes ES71, who reported noticing his SM interest at the age of 12, half of the depressed subjects were already on that path of sexual development before the usual age of puberty, some from the ages of 3, 4 or 5. The picture is, in fact, not very different with respect to the nondepressed subgroup where 47% were heading in that direction before the usual age of puberty, some, again, from as young as 3, 4 or 5.

Table 8.6. The Extent to which Love is Associated with (1) Tenderness, (2) Teasing, (3) Pain, (4) Betrayal, as Reported by all 15 Sadomasochistic Subjects Responding to Questionnaire 4.

Love associated with	Not at all	Somewhat	Largely	Completely
(1) Tenderness	0 (0.0)	2 (13.3)	8 (53.3)	5 (33.3)
(2) Teasing	4 (26.7)	10 (66.7)	1 (6.7)	0 (0.0)
(3) Pain	3 (20.0)	7 (46.7)	4 (26.7)	1 (6.7)
(4) Betrayal	10 (66.7)	4 (26.7)	0 (0.0)	1 (6.7)

Scoring: Not at all = 0, Somewhat = 1, Largely = 2, Completely = 3.
Extent of association of love with (1) Tenderness = 33, (2) Teasing = 12, (3) Pain = 18, (4) Betrayal = 7. Depicted visually as Fig. 8.4.
For wording of Questionnaire 4 see Appendix 5. Numbers given are actual numbers of subjects making the report, with percentages in parentheses.

The other information gathered on Questionnaire 3, in response to questions 2–8, was too diverse to be meaningfully tabulated. It will, however be summarized and simultaneously discussed in the next section.

QUESTIONNAIRE 4

This questionnaire (for wording see Appendix 5) was completed by 15 out of 20 sadomasochistic subjects, selected for their apparent articulateness. Only question no. 5, 'To what extent do you associate love with tenderness, with teasing, with pain, with betrayal?' lent itself to numerical scoring (Not at all = 0, Somewhat = 1, Largely = 2, Completely = 3). The responses to this question are presented in Table 8.6 and depicted visually in Figure 8.4. It can be seen at a glance that these 15 sadomasochists, as a group, associated love chiefly with tenderness, then with pain, then with teasing, then with betrayal, in the respective proportions 33 : 18 : 12 : 7.

With respect to question no. 6, 'Did you ever witness sexual intercourse as a child and take it to be an aggressive act?' none of the 15 respondents reported witnessing sexual intercourse in childhood, and most answered with a simple 'no'.

The other questions, being open-ended, are dealt with in the next section, where information gathered from them is reported and simultaneously discussed.

FURTHER NONNUMERICAL INFORMATION AND DISCUSSION

One of the aims of this section is to present, using the material acquired by questionnaire, a type of profile of the depressed subgroup of

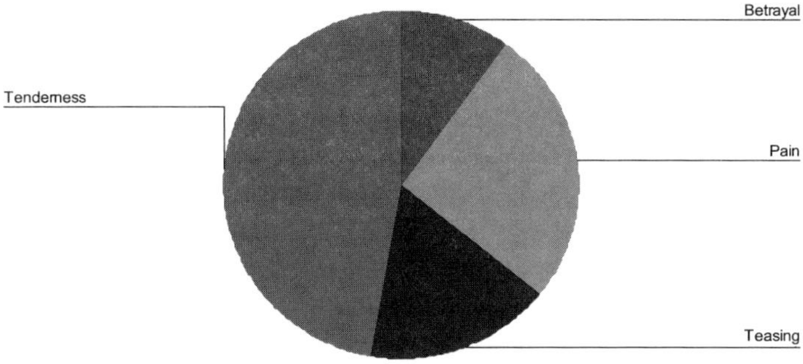

FIGURE 8.4. The extent (see Table 8.6) to which love is associated with tenderness, with teasing, with pain, with betrayal, as reported by all 15 sadomasochistic subjects responding to Questionnaire 4 (see Appendix 5).

index subjects, since it was this subgroup which struck me as important to the characterization and understanding of masochism. First, however, the four questionnaires will be further reported and discussed separately.

QUESTIONNAIRE 1

The proportion of subjects whose sex life nearly always involved SM activities was 31.3% in this study (Table 8.1). This proportion is almost identical to that of 32% found by Gosselin *et al.* (1991), even though their sample was one of sadomasochistic women. Considerably more subjects preferred to adopt a submissive role rather than a dominant role (56.3% vs 43.8%). These proportions are also almost identical to those quoted by Gosselin *et al.* (1991): 57% vs 41%. Here, however, the two reports diverge, though proportions remain similar in some cases, for instance, in the large proportion of subjects responding that they engage in SM activities for 'a sexual turn-on': 64.6% in this study, 53% in Gosselin *et al.* (1991). Some divergence is only to be expected, not only as a result of individual differences but also when the constitution of the two samples differs so radically as to gender (the sample under present investigation is preponderantly male) and as to the length of time there had been involvement in the SM 'scene' (83.3% of the present, predominantly male, group had been involved for more than six years, in contrast to the 34% reported by Gosselin *et al.* for their female group).

The explanations brought forward by index subjects in response to the question, 'Why do you think you developed SM interests?' (Table 8.2) invite comparison with the possible causative factors listed in Table 5.8 and in Appendix 3. Apart from ill-treatment in childhood, they were very different. They were generally, in fact, neither particularly insightful nor particularly plausible. Above all, they did not really address the question 'why?' Many subjects simply stated what attraction SM activities held for them, the benefits and pleasures they provided.

ES7 pointed out that when buying fetishistic materials (rubber, leather or PVC clothing) magazines were on offer on subjects such as domination/submission. His interest thus deepened by reading about other aspects of SM. ES39 roughly endorsed this account. Although not stated specifically in reply to Questionnaire 1, fetishism was quite commonly the introduction to the SM 'scene'.

ES29 cited an inability to form 'normal' relationships, and explained that he meant 'loving', not sexual, relationships.

ES7, ES27 and ES40 all spoke of an initial urge to 'cross-dress', often in garments belonging to their mothers or sisters. It would seem more than fortuitous that their mothers had wanted a girl-child. ES40 explained that he could not accept his behavior so had to fantasize that he was tied up and compelled to wear female garments.

ES80 felt that he was seeking a comforting mother-child relationship in which he could be dependent again.

Although he offered no explanation as to *why* he had *originally* developed SM interests, ES11 wrote a miniessay in response to this question, with paragraph headings: Sense of mutual communication, The visual aspects, The unknown, The innovative, The forbidden, People. The nub of this eloquent defence was that SM involvement was a positive vehicle for communication and trust.

ES37 attributed his SM interests to being spanked in front of the other family members. The presence of onlookers seemed to be of importance to several subjects and surfaced again in the 'favorite fantasies' described at the end of Questionnaire 2. This need for onlookers is, in my view, a combination of Theodor Reik's 'demonstrative factor' (Reik, 1939) and the conversion of a moment of intense shame into mastery of the situation: "I will gain pleasure out of being made a spectacle!"

ES50 expressed a very common attitude: "... if my partner *demands* sexual services, I am not responsible—I am doing just as she wishes and I am then free to enjoy the sexual realease [*sic*] without guilt." The requirement to be compelled to perform sexual acts would appear to stem directly from an inhibited, puritanical attitude towards sex in the childhood home. No acknowledgment, no information, no advice was forthcoming from a prudish mother or an embarrassed father. Sexual activity (usually masturbation) was dirty, dangerous and quite properly associated with guilt. How being urinated or defecated upon can be seen as less offensive remains one of the puzzles of masochism—presumably because the humiliation is dictated by the recipient and takes him back to the indignities and defiance surrounding 'potty training'!

ES63 noted the accident which befell him as a small child (when he was one-and-a-half years old he was badly scalded). He was asked to expand this but, rather than drawing any inference about the pain involved, he recalled a rubber sheet on the hospital bed. It seems possible that an intense physical stimulus, such as pain, might sometimes lie at the root of a fetish. "The factor of intensity, in the case of pain, is not a matter of complete indifference," Freud observed, "... in the case of a great number of internal processes sexual excitation arises as a concomitant effect, as soon as the intensity of those processes passes beyond certain quantitative limits" (Freud, 1905, S.E. *7*, pp. 204–205). The endogenous opioids produced as a result of protracted pain might cause rubber to become part of an addiction, a little like the syringe and other paraphernalia of exogenous opiate addiction.

ES74 mentioned the excitement he remembered, stemming from the sense of enclosure in his childhood cot. This was in his parents' bedroom, causing him to be jealous of their sexual relationship.

ES75 thought her interest was genetically determined. Blithely, she said she had noticed it in her son—she had seen him bind his wrists. As can be seen from Table 8.2, the idea of an inherited predisposition was more popular with the nondepressed than the depressed subjects. Presumably it absolved them of any need for heart-searching. There was, after all, nothing to be done about inborn inclinations—one might as well banish recriminations from one's mind.

Specific occasions were cited as causal by two subjects. ES10 became sexually excited whilst watching an escapology act around the age of seven or eight; ES77 was tied, naked and spreadeagled, to the ground whilst camping as a twelve-year-old (he did, however, also mention the effect of skintight clothing as a ballet pupil). These are the concrete interpretations likely to be made where theory of mind is lacking. In general, the index group was not at ease with the question '*Why* do you think you developed SM interests?' Of course, anyone, not only a sadomasochist, might find it difficult to explain his own sexuality. Is this lack of psychological insight in any way specific, therefore, to this SM group? In some ways, yes, (a) since their sexuality figured so largely in their interests and concerns, (b) since most showed signs of an ambivalent attitude, a degree of unease, regarding their deviance, (c) since they had elected to come and talk about it in a Department of Psychology, (d) since many of them had expressed an interest in understanding it in their initial communication. All these considerations might reasonably be expected to act as incentives towards a measure of prior introspection. But there were scant signs of genuine self-scrutiny in response to this question 'why?' which offered, after all, an opportunity to assume the knowledgeable role. At least, some respondents had the honesty to state that they had not the faintest idea. These were mostly in the rather more dismissive, nondepressed subgroup.

Questionnaire 2

This questionnaire's main area of investigation was the relative prevalence of four sadomasochistic themes. The results showed conclusively (a) that 'whipping', 'bondage', 'forcing', 'hurting' represented a descending order of popularity in both fantasy and reality; (b) that, overall, fantasy scores were higher than scores for enactment in reality (across all 48 subjects, mean Fantasy Sum = 12.10, S.E. 0.73; mean Reality Sum = 10.38, S.E. 0.75); (c) that, overall, masochistic themes were more espoused than their sadistic counterparts (for all 48 subjects, mean Masochistic Sum = 13.08, S.E. 0.82; mean Sadistic Sum = 9.40, S.E. 0.99).

Whipping and bondage are, of course, the two themes most readily traced to actual childhood experiences. It should be remembered that these sadomasochistic subjects *all* had less than optimal childhoods in one way or another. It is only necessary to compare the mean AAI scores for probable childhood experience of index versus control groups, set out in Table 5.2 of Chapter 5, to remind oneself of that fact. Not one single individual in the index group received a primary 'F' (Secure) classification. It is not, therefore, difficult to discern that the entity who is administering the whipping is most frequently a stern mother figure, occasionally a composite of parent, nurse or teacher. A desire for bondage would seem, for the most part, to go back to actual physical memories of the restriction of movement in early childhood.

Responses to the last question, at the foot of Questionnaire 2, regarding any favorite fantasies which might have been omitted from the list above, were informative, though hardly unexpected. One of the most striking features was the frequency of fetishistic material. For example, ES7 fantasized that he was a slave, dressed in rubber, licking the high-heeled boots of a 'dominatrix'. At least 10 other subjects (ES8, ES15, ES18, ES19, ES20, ES26, ES27, ES28, ES39, ES76) described fantasies with a fetishistic content. Many concerned 'cross-dressing' (e.g., ES26, ES74) with obvious implications of (fear of) homosexuality. The typical transvestite claims adamantly to be heterosexual but 'the lady doth protest too much, methinks'.

Several favorite fantasies concerned bondage (e.g., ES10, ES13, ES42, ES76) but notably, there were only two which concerned real pain, as a definite goal, rather than as a by-product of being beaten: ES2 wrote "electrical torture" as his response, and ES52 wrote, "Being severely tortured by a loving partner (not life-threateningly—sensually)." Both men were academics (!) but in the latter case, there was apparently no perception of any implicit contradiction in a *loving* partner who metes out severe *torture*. No misgivings, no uneasy or distressed mental state is attributed to her, because she is evidently a mindless object dispensing a strange brand of pleasure.

As already mentioned, several favorite fantasies, such as those involving whipping or caning (e.g., ES1, ES19, ES22), would obviously also be painful, but more involved humiliation, mostly implied but sometimes explicitly stated (e.g., ES8, ES15, ES24, ES28, ES40, ES42, ES51, ES81). There was a childish greediness about some of them (e.g., ES11, ES27, ES62, ES77)—they wanted everything, including the kitchen sink! ES11 indulged himself with "all of the themes listed above over 8–10 hours, possibly up to 48 hours, in a sensual and sensitive manner." ES58 wrote "Lots!" but did not go on to specify. She also twice wrote "*N.B.* with consent only," against 'Forcing someone to do something' and 'Hurting a partner', but consent is hardly plausible in the case of fantasy, and why, after all, should it be necessary?

Onlookers were often a requirement (e.g., ES28, ES50, ES62). In his fantasy of tying up a female partner, ES13 required another female as an assistant, also dominating the 'victim' (quite a parental pair with sex-changed offspring, one might speculate!). ES22 was observing a woman being spanked. ES36 was observing chain gangs of males and females. These fantasies involving onlookers create the strong impression that they arose as a result of real incidents of public humiliation in childhood and, indeed, several subjects actually described occasions when they were deliberately punished in front of relatives or friends.

Some fantasies were highly specified, had possibly been honed over a considerable period. ES19 stipulated whipping or being whipped in appropriate fetishistic clothing and, when this was probed, he explained that a woman partner should be in exotic *lingerie* of black leather or PVC, looking 'tarty' and dominant in stiletto heels, whilst he, himself, when in submissive role would be skimpily clad in one item of underwear; if he was dominating he would be in a conventional suit. ES15 specified the following chain of events: being forced to dress in female clothing, being told he looked like a whore, being told he would have to 'service' punters, being punished.

The favorite fantasies described in response to this last question of Questionnaire 2 were, thus, often elaborate but they were also often stereotyped, as, for instance, the response written by ES20: "Females dressed in SM clothing, torturing men in a dungeon and having female slaves giving them (the women) oral sex." Some were simply vague, like ES17 whose fantasy was "dominating a partner who wishes to be submissive."

There were 13 subjects (ES4, ES21, ES23, ES29, ES34, ES37, ES41, ES57, ES61, ES63, ES65, ES66, ES69) who stated that they had no favorite fantasy to add to those listed on the questionnaire, but only 2 of these subjects (ES29 and ES61) belonged to the depressed subgroup, where sexual release depended so much on fantasy. ES80 had likewise stated that he had no fantasy to add, but when queried about what he precisely envisioned under 'being forced to do something' (his most exciting fantasy), he opted for being forced to do domestic duties, to stand in the corner. Also of this depressed subgroup, ES71 evidently had a favorite fantasy but he stated, chillingly, that he would rather not indicate it.

Questionnaire 3

It can be seen clearly from Figure 8.3 that sadomasochistic interests often dated from an early age (22 out of 48 subjects noticed them before the age of 12, another subject actually at the age of 12, some reporting them from the first five years of life). This links up with the general precocity of sexual development which was alluded to by several subjects (ES58, for instance, experienced the menarche at 10 years of age) and which could be deduced in many cases, even when not stated explicitly. Together these facts point to the process of erotization of emotional trauma on the one hand, and of depression, boredom and loneliness on the other, already postulated in Chapter 7.

Responses to the second question, asking what happened on the occasion which brought first awareness of sadomasochistic interests, were all individual, of course, but they might be summarized under the following headings: excitement on first encounter with rubber, or on first purchase of fetishistic clothing, or on first putting on mother's clothing, particularly underwear, masturbation or, at least, erection following pornographic reading, mostly, but not always, a subculture magazine, occasionally a sadistic film sequence, even excitement caused by sadistic material on the radio, sexual arousal connected with childhood beatings which were either experienced, witnessed or described, excitement about caning at school or the threat of caning, or as a result of being tormented at school, childhood games involving tying up, masturbation associated with some form of physical restraint, spanking someone who enjoyed it, excitement confused with a need to urinate. ES20 described sexual excitement on smacking a dog. He also alluded later to burning and decapitating pigeons, but maltreatment of animals was certainly not typical of the people I interviewed. On the contrary, ES58 shed genuine tears about the death of a Great Dane that had been her main childhood companion.

In rare cases, the subject first noticed the unusual nature of his own fantasy: ES21, for instance, fantasized at the age of 8 that he was kept in a cage in the school hall where the girls would pay attention to him and be caring. It might be argued that the assessment of a fantasy requires metacognition and could help a child to arrive at the distinction between appearance and reality (Flavell *et al.* 1983). The marked proclivity of the sadomasochist to fantasize leads, however, neither to a developed metacognitive faculty nor to a perception of reality. It invariably ends in stereotypy and a disregard for reality. If one searches for the reason why this is so, it probably lies in the association with sexual excitement, in the extreme coercive power of the sex drive and of deviant sexual aims in particular, for the latter are the 'polymorphously perverse' aims of infancy which insists on endless repetition. There is no freedom of the imagination in sadomasochistic fantasy. Its very subject matter is doom and bondage. Its themes are hackneyed.

Answers to question 3, which asked how the subject felt about it when he first became aware of his SM interests, fell into 4 main categories: 'I liked it' (17 responses), 'Guilty' (15 responses), 'Excited' (14 responses), 'Puzzled' (9 responses). Five subjects said they felt embarrassed, three replied explicitly that they felt they wanted to repeat the experience, two reported that they felt frightened. Many subjects responded with a dual, usually conflicting, reaction. ES17, for instance, said that he felt "physical pleasure but mental guilt". ES26 replied that he felt pleased when, at 14, he dressed in his mother's clothes but relieved when, at 17, he saw men being submissive to women in a magazine and realized he was "not the only one". The adopted subject, ES69, said: "It was where I'd been trying to get all my life." When he was 10 years old, ES52 was tied to the bed in his school dormitory and tormented. He did not admit enjoyment—this was his response to question 3. He was certainly one of those subjects who did not accept their deviant sexuality and, of course, he belonged to the depressed subgroup. The impression he made was of being 'uptight', continually pulling away from one as he sat in his chair.

Question 4, enquiring which activities the subject preferred, acted as a check on what he had written down himself in response to Questionnaire 2, particularly with respect to the sadomasochistic theme found most exciting in reality. There appeared to be no glaring discrepancies. These people who had come forward for interview were prepared to be honest and, more than that, were eager, for the most part, to tell someone about their deviance. Thus, relative preference (see Figure 8.1) for the main activities remained roughly the same: Whipping (25 responses),

Bondage (21 responses), Domination/Submission (13 responses). Again, subjects often cited more than one activity in response to this question. Some subjects also expressed preferences for fetishistic materials or transvestite interests: rubber/leather/PVC (8 responses), cross-dressing (3 responses). The latter were explicit responses to question 4 but they underrepresent the prevalence of transvestism, particularly if account is taken of the frequency with which subjects, as they reported at other points in their interviews, donned their mothers' corsets, stockings, rubber macs and high-heeled boots! Yet ES7, when expressing a *penchant* for being tied up as a slave and punished with whip, tawse, strap or hand, stipulated rather primly, "by a woman *only*"! ES52 included 'electricity' and 'piercing' amongst his favorite torments. The only other subject to mention 'piercing' explicitly was the female subject, ES58. 'Humiliation' was only mentioned specifically by ES35 who said he was "not too much into pain"—what he liked was submission and to be "deduced, decoded, found out." He used to fantasize that he was caught in the woods, masturbating, by a woman and exposed, even blackmailed. ES74 said that what delighted him was role play, theatre—violence was now secondary. It will be recalled that two subjects claimed that they only fantasized, never performed any sadomasochistic acts in reality. The 64-year-old, depressed subject, ES71, said of his fantasies of torture leading to masturbation that they only occurred twice a week now, where they had formerly occurred 4 or 5 times a week. The younger (44-year-old) ES76 fantasized that he was being restrained under the control of a female partner, wearing shiny plastic, more than once a week either for masturbation or whilst making love to his wife.

Frequency of occurrence was, in fact, probed with question 5. The chosen ritual appeared to be enacted regularly, but at various intervals: once a month (11 responses), once a week (9 responses), every 2 months (7 responses), every 2 or 3 weeks (also 7 responses), once or twice a week (5 responses), 3 times a week (4 responses), every day (also 4 responses), every 3 months (1 response). Four subjects were reluctant to indicate specifically and confined their reply to a noncommittal "not very often". Several stated that their SM activities had been more frequent in the past than they were at present. ES34, for instance, pondered wistfully how often he caned his wife: "Once a month or once every six weeks—of course, there'd be straight sex going on in between—but it used to be 2 or 3 times a week." Sadomasochistic rituals would seem, therefore, to suffer the same ultimate decline in frequency as ordinary sexual relations (dubbed 'vanilla sex' by SM practitioners). Partly due to the prominence of masturbation, the overall impression was, however, one of more-than-average preoccupation with their own sexual gratification. This impression was, of course, reinforced by the statement of 22 out of 48 subjects on

Questionnaire 1 that their SM activity was mostly for their own enjoyment (Table 8.1).

Question 6, asking when the SM activity was last engaged in, brought a similar spectrum of statements: last week (18 responses), 3 weeks ago (8 responses), 3 months ago (6 responses), 2 months ago (5 responses), 1 month ago (4 responses), this morning or last night (also 4 responses), this week (3 responses). It would have been desirable to ascertain the last occasion with more precision but persistent probing would probably have caused offence without much improvement in accuracy.

The enquiry moved with question 7 to what the subject got out of these activities. The question had really already been put in 'forced choice' form in Questionnaire 1, possibly concentrating the mind to some extent, but further information was often volunteered in response to this open-ended wording. Several types of reward were mentioned by the same subject in many cases: a sexual 'turn-on', i.e., intense sexual excitement and sexual pleasure (25 responses), a mental 'high', i.e., elation and heightened perceptions (19 responses), a sense of power or control (9 responses), mutual enjoyment or a thrill from the partner's enjoyment (3 responses). It will be noted that although the proportions of these responses are similar to the proportions emerging from subjects' 'forced choice' responses to question 7 of the first questionnaire, reported in Table 8.1, they are not the same, since subjects here gave a fuller description and in some cases shifted the emphasis from one reward to another. Some subjects introduced other considerations, such as sexual relief and relaxation afterwards (6 responses). Each of the following received 3 mentions: intense communication or intimacy, unloading of responsibility in becoming helpless, like a baby, a sense of achievement at doing the forbidden. It was also stated by 3 subjects that there was not necessarily any orgasm during the enactment—orgasm was not important.

Some individual replies are worth quoting for the light they cast on the nature of the deviance, whilst being for the most part self-explanatory. ES28 said: "It's not to do with making love," and 77-year-old ES40: "Fantasies get more extreme with time." ES36 stated that he found SM fantasy necessary for sex—at the age of 44 he could only remember 'straight' sex, without SM fantasy, on three occasions. When he was caned, ES22 felt that he was given something he had always wanted. ES8, at the age of 75, stated that he no longer had any orgasmic pleasure—"the woman gets me to suckle at her breast—it gives her pleasure to inflict pain" (probably a dubious and wishful assertion). ES10 enjoyed the opportunity to "lie back and have things done, with no responsibility for a partner's enjoyments." On the other hand, ES1 felt there was "a responsibility not to abuse the submissive," and rather poignantly, ES80 felt "a sense of belonging to the partner, even though it was a business relationship."

The reports of a mental 'high' strongly suggest the secretion of enkephalins and endorphins and, I would submit, support the hypothesis of physiological addiction to pain and stress advanced at the beginning of this section. ES11 described "afterwards, great peace and tranquil well-being lasting for up to a week," ES37 spoke of "a mental 'high'—euphoria lasting over days," and ES61 reported "a mental 'high', longer lasting than orgasm." ES75, who declared herself a 'love slave', said it was "like orgasm in the head, with exploding colours." The rewards ES21 described were a sexual 'turn-on', a mental 'high' and, he went on, he would "refuse to orgasm for many hours afterwards" (precisely the tendency to prolong described by Reik (1939)). The response to this question 7 of ES35, which the uncharitable might call pretentious humbug, ran thus: "Catharsis. Soul-baring. Religious, ritualistic devotion. Genuflection to a certain image of woman—the Madonna-whore." Even the charitable might, I imagine, detect a whisper of self-indulgence, if not self-deception, and catch a whiff of hypocrisy.

Question 8 asked subjects for a description of their *physical* sensations. It was difficult to persuade them to confine themselves to the physical in answering this question, since physical and mental phenomena are frequently confused by these subjects. The physical is, in fact, often acting as proxy for the mental, but they sometimes, as in the case of ES27, for instance, point to the large visual and mental input in SM ritual as the explanation of its giving more intense pleasure than 'straight' sex.

The accounts subjects gave of their physical sensations during SM rituals again supported the hypothesized involvement of endogenous opioids (Turner, 1991, pp. 412–416). Twenty-one subjects reported that, after experiencing initial pain from a beating, the pain would distance, would go over into a sort of pleasure—several subjects reported a pleasurable tingling. Nine subjects stated explicitly that they considered these sensations were addictive, that they had, in fact, an addiction to pain and stress. Two subjects (ES62, ES81) spontaneously mentioned endorphins. Seventy-year-old ES61 said: "Pain goes over into 'all-over' pleasure," and 65-year-old ES18 explained: "A tolerance level is reached—beyond, one is suddenly not feeling pain any more. It is addictive—you want stronger medicine." (Several of the most characteristically masochistic remarks which have been quoted come from the depressed subgroup of index subjects, shortly to receive special attention.) ES51 responded: "It is a psychological addiction—orgasm is not the end, the well-being continues." The female subject ES58 remarked: "Cathartic ecstasy is addictive." ES1 became anecdotal: "I'm not in any way religious, but I remember one almost mystical experience. I had just finished beating my earlier girlfriend at a party. She said, 'Shall we dance?' As we were dancing she had a mental orgasm, her legs gave way under her and I had to carry her off the dance-floor." These flowery and fervent interpretations do not, however, preclude the involvement of endogenous opioids.

The tendency to prolong forepleasure and delay or avoid end-pleasure, so accurately portrayed by Reik (1939) was confirmed by the fact that 24 subjects reported erection, but 10 stated that sexual excitement would not necessarily lead to orgasm; 9 subjects said that anticipation of punishment and retrospective replay were pleasurable. For some subjects, for instance ES15, the 'suspense factor' had already reached the end stage described by Reik (1939) and, indeed twenty years earlier, by Freud (1919, p. 197)—impotence. ES30 remarked: "Fear gives relish," and ES10 explained that the frustration of bondage added to his sexual excitement. Light was cast on one attribute of the fetishistic materials, often overlooked, which contributed to their attractiveness: ES24 enthused, "Rubber and leather—the feel, the texture—their *restraining* qualities," and ES76, "Plastic touching the skin all over—the smoothness—encapsulated in it—*restrictive*." (As already mentioned in the Discussion section of Chapter 6, the forty-year-old stockbroker described by R.D. Laing (1976) felt, not only newborn but 'mummified' when covered in leather.)

The quintessential masochistic scenario is perhaps captured in the account given by ES80. He would obtain an erection from the anticipation of being tied up. Orgasm was not important—he would masturbate at home afterwards, reliving the scene. When forced to kneel for an hour, pain remains pain but the erection remains also, and therefore the pleasure. It was addictive in the sense that he would like to move in with this prostitute. His mind goes onto "her in control."

Questionnaire 4

The first question, asking in what way feelings towards an SM partner differed from those aroused by other people, brought various answers from the 15 index subjects who completed Questionnaire 4, without compelling overlap. The largest consensus was formed by the 3 male subjects who declared they felt completely submissive before a genuine authority figure—never her equal. ES15 adopted a slightly different attitude—that his SM partners (significantly placed in the plural) were the only people he was prepared to obey or be subservient to, "including cabinet ministers, royalty, etc ..." Two subjects agreed that there was greater bonding and communication, two agreed that there was absolute trust to be found in the SM relationship. In contrast, ES19 stated rather cynically that he doubted whether there was much liking involved, simply SM interests in common. Other responses mentioned admiration for a person with the ability to break through the conventions of acceptable behavior, the partner as a source of pleasure, intimacy of the mind as well as physical intimacy. (My own view is rather that physical intimacy must perforce serve as proxy for intimacy of the mind for these subjects.) ES75 brought it all down to earth when, after describing her 'Master' as kind, caring and loving, she concluded "and he gives me the best orgasms I have ever experienced"!

Question 2, asking to what extent the subject felt that his sexuality was focussed in the genitals, was testing the Freudian theory of erotogenic zones. Freud (1905, p. 169) suggested that in sadomasochism, the skin assumed the role of an erotogenic zone. ES75 considered her anatomy in some detail and then wrote: "I quite often say that I have only one erogenous zone—my skin." ES19 replied that his interest focussed on the buttocks "and I also enjoy anal stimulation (giving and receiving)." Three subjects stated that their sexuality lay 50% or more in the mind. The bondage practitioner, ES51, wrote: "A more powerful focus is to be found in the brain. There are certainly endorphin releases during sexual acts and the S/M participant may experience more heightened responses due to the greater involvement of all the senses." He illustrated this with a glowing account of the various physical and psychological effects achieved by a blindfold. Only two of these 15 subjects considered that their sexuality was focussed substantially and at all times in their genitals; two others replied that it was at some times and not at other times; ES2, with characteristic precision, specified that it was only when masturbating. Four subjects gave the explicit response that their sexuality was focussed very little in their genitals. These responses tend, therefore, to confirm the Freudian model of sexual development, in that they suggest fixation at, or regression to, a pregenital stage of infantile sexuality. One's interpretation depends largely on whether or not one accepts the Freudian model. My personal view is that, particularly with respect to sadomasochism, it is as useful as any other model.

There was some division of opinion as to whether there might be an element of revenge in SM practice (question 4). Six subjects considered there was not; six considered there might be some element of revenge springing from a feeling of having been abused by the opposite sex. Three of these latter informants singled out dominant women. They included ES75 who, it may be remembered, styled herself a 'love slave'. She wrote in a censorious tone: "Dominant women, on the other hand, seem to have little or no regard for the feelings of their partner, and are likely to be more severe and unrelenting. I could imagine some of the dominant women I know exorcising all their frustrations against the male chauvinists they meet in real life by venting their anger on some male sub's [submissive's] backside." Only ES11 appeared to consider the effect of an unhappy childhood, and that in a rather formal manner: "I'm not overly conscious myself of this being a vital element, although I suspect that it might be in there somewhere, connected with some dimly perceived imbalance of power at an early stage of development."

The last question (see Appendix 5), similarly, brought little enlightenment. In February 1994, James Rusbridger, the controversial writer on intelligence matters and former spy, was found hanging from the loft of his Cornish cottage, wearing a gas mask and a black oilskin, surrounded by pornography. His definition of masochism, quoted in question 7, ran: "Masochistic pleasure occurs when the masochist voluntarily *suppresses* a reaction to a situation that they would tend to react strongly to, if that situation also contains exposure to a sexual stimulus" (my italics). It was taken from his article entitled "Why?" in a subculture magazine, *Dressing for Pleasure*, generously supplied to me by ES15. The latter interpreted it as meaning that a masochist is willing to suppress his objections to pain and humiliation provided "a 'mistress' creates a sexually stimulating situation." ES19, ES37, ES51 and ES61 broadly concurred in this interpretation. ES2 objected both to Rusbridger's assumption of a necessarily *sexual* stimulus and to his assumption of suppression: "When, for instance, one is being caned, what is being suppressed?" The pain may be transformed so that it becomes desirable, not suppressed. ES62 similarly thought 'supresses' was the wrong word since she felt everyday reactions do not occur in the calm, the pleasure, the communication of an SM situation, and therefore need not be suppressed. ES76 made more or less the same point. Altogether, the responses to this question 7 reminded one of Sacher-Masoch's own 'scientific' theories, often disrupted, as Lenzer (1975) pointed out, by the primary (unconscious) processes.

The real lack of coherence emerged, however, in response to questions 3 and 5, concerning subjects' attitudes to cruelty and to love. Love was associated primarily with tenderness by the 15 respondents as a group and, in fact, by every individual except five (ES2, ES58 and ES75 associated love with tenderness and pain equally; ES41 with tenderness, teasing, pain and betrayal equally; ES15 with pain and betrayal more than tenderness). Not one of these respondents, as it would appear, saw any implicit contradiction between sadomasochism and tenderness (the response of ES15 was, one felt, in keeping with a somewhat theatrical personality).

Of course, it depends on what you mean by 'love'. The same striking lack of coherence is, however, visible, in fact even more marked, in their unanimous condemnation of cruelty. This surely amounts to 'doublethink'. It is precisely at this point that one can begin to be at cross purposes.

By 'SM' they do not necessarily mean what most people mean by 'sadomasochism', and therefore they do not define 'S-for-sadism' as 'cruelty for sexual pleasure'. Information supplied by ES2 and summarized at the end of this discussion will, it is hoped, help to elucidate this conundrum.

A Profile of the Depressed Subgroup of Sadomasochists

This profile is based solely on self-reported questionnaire material, Beck Depression Inventory scores and scores on one scale, Passivity, of the Adult Attachment Interview. It is a sort of statistical photofit—the temptation to smooth it and round it by introducing supplementary material gathered in informal discussion has been resisted.

Overall, 21 index subjects styled themselves dominant, 27 submissive, but of the self-styled dominants only 3 were in the depressed subgroup and of these 3, ES71 insisted he only fantasized—he was only dominant, therefore, in fantasy. The depressed subgroup was predominantly masochistic and 8 out of the 14 in this subgroup could not 'switch' roles or could do so only with difficulty. Only one (ES61) admitted to being bisexual; all the others were adamantly heterosexual. A sexual 'turn-on' was the stated incentive of 12 of these 14 subjects, the only exceptions being ES20 who reported a mental 'high' and ES10 who apparently gained a sense of power from SM activity (he was one of the three claiming to be dominant and the only one claiming to be able to switch roles easily).

Already we have a contrasting picture with the 34 nondepressed subjects, of whom 18 asserted they were dominant, 13 reported they could switch roles easily, 4 stated they were bisexual and one (ES2) even stated straightforwardly that he was exclusively homosexual. (This was the only individual to make the declaration in the entire group of 48 sadomasochists, when there is much evidence, from Freud onwards, for a homosexual vein running quite generally through male sadomasochism.) Although a sexual 'turn-on' was the reward sought also by 19 out of these 34 subjects, as many as 10 seemed happy with a mental 'high'.

It will be recalled from Chapter 7 (Table 7.3) that for the depressed masochistic group alone, out of all groups of respondents to the Beck Depression Inventory, depression was *negatively* correlated with 'loss of libido' ($r = -0.248$). The fact that 7 out of 14 depressed subjects rated their sex life as unsatisfactory is hardly surprising in view of their depressed state, but when only 5 out of 34 made this report in the other subgroup, it suggests a difference in behavior. I would submit that the difference between their mean scores on the Adult Attachment Interview scale for Passivity (5.07, S.D. 1.68, and 3.14, S.D. 1.79, for depressed and nondepressed, respectively; Table 5.2) may provide a clue to the nature of this difference. It was suggested as part of a tentative interpretation of the significant interaction, displayed as Fig. 5.2*e*, between sadomasochism and depression with respect to passivity, that the more active sadomasochists were perhaps less depressed in proportion as they externalized anger emanating from their childhood grievances, possibly frequenting SM clubs. In other words, the nondepressed subjects might be somewhat more open, more accepting, less guilt-ridden about their sexuality. This observation was, in fact, made in the larger study (reviewed in detail in Chapter 3) by Spengler (1977).

Turning now to the correlations displayed in Table 8.5, it is interesting that the strengths of association between the Fantasy Sum, the Reality Sum, the Masochistic Sum and the Sadistic Sum calculated from Questionnaire 2 are reversed when one looks from the depressed to the nondepressed subjects. The group we are particularly interested in, the depressed masochists, appear to be considerably more sadistic than masochistic in their fantasies and, as one would expect by definition, more masochistic than sadistic in their actualizations in reality. The opposite is apparently true in the case of the more dominant, nondepressed group. Fantasy and reality are, of course, themselves correlated for both subgroups but depression, represented by BDI total scores, is only correlated with masochism in the group we have been attempting to characterize. In Chapter 4, when setting down my own views, before commencing this empirical investigation, on the essential characteristics of masochism, I mentioned passivity, rigidity and hypocrisy as three of them. I submit that this profile of the depressed subgroup, constructed from self-report, may go some way towards supporting these assertions.

Information Given by ES2

ES2 was an extremely collaborative subject who gave generously of his fund of knowledge, accumulated over many years of active participation in SM activities. His attitude to his subject lay somewhere between academic absorption and religious piety. In his own circles, he was admired and respected, giving lectures and demonstrations of safe techniques. He seemed unlikely to pose a threat or a danger to anyone and, whatever his motives, the assistance he afforded my research was magnanimous. Besides being a prolific writer of SM stories, he compiled a scholarly exposition of SM attitudes with a reference list and glossary of SM terms. The abstract of this document states that "S/M has no relationship to either sadism, masochism or sadomasochism" and proceeds to the definition: "S/M covers activities between consenting, caring participants which involve giving and receiving pleasure by playing the roles of dominant and/or submissive possibly with the involvement of one or more of stimulation, pain or bondage." The true sadist is not interested in giving pleasure—his partner is at best an object on which to vent anger, at worst an enemy. S/M is not a perversion but a normal part of human behavior, which can vary, like love, from absent to an obsession. The term may, in fact, be an abbreviation of 'slave/master' or 'slave/mistress', of 'sex magic' or 'sensuality/mutuality'. Gentle flagellation with rods or nettles was practised by the Romans; bites and punches figure in the Kama Sutra; bondage and discipline was rife in Victorian England.

The historical background is presented tendentiously but some fair points are made, such as the observation that during periods when sexual activities were restricted, "acts and images of extreme violence flourished." During such periods (actually left unspecified), stories and images of martyrs became popular, the image of Christ in Majesty was replaced by The Suffering Christ, and those most proud of their sexual abstinence were foremost in cruelty. Coming to the present day, the symbols of S/M are to be found everywhere in fashion and the arts. Models are photographed in leather collars, holding whips—films are about people falling in love with those who have insulted and mistreated them. With the discussion of the prevalence of S/M practices in our contemporary urban populations and the introduction of statistics, tendentiousness, not surprisingly, increases! He arrives at an estimate of 500,000 Londoners with some experience of S/M.

The next section reviews the range of S/M activities, starting with a recognition of the role of imagination and a warning to the feckless: "It does not matter how skilled the practitioners are or how advanced is the equipment used, if the imagination is interrupted because the participants are distracted the scene fails." It is, thus, play-acting, in uniforms, in rooms designed like stage sets. Domination and submission are the commonest actions, as they are in life, only the usual roles may be reversed and exaggerated. The dominant may dress as an army officer while the submissive may wear a slave collar and act the part of a dog, but the dominant is seldom the controller of the scene. The submissive sets the limits of the scenario he has chosen and is often casting off the responsibilities of a director in his real work. The dominant in the S/M scene must take on responsibility for his mental well-being and happiness, as "awesome" a responsibility as parenthood. "The submissive has to trust the dominant like a child trusts a loving parent and like a child the submissive believes this trust will be justified." (A poignant statement in view of the actual childhood experiences related by so many of the "S/M practitioners" (Chapter 5). Even more poignant, perhaps, is the solemn reverence emanating from ES2, who did not accept any flippant approach to his belief system.) In the glossary, the entry 'Daddy scene' is defined: "An S/M fantasy scene in which adult participants play father and child respectively. May involve humiliation and spanking." One must presume that theoretically, therefore, this would reenact a scene where trust was originally lost and to which, in replay, it was now restored.

Bondage may or may not be associated with the application of pain and may vary from a person holding a partner's wrists, through blindfolding and tying hands and feet to bedposts, to complete immobilization (mummification). It may involve suspension, imprisonment in a dungeon or a box. ES2 points out that bondage and confinement are a part of everyday life, the former figuring in various types of restrictive clothing, the latter in the restriction of movement imposed by schools, prisons, the army and religious institutions. It is worth quoting his gloss upon the latter because it captures the characteristic prevarication of the sadomasochist, from Sacher-Masoch himself onwards: "...it is more likely that this is actually sadism, although one or both of the participants may experience S/M pleasure." This is precisely the equivocation, the double-talk, that made me cite hypocrisy as an essential feature of masochism at the end of Chapter 4. And it continues when ES2 makes a preliminary mention of pain: "... the giving of undesired pain and the practice of torture have not, and have never had, a part in S/M activities. Indeed the pain involved in S/M activities could often be better described as stimulation." A likely story! Well, the indefatigable ES2 tackles it: why should one believe that S/M films are not *really* violent? Well, "the same argument could be used against those who practice non-S/M sex and also read, see and hear about extreme violence." Observation at S/M meetings reveals few people with any outward signs of injury, whereas there are obviously many people who obtain sexual pleasure from giving or receiving nonconsensual pain in the course of their professional activities. There are boxers and wrestlers; there is the prewar judge who ejaculated each time he sentenced a young man to hanging. Less dramatically, there are those who inflict pain on themselves by bodybuilding and jogging.

After a mention of voyeurism and exhibitionism in the same vein—watching and displaying violence are common phenomena—and a few more statistics relating to the nature and prevalence of S/M practices, ES2 gets his teeth into his main interest—pain.

His first point is that pain has more uses than simply causing the organism to change a situation in such a way as to diminish the pain and avoid damage. It draws attention to the location of a stimulus, so that a dog can, for instance, deal with a flea. It is used as a teaching aid and as a means of establishing a hierarchy in higher animals. What detracts from the efficacy of a judicial use of pain for these purposes is, however, the invariable delay before punishment and the impersonal nature of the punishment. Pain in childbirth may help bonding, and pain associated with the sexual activities of higher animals may have the same effect. Finally, there is all the weight of psychological and religious evidence to support the view that punishment relieves guilt. This may explain the extremes of self-mutilation and suicide. ES2 makes the valid extrapolation: "In countries where guilt is strongly associated with sex it is understandable that some people may only be able to function sexually after the removal of that guilt." One might narrow the boundaries from country to home, where a prudish mother can produce the same effect (Table 5.8).

Some authors claim that pain during S/M rituals is simply normal pain; others maintain it is scarcely felt due to excitement. Both views are erroneous, according to ES2. The term sensualized or eroticized pain has been used but he would prefer *spiritualized* pain (abbreviated to S-pain) on account of its relatedness to the pain experienced by the Christian flagellants of the period of the Black Death, Indian fakirs taking Kavadi, and Amerindians undergoing initiation rites. Further evidence of the difference between this S-pain of individuals using pain to enter higher spiritual states and ordinary pain is the fact that an S/M participant quite happily accepting heavy S-pain will complain bitterly about an accidental splinter in the hand.

ES2 evidently felt that he had a few more observations to make and sticky problems to raise before proceeding to his conclusion. He observes that the ability to stand pain is probably still regarded as a desirable quality in some spheres of activity. Army training, for example, reflects this. The sticky problems he disposes of perfunctorily: the physiological effects of pain are "extremely complicated and should not be reduced to vague statements about the release of opioids"; the giving of pain to relieve anger may occur "in certain instances of sudden random violence but is ... almost unknown in the S/M context." In the opinion of ES2, the giver of 'stimulation' (minor pain) or S-pain "either obtains pleasure vicariously or else simply enjoys giving a partner the same pleasure that he or she enjoys from receiving stimulation or S-pain." (Metacognitive monitoring has broken down, and the primary processes have broken through again with Sacher-Masoch's 'witch-algebra' (Lenzer, 1975), for apparently he does not notice that he has just said the same thing twice.)

As a preamble to his concluding definition of S/M, ES2 reviews 14 others, previously published in the psychological, sociological and subculture literatures. One of the more interesting comes from Pat Califia, a venerated figure in the S/M scene, to the effect that it "focuses on whatever feelings or actions are forbidden, and searches for a way to obtain pleasure from the forbidden." (What clearer picture of the masochist who "wants to be treated like a small and helpless child, but, particularly, like a naughty child" (Freud, 1924*a*, p. 162), or indeed, of the infantilism posited at the beginning of this section?) ES2 underlines the limiting parameters of the S/M scenario: firstly, it should be with the full consent of the participants (and what about the women involved simply to gratify their men, as discovered by Litman & Swearingen (1972), for instance?); secondly, it should be "within a caring (or loving) relationship, even if the caring is only for the period of the session" (a somewhat specious accommodation, one feels!) The first excludes animals, since they cannot give consent; the second excludes all 'unsafe sex' and dangerous practices. A safe word or halt word is agreed which will stop activities. These limits indicate that S/M people are neither sadists nor masochists but "independent-minded, freedom-loving, caring people". With this comforting assessment, ES2 restates the definition of S/M he put forward in the abstract with which his document commenced, but with the *caveat* (the ironic appropriateness of which appears to have escaped him) that a definition should not become a strait-jacket: "... nothing in either the definition or in this paper is intended to suggest either what should or should not be done or what should be allowed to be done." One is likely to feel too uneasy about the vistas opened up by this statement to bother much about the fact that he has once again said the same thing twice.

CHAPTER 9

GENERAL DISCUSSION AND CONCLUSIONS

SUMMARY

The etiology of sadomasochism is presented as diverse. In some cases, a form of physiological addiction may result from protracted pain or stress in childhood. Traumatic experiences or insensitive parenting have often permitted little opportunity for the development of a theory of mind.

It would seem useful to start this discussion with a summary of findings up to this point. In Chapter 4, a multicomponent model of masochism was put forward, chiefly based on psychoanalytic theory but having also a physiological dimension. The latter postulated that prolonged pain or stress in childhood, resulting in the production of endogenous opioid peptides, could create a form of addiction to painful and stressful situations. In Chapter 5, the attachment theory of John Bowlby, Mary Ainsworth, Mary Main and co-workers was brought into the empirical investigation of sadomasochism. The analysis of verbatim transcripts of the Adult Attachment Interview (all, it may be recalled, transcribed over many months by myself and therefore studied in considerable detail) revealed that sadomasochistic subjects had, without exception, received an upbringing which was damaging in one way or another and which had led them to develop insecure internal models of personal attachment. They possessed, on average, significantly less coherence and metacognitive capacity than controls, whether depressed or not depressed. In Chapter 6, the 'emotional' Stroop task was used to demonstrate a sadomasochistic mind-set, and this was confirmed by an analysis of the free recall of words included, or thought to have been included, in the Stroop presentation. Chapter 7, reporting on the Beck Depression Inventory, considered the difference and the overlap between depression and masochism. It included a scrutiny in this context of the small number of female subjects participating in the study. Loss of coherence could be one of the prices index subjects paid for their defensive erotization of psychological pain since depressed control subjects possessed, on average, significantly more coherence of mind. Chapter 8, presenting results gathered by questionnaire, demonstrated differences in attitude and behavior within the sadomasochistic group. These differences probably revolve around self-acceptance and openness with respect to the deviance. The more passive and depressed subgroup of males were posited as more quintessentially masochistic. In the interests of fairness, the last word was deliberately given to an index subject with an academic background who distinguished at length between 'consensual' SM activity and sadomasochism. The present chapter seeks to move forward to provide a model which will permit the integration of the experimental data and the individual case material reported in Chapters 5 to 8. In seeking such a comprehensive interpretation of the findings of this section, what emerges as a major feature, distinguishing sadomasochistic subjects from controls and accounting for their diminished metacognitive capacity, is an early background which afforded them little opportunity for the development of a theory of mind and which therefore left them preoccupied with the physical.

To discuss the development of a theory of mind, one might well go back to Hegel's *Phänomenologie des Geistes* (Phenomenology of Mind, 1807) and, with ironical appropriateness to this particular investigation, to the section 'Herrschaft und Knechtschaft' (Lordship and Bondage): "Das Selbstbewusstsein ist *an* und *für sich*, indem und dadurch, dass es für ein anderes an und für sich ist; d.h. es ist nur als ein Anerkanntes" (self-consciousness exists in itself and for itself, in that, and by the fact that it exists for another self-consciousness; that is to say, it is only by being acknowledged or 'recognized' as existing). In their work on Reflective-Self Functioning, Peter Fonagy and colleagues (Fonagy *et al.* 1991*a*) relate the development of a capacity to understand mental states, or to 'mentalize', to the young child's interactions with parents. In many fortunate instances, it is the mother who acts as a mirror wherein the child can read his own emotions and learn to regulate them. It may be in playing, in an atmosphere of warmth and security, with father or elder brother, in 'pretending' together, that the foundation of the appearance-reality distinction is laid. The child is *recognized* as an *intentional* being and begins to perceive the desires and beliefs of others. A different development, in circumstances of rejection, neglect, abuse or smothering, is bound to entail defence mechanisms, such as dismissal or denial, which may be adaptive for the time but are bound to be maladaptive in the long term. To attribute mental states to persecutors becomes too painful.

Even where parenting is 'good enough,' the rate of development of a child's capacity to grasp the viewpoint of another is influenced by whether his parents, in their dealings with *him*, take account of *his* viewpoint. As pointed out by Light (1979), in judging that an adult's behavior is egocentric, it seldom occurs to us that he simply may not know that other people have differing perspectives from his own, that he has never developed the capacity to take account of this. We are more likely to assume that he possesses the mental capacity but that it is not his habit to use it, that he simply does not bother to use it.

At the heart of selfishness, then, lies the absence of a theory of mind. If there is no capacity for empathy, there is no sympathy, no capacity for attachment on a free, reciprocal basis. People are not *intentional* beings—they are baffling, unpredictable objects and relationship with them is similar to the use of addictive substances. It is likely to be on a concrete level: if, having blindfolded, gagged and bound them, you start piercing them, you can make a fair guess at what they are feeling! The physical has become the means of communication, with pain the most reliable and unambiguous language.

The absence of a theory of mind leads, therefore, directly to an inner life centred around the physical. Hence the sadomasochistic interest in the fetish, in 'body modification' by piercing, scarification and tattoos (there is even academic work being conducted in this field by Dr Milton Diamond of the University of Hawaii) and hence the marked concern displayed by sadomasochists about body image changes with age. In responding to the Beck Depression Inventory, 26 out of the complete group of 48, including some in their twenties and thirties, said they were worried that they were looking old or unattractive.

A lack of a theory of mind presumably lies behind the faceless woman fantasized by ES30 or the female torso which obsessed ES35. The emphasis in this anatomical puppet-theatre is on bare breasts and bellies, most likely of maternal origin, sensual memories from infancy. But let us not forget that the masturbation fantasy of ES71, in his loneliness, was that he was *torturing* the breasts of a faceless woman who was only breasts, that ES74 fantasized *butchery* quite commonly at the age of seven or eight, the *mutilation* of young girls at his school. What makes sadomasochistic fantasy different from the wishful daydreams produced by almost everyone is the compulsive negativity of its subject matter. One surmises that Kenneth Grahame had in many ways a disrupted, sorrowful and deprived childhood but he escaped into *The Wind in the Willows*, not into a world of torture and mutilation. Was this because he had received love and recognition from his mother until her early death?

There is an obvious line of defence open to those questioned about the reason for their sadomasochistic activities and, indeed, fantasies: we are simply acknowledging and expressing the cruel and depraved impulses which are dormant in everybody, and we are thereby purging ourselves of cruelty and depravity. Strangely, none of the index subjects adopted this rationale of catharsis, although all 48 of them were questioned. ES1, who was an articulate and intelligent person, as were many others, took the line: it's a relative matter—any girl on the street would probably enjoy a little light spanking—some want to take it further—that's all. Note that the defence is pleasure—there is no perception of any need for moral justification. Only ES58 came near such a perception in her response to the question on Questionnaire 4: 'What are your thoughts on the subject of cruelty?' She wrote: "That it is an abomination when unconsenting and probably an abomination even with consent!" 'Consensual' is, of course, a 'buzzword' in the subculture literature. For the 14 other respondents to this question, cruelty apparently had little or nothing to do with sadomasochism.

The lack of coherence is perhaps at its most striking when sadomasochists are speaking of their sexuality in psychological, or more accurately pseudopsychological, terms. Unassailed by any sense of paradox, ES26 asserted, for instance, that sadomasochism was about trust and openness; ES28 echoed that he longed for trust. In her response to the last question of Questionnaire 1, 'Why do you think you developed SM interests?' ES42 wrote (amongst other considerations such as self-confidence, trust, being admired): "Therapy—to explore humiliation and by looking at it, to gradually heal it." The submissive mind-state was described by ES26 as like a switch being flicked, so that you would do anything for the dominant person, freed from the responsibilities and the codes of conduct of real life. This has little to do with Hegelian 'spiritualization', of course. What is in question here is rather a means of escaping from sexual inhibition to attain the ultimate goal of physical pleasure. As noted in Chapter 8, ES2 spoke and wrote at length of 'spiritualized' pain, occasionally adopting the term 'transformed' which he considered less emotional, but I am inclined to interpret this on a physiological level. It is possible that endogenous opioids, released in response to prolonged pain, produce what may be perceived as a different state of consciousness.

So why no theory of mind? Why, in its place a sadomasochistic mind-set? The concrete world just grew, like Harriet Beecher Stowe's Topsy, by processes of natural selection. The human individual, if he is to escape insanity, has to weave meaning into this kaleidoscope, to interpret it as a coherent story. But he has at his disposal only the representations formed from what he has received. If no one has been sensitive to the signals he has sent out in his helpless infancy, if no one has interpreted his intentions, if no one has helped him to recognize and regulate his feelings, he has to construct a model of the world with clumsy infant's hands, as best he can from the concrete objects, animate and inanimate, impinging on his senses. Without loving help he is not likely to move forward and leave the bizarre interpretations of early childhood behind. The harsh, frightening world through which he moves is the only one he has—at least it is familiar. If he builds an imaginary world, it is no escape, it is the same—the only respite from reality it can give is by being worse. This account is, of course, exaggerated. No human being is only a sadomasochist; no mind-set is unrelieved; a theory of mind is for everyone only relatively present or relatively absent. However, to seek the etiology of masochism is not reassuring. The slights and cruelties of infancy begin to form representations of self and of others in childhood which grow, fractal-like, into working models operating for a lifetime. It only requires a small insult or injury to inscribe the formula which will set the process in motion and ultimately form a masochist.

MULTIPLE MODELS OF ATTACHMENT

"Models once established prove very hard to change" (Bowlby, 1980, p. 241). This difficulty is compounded "when a person finds himself unable to review the representational model(s) he has built of his attachment figures(s) because to do so would infringe a long-learned rule that it is against one or both his parents' wishes that he study them, and their behavior towards him, objectively" (Bowlby, 1980, p. 56). There was often word-for-word repetition in the way ES71 described his upbringing at various stages of his interview: "... we were taught to say 'please' and 'thank you' and always give up our seat on the bus if there was adults standing ... it was church on Sunday—church in the morning, church in the afternoon and church in the evening ... we knew what was required of us." Small wonder that this 64-year-old, quintessential masochist, who had never been married, when asked the final question of the interview as to whether he felt he had learnt any particular thing, above all else, from his childhood experiences, replied: "No, I think if I had children, I would bring them up very much the same as my parents brought me up."

INFANTILISM

In summarizing my own views on sadomasochism before commencing this empirical study, I mentioned infantilism as a key characteristic

(Chapter 4, subsection iii), using the Freudian concept of fixation. Whilst standing by this and considering it amply confirmed by the fantasized rituals described by the sadomasochistic subjects who came for interview, I would like to expand it. (Models of the mind come and go; most of them have their own worth and, in my opinion, it is regrettable that the Freudian model should be thrown out like the proverbial baby with the bath-water. I therefore devote the next subsection to its defence.)

John Bowlby, in considering the development of behavioral systems which takes place in the human child during his first years, links the mental with the physical, and specifically, with the development of the central nervous system: "Without the necessary neural equipment, behavioral equipment cannot be elaborated; and, until it is elaborated, behavior remains more in keeping with the pleasure principle than with the reality principle" (Bowlby 1969, p. 156). It is precisely at this stage that the sadomasochist is, in Freudian terminology, 'fixated' and to which he constantly strives to 'regress', in his rituals, in his dreams and, ultimately, in his ageing.

Of course, it is during the personal interactions of these early years that the images of self and others are created. It is worth reiterating Bowlby's observation at this point (it was already alluded to in Chapter 6) that psychopathology ensues from representational models which are either out-of-date or confused and inconsistent. In order to remain serviceable, models require revision but "revising, extending, and checking of models are ill done or done not at all unless a model is subjected from time to time to whatever special benefits accrue from becoming conscious" (Bowlby, 1969, p. 83). In other words, metacognition, and metacognition is precisely what is lacking in the case of sadomasochists, as evidenced in the present study by their interviews.

An impression of infantilism is also created by the physical clumsiness displayed by sadomasochists. In expounding his concept of 'the demonstrative feature' as quintessential to masochism, Reik (1939) writes: "In place of bodily hurt or pain these people often put on a shameful or degrading exhibitionistic display of bodily or psychic awkwardness which in their imagination has a stimulating effect. The 'embarrassing situation' is enjoyed with the same anxious-pleasant feeling which accompanies bodily punishment" (p. 51) ... "The attention of others must be drawn to the ego through clumsiness" (p. 56). It is a weapon of provocation, but, in the case of several index subjects (e.g. ES61, ES71), it seemed also a somatic manifestation of depression, of low self-esteem.

The predilections for being beaten and for bondage (Figure 8.1 of the previous chapter) amongst sadomasochistic rituals can also be traced directly and obviously back to infancy. Many of my interviewees actually

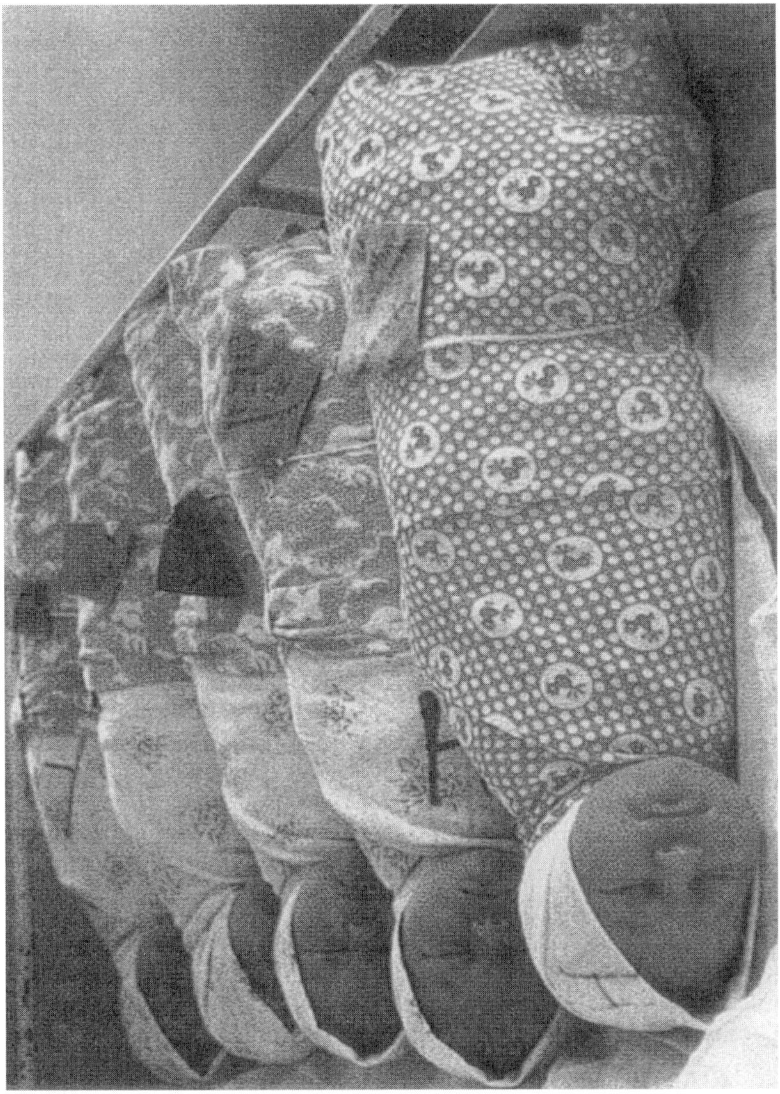

FIGURE 9.1. Five newly born babies in a St Petersburg hospital in 1994. Babies were usually separated from their mothers within moments of birth. Fathers were not able to see them until, at a week old, they were handed over in a ceremonial 'discharge room'.

stated that being beaten represented the loving, concentrated attention their mothers had either not given or given too much. Bondage was warm, comforting, and above all, secure—tucked up tightly, blissfuly relieved of all responsibility, like the Russian infants in Figure 9.1. With earliest bodily memories such as theirs, one can only suspect that there must be bondage practitioners in the making!

Like young children, sadomasochists seek repetition of behavior and situation. They are, it seems, unaware of the stereotyped nature of their dress and their scenarios. They have a child's anxiety that all details should be fitting. For subjects such as ES8, simplicity is preferable to complexity—the complexity of adult life is troublesome. Effort is required to navigate through it and at any moment one may wreck the vessel, one may fail. The infant's life is in one crucial respect simpler—security lies with mother. She provides, defends, consoles and explains. Of course, having all the eggs in one basket is perilous. If she does not fulfil this all-round, one-person service, the future may not be a 'normal' or happy one. The longing for such a delightfully simple security remains with most of us but with some quite addictively, hence the Adult Baby Clubs and poignant rituals of men in frills being scolded for 'naughtiness' or men in diapers being tucked up in cots. For them infantilism is a desperate and addictive return to simplicity, to one all-loving, all-powerful protector who bestows relief, for a time, from the complexities of life.

THE RELEVANCE OF FREUDIAN THEORY TO AN UNDERSTANDING OF MASOCHISM

John Bowlby rejected certain aspects of Freudian theory when he developed his own conceptual framework of the attachment behavioral system which enabled him to forge links with evolutionary biology, with neurophysiology and with cognitive psychology. He claimed that this new approach could be tested empirically and that certain 'abstract' concepts such as psychic energy and drive could be dispensed with. "Psychopathology," he wrote, "is regarded as due to a person's psychological development having followed a deviant pathway, and not as due to his suffering a fixation at, or a regression to, some early stage of development" (Bowlby, 1980, p. 41).

On the one hand, one might point out that a developmental *pathway* suggests strongly that it might be traversed in both directions. What, indeed, has taken place in the second childhood of extreme old age? On the other hand, most of the paradigms and models of psychology are, in the end, metaphors. They are constantly being challenged, revised or overturned. Their respective values lie surely in the understanding they are able to promote, in their power to elucidate problems. Bowlby's work was not concerned with the phenomenon of masochism. The word does not even appear in the index of his 3-volume *magnum opus* (Bowlby, 1969, 1973, 1980). Freud, however, was supremely concerned throughout his professional life with the problem of masochism. Like Theodor Reik after him, he knew it through and through. In view of the fact that infantilism is so prominent a feature of masochism, the Freudian concepts of fixation and/or regression would seem appropriate and meaningful. Remember there is that adhesiveness to account for! And, incidentally, what more useful way of considering what appears to be the pathological laziness of many masochists, their lethargy and their sloppiness, than in terms of psychic energy? Bowlby himself, when reviewing the experiments of Hilgard (1973, 1974) on information processing under hypnosis, writes: "Thus Hilgard's findings show that the exclusion of information that would normally be accepted is an active process requiring effort" (Bowlby, 1980, pp. 57–58). As postulated in chapter 4 under the subheading 'Passivity', the masochist is drained of energy by the necessity to keep material out of consciousness, to sustain a constant self-deception—a fundamental economic concept of Freud's.

How well does Freudian theory stand up in the light of some of the statements made by self-declared masochists, reported in Chapter 8? The bisexual subject, ES74, whom Freud might well have called 'polymorphously perverse', wrote in reply to the question, 'Why do you think you developed SM interests?': "My parents and I shared a room until I was seven. As a result I was jealous of my parents' sexual relationship. I found it hard to be physically affectionate with my father, and he with me. We did however fight, but verbally, not physically. I was very angry with my parents, partly because they denied me the sexual relationship with them I craved." Surely there could hardly be a clearer confirmation of the process, outlined in *'A Child is Being Beaten'*, whereby masochism derives from an inverted oedipal situation (Freud, 1919, pp. 198–199; see Chapter 1).

The 'spiritualized' pain, described with veneration by ES2, immediately recalls the observation in *Three Essays on the Theory of Sexuality* (Freud, 1905, p. 204) concerning the erotogenic effect "attaching even to intensely painful feelings, especially when the pain is toned down or kept at a distance by some accompanying condition". The "accompanying condition" in Freud's mind at that point was "its occurring in an imaginary world, in a book or in a play", or, one might add, in an SM scenario. The main point is that it would probably be more accurate to call it 'eroticized' rather than 'spiritualized' pain.

SADOMASOCHISTIC WOMEN

Recently a 60-year-old dominatrix spoke of her life on UK television (10.45pm, 11 February 1998, BBC1). Her story held several features worth noting. Her father had gone out of her life at an early age. Her mother had idolized her brother whilst meting out deliberate cruelties to her. She had tied her, for instance, to a pitch-dark staircase for several hours. She thought she had acquired much of her own technique, in fact, from her mother. She would use her mother's words to her clients: "Don't try to lie to me, because if you are telling lies I shall know!" For many years this woman, who now related events with a winning honesty, had led a double life as a housewife, a mother and a prostitute, saving enough money to leave her husband and 'come out' as a 'butch' lesbian. She considered that the sudden death of her 10-year-old daughter had hardened her, but she had no contempt for the men whose various needs she catered to, deriving enjoyment, herself, in the process. Her mother would have been incensed but there was now nothing her mother could do to her—*she* was in charge now! Significant features of this account are (a) the loss of first her father, then her daughter, leading to a partial deactivation of the attachment behavioral system (Bowlby, 1980, pp. 65–70); (b) the intergenerational cycle of abusive behavior unfolding between her mother and herself (Main & Goldwyn, 1984); (c) her lesbianism which demoted men to paying clients whom she had dealt with, from the first, with her thoughts elsewhere and sent on their way as swiftly as possible.

The sadomasochistic women who came forward to take part in this study are too few to justify any general statement but it is noteworthy that 3 of the 5 accorded with this last point (c). ES42 became aware around the age of ten that she was thinking like a boy—she would even take her shirt off at games—and she went on, in her own assessment, to develop male attitudes to sex. ES58 was a professional dominatrix and bisexual. ES62 was a lesbian, currently involved in two serious relationships with women, who had loved wrestling with boys at school and holding them down. Even ES41, in her avid reading as a child, had been fired particularly by images of heroism, of fighting against odds. With respect to point (a) above, ES42 had lost her mother before the age of two. As to an intergenerational cycle, point (b) above, ES75 had noticed her son binding his wrists, though she interpreted his interest in bondage as an inborn predisposition rather than learned behavior.

I outlined the television interview as a yardstick against which to take the measure of my small group of female index subjects, but gender was irrelevant to what was probably the most telling remark and the note on which the interview ended: "I'm in charge now!" As already stated, the five women I interviewed all asserted themselves from the outset and guarded their position warily, but control is a preoccupation of sadomasochistic men and women alike. It soon becomes clear that what they are all involved in is the re-enactment of situations, long past, in which they were helpless but which they now master. Control, as an ever-present issue, is taken up again in the following discussion of the etiology of masochism under the heading 'Incomplete individuation' and considered at greater length in Part III.

THE THREE CONTROL SUBJECTS UNDER SPECIAL SCRUTINY

As mentioned first in Chapter 5, much consideration was given to the problem of three control subjects who appeared to have deviant tendencies. In conversation following the Adult Attachment Interview and the 'emotional' Stroop task, CS125 stated that his partner sometimes liked him to slap her. Actually in response to one of the AAI questions, CS175 spoke of a long-standing pattern of failure just as success was within his grasp: "There is a part of me that wants to fail." Finally, NS269 confessed in discussion after the Stroop task that his fantasies were sometimes sadomasochistic. The problem was to decide whether to remove these three men from the control group, and the decision taken was to leave them in that group, for the reasons given in Chapter 5: (a) a control sample should represent the general population, and the features displayed by these three individuals could easily be observed in that population; (b) the control group should, in principle, not be manipulated but as randomly recruited as was possible, given the need for a sufficient proportion of depressed subjects to make comparison with the index group meaningful; (c) the tendencies manifested by the subjects under scrutiny did not meet DSM-III-R criteria either for sexual sadism, sexual masochism or self-defeating personality disorder; (d) discriminant analysis showed that these three subjects were correctly assigned to the control group. Belatedly, one further argument might be added to this rationale: any erosion of difference between index and control subjects could only militate against the erroneous adoption of an alternative hypothesis under test, pulling in a conservative direction for retention of the null hypothesis.

However, misgivings about the control status of these three men were not entirely unjustified in the event. In their performance of the 'emotional' Stroop task, all three were found to have increased response latencies for sadomasochistic-content words (Chapter 6; Appendix 4). The lists of words written down in 3 minutes of free recall by CS175 and

NS269 had a distinctly sadomasochistic flavour (Table 6.8*c*). It is notably these two who show signs of a mind-set rather than CS125 who, if he is to be believed, slapped his partner not for his own pleasure but for hers. The fact that all three men have reached their 40s without apparent escalation of sadomasochistic interest or, in the case of CS175, without proliferation of self-defeating behavior patterns, suggests that they might still, realistically, be more representative of the general population than candidates for the index group. Realistically, that is, when one cannot now push one's trolley around a supermarket without encountering people with rings through their noses, lips and eyebrows, when the circulation of *Skin Two*, as only one of many glossy subculture magazines, stands at around 30,000 (*Sunday Times Style Magazine*, 27 April 1997, p. 8), when self-mutilation in the film *Sick: The Life and Death of Bob Flanagan, Supermasochist* is awarded a special jury prize at Robert Redford's Sundance film festival and is considered a prime contender for a documentary Oscar (*Sunday Times*, 7 December 1997, p. 22).

Sadomasochism has frequently been described as a continuum (e.g., Kernberg, 1988)—a spectrum would be another metaphor, with feckless theatrical games at one end and sadistic serial killings at the other. My personal impression of the self-declared sadomasochists I interviewed was that they were not dangerous. In talking to them, the main difference I noticed between them and depressed controls was that they were reluctant or unable to look at reality, whereas depressed control subjects were, for the most part, gloomy realists. The mentation of these index subjects was often wishful—they seemed still to believe in what Freud called 'the omnipotence of thoughts'—whereas depressed controls, despite distorted perceptions with reference to themselves, retained a capacity for logical thinking. Finally, there was a marked preoccupation with sex in the index group which was not to be found in the interviews of depressed controls.

The danger comes when preoccupation with immediate physical pleasure takes over and a theory of mind is totally absent, when other human beings are only insensate means of sexual gratification, and this is indissolubly linked with domination, as it was, for instance, in the case of Frederick West, who committed suicide in his prison cell on January 1, 1995, while awaiting trial on 12 charges of murder. Another such case was that of Peter Moore whose brutal attacks on lone men in North Wales culminated in four murders in 1995 (British TV documentary entitled *A Very British Murder: Dressed to Kill*, 10pm, 26 September 2000, Channel 4). In the spring of 1992 the former children's entertainer John Wayne Gacy was interviewed in prison, thirteen years after he was convicted of murdering 33 young men and boys, mostly in the Chicago area. His first murder by stabbing was messy so thereafter, between 1972 and 1978, his victims were sexually abused, tortured, then strangled. They were to blame, they attempted to seduce him. He admits to the killings but not to his own guilt. He shows no remorse. He even draws a plan indicating where he buried some of the 29 bodies in his basement. He claims that his father was abusive but that he himself was always a good father, a concerned citizen and a dedicated contributor to the life of the community. On May 10, 1994, still unassailed by the realities of his life, Gacy was finally executed by three lethal injections (documentary produced by Cinetel Productions, Knoxville, Tennessee, in association with Courtroom Television Network, shown on British television as part of a series examining the lives of serial killers, 9pm, 30th October 2000, Channel 5). The self-declared sadomasochists I interviewed seemed, on the whole, immature and therefore inoffensive. They seemed to bear little resemblance to the Moors murderers, Ian Brady and Myra Hindley, who were jailed in 1966 for three sadistic murders and confessed in 1987 to two more. Nevertheless, it has to be said that, at certain points, Hindley's letter to *The Guardian* after thirty years of imprisonment sounded some familiar notes. There, in its length and its 'psychologizing', was the 'demonstrative factor' (Reik, 1939), springing from a problem of personal identity, yet the long 'explanation' of her personality and her behavior contained no insight into why she was impelled to commit these murders. Why, indeed, were she and Brady impelled to tape-record their victim's cries? Hindley's description of her own mind was one of compartmentalization: "I knew that what I was involved in was indefensible ... I locked these feelings away" (*The Guardian*, 18 December 1995, p. 10).

That, at the other end of the spectrum, everyday human relations are shot through with covert sadomasochism is a point made by most intellectual apologists for a bigger, brighter, better SM world (e.g., Jacques, 1993). It is, of course, as irrefutable as saying that *homo sapiens* is a dangerous species. What sexual deviants of no matter what ilk wish to claim, above all, is normality.

THE ETIOLOGY OF MASOCHISM

Masochists are, like other human beings, individually different. If their sexual aims give them characteristics in common, the adoption of these aims has often come about in different ways, as can be inferred from Table 5.8 and, even more clearly, from Appendix 3. Their masochism is often, in Freud's usage of the word, overdetermined. For ES27, for instance, the dice were heavily loaded against a 'normal' sexual development. Besides preventing him from crying, his mother dressed him in girls' clothes because she had wanted a girl child and, as an adult, he made a strong impression of latent, unacknowledged homosexuality. At 4, his back teeth were extracted under gas, then his tonsils were removed, both situations of helplessness also signifying betrayal to him. He suffered the pain of a broken arm at 10, of a broken leg at 11, and chronic rheumatic pain. He arrived at puberty prematurely. He was jealous of his younger brother, and at school, all the girls were taller than he was. He laid his short stature at the door of his mother who had smoked 30 cigarettes a day during his gestation.

Incomplete Individuation

Mervin Glasser (1979, 1996) has, out of his extensive clinical involvement with sadomasochism at the Portman Clinic, London, put his finger on an important and frequently encountered etiological factor. His 1979 exposition of a 'core complex', reviewed in Chapter 2, remains basically unchanged in his revised contribution to the 3rd edition of *Sexual Deviation* (1996, edited like the 2nd edition by Ismond Rosen): "a deep-seated and pervasive longing for an intense and most intimate closeness to another person, amounting to a 'merging', a 'state of oneness', a 'blissful union'", which persists through all later stages of development and invariably awakens the fear of a permanent loss of self—what Glasser calls 'annihilation anxiety'—as soon as closeness is offered. The flight to a safe distance brings a sense of isolation and, in a vicious circle, the return of longing for union. Naked, destructive aggression, aroused by this threat of obliteration, cannot be directed towards the potentially engulfing person (originally the mother)—it may, however, be focussed on the self, and it may be sexualized and the relationship preserved in sadomasochistic mode.

Many observations made in the course of the present investigation confirmed the validity of Glasser's 'core complex', persisting from an early and primitive epoch of childhood. The majority of sadomasochistic subjects evinced a yearning for intimacy, for communication and trust. Most of them had poorly defined personalities in the sense that cliché and stereotype abounded in their discourse and their attitudes and went unrecognized. Particularly, those subjects whose Adult Attachment Interview transcripts were assigned an E1 classification seemed to lack a sense of personal identity. Such a lack of any identity apart from that of the family or the childhood background is, indeed, one of the criteria on which 'E' (entangled/preoccupied), as an overall classification, is awarded, and in Chapter 6 'E' was shown to be the model of attachment most strongly associated with sadomasochistic mental processing (Table 6.5). What the E1 classification, in particular, implies is that any struggle for autonomy which may have started, perhaps with adolescence, has failed. ES8, for instance, at the age of 75, belonged to an Adult Baby Club. Although away in the Forces for 6 years, he only left home when he married at 32. ES50 lived with his adoptive mother until her death when he was 41. When asked which parent he felt closer too, he replied: "I felt close to them both but I always had this overwhelming feeling that there was some unresolved emotional thing between my mother and myself ... I always felt that I really couldn't leave home, couldn't leave her." He described an experience he had some time between the age of four and six which was a compelling manifestation of Glasser's 'core complex': "There's an episode which—I don't know—I have a feeling probably affected my sexuality, and that is at one point she was—she was lying on the floor, when I was very young, and I was sort of jumping on her and we were playing, and she sort of enveloped me in a big cuddle or something and I had a very sudden, quite overwhelming feeling of revulsion somehow, that she was going to swallow me up or something and I sort of rebelled against that and I felt it physically affect every nerve in my body, made me sort of tingle ... "

In outlining their sexual activities as adults, several index subjects said that an orgasm was not necessary. Not only did they have an obvious reluctance to achieve satisfaction in conventional sexual intercourse with a partner, which might have been a reluctance due to a sense of guilt, but they even feared such a loss of control as the culmination of a punishment ritual. They would rather masturbate alone afterwards. This again confirms Glasser's interpretation that the masochist needs to regulate his moving towards or away from his partner, ensuring that he does not lose control of the situation in her presence and expose himself to the danger of being engulfed (Glasser, 1996, p. 292). This terror appears to emanate from the earliest years—that period designated in the jargon 'separation-individuation' which the masochist has never completed.

Sadomasochism as a Physiological Addiction

Perhaps one of the most striking confirmations of this hypothesis, put forward at the end of Chapter 4, came with the 41-year-old subject, ES17, who showed me his hands and said: "I've got hands like a sixty-five-year-old according to the doctors." The cause he had already explained: "I had severe eczema—and I mean severe, over every inch of my body except my face ... So I just bled and stuck to the sheets." Incredibly, in his late 20s he had himself tattooed on both shoulders and thought of this as a defiant reaction to victimization because of eczema—it was a different pain, he said, from eczema.

In a study of T.E. Lawrence, published under my maiden name (Turner, 1991), I discuss the probability that in cases of prolonged illness or severe injury, the endogenous opioids produced as a biological response to these situations may create an addiction to pain and stress, for they have been reported as being many times more addictive than morphine and other exogenous opiates ('Note on endogenous opioids', pp. 412–416.) As I already pointed out, their existence was deduced by Freud. *Project for a Scientific Psychology* (1895, though he himself did not settle on any title for the work) was Freud's heroic attempt to forge a link between neurology and psychology. He abandoned the draft as unpublishable and formulated his insights thenceforth in psychological terms only. But the intense analytic scrutiny behind the *Project*, his study and use of cocaine and his clinical familiarity with morphine must all have led him to the conviction that neuronal transmission was a strictly quantitative electrochemical process. In formulating the pleasure/unpleasure principle, the quantitative factor was there from the start (e.g., Freud, 1895*a*, *1*, p. 312). It was restated (1900, *5*, p. 598), critically examined (1915*a*, *14*, pp. 120–121), qualified but nevertheless reendorsed (1920*a*, *18*, pp. 7–8):

> We have decided to relate pleasure and unpleasure to the quantity of excitation that is present in the mind but is not in any way 'bound'; and to relate them in such a manner that unpleasure corresponds to an increase in the quantity of excitation and pleasure to a diminution.

The unravelling of the pleasure principle, the reality principle (which should moderate the pursuit of pleasure in the interests of self-preservation) and the Nirvana principle or principle of constancy was attempted in 1924, perhaps significantly in *The Economic Problem of Masochism* (*19*, pp. 159–161). The basic neurological concept of pleasure/unpleasure corresponding to diminution/increase of excitation was again only modified by the hypothesized temporal factor (rhythm of change). It is upon this quantitative aspect of the pleasure/unpleasure series, to which Freud adhered throughout his life, that I wish to focus.

On the chemical nature of neurological processes Freud observed presciently:

> ... it is a fact that there are foreign substances which, when present in the blood or tissues, directly cause us pleasurable sensations; and they also so alter the conditions governing our sensibility that we become incapable of receiving unpleasurable impulses. The two effects not only occur simultaneously, but seem to be intimately bound up with each other. But there must be substances in the chemistry of our own bodies which have similar effects ... (1930, *21*, p. 78)

These endogenous morphine-like substances, variously referred to as opioids, opiates or opioid peptides, were reported definitively by Kosterlitz and Hughes in 1975 in *Nature* (Hughes *et al.* 1975). The complete January issue of the *British Medical Bulletin*, edited by Hughes, was devoted to them in 1983, whilst Olson *et al.* (1980–1987) conducted a series of annual reviews of the on-going research in the field in the journal *Peptides*. The interest, the controversy and the literature generated by these neuromodulators have, in fact, been immense. The endogenous opioids most frequently investigated were the pentapeptides, met-enkephalin (amino acid sequence: tyrosine-glycine-glycine-phenylalanine-*met*hionine) and leu-enkephalin (tyrosine-glycine-glycine-phenylalanine-*leu*cine), β-endorphin, with a 31-amino-acid-sequence which arises from a different gene but contains the enkephalin chain, and the dynorphins from yet another gene, but many potent and long-lasting analogues have since been discovered. The receptors (mu, delta, kappa, epsilon and others, which are thought by some to be one basic receptor with multiple binding capacity) to which these neuromodulators bind have been found in many parts of the human body but are chiefly located in pain pathways and limbic parts of the brain. The inhibition of neuronal transmission which they effect may be achieved both presynaptically and postsynaptically, and the time course of action of opioid peptides is long in comparison with neurotransmitters such as acetylcholine. Their action has been reported as dose-dependent and, in some cases, biphasic. It is classically naloxone- or naltrexone-reversible. They have been implicated in eating, drinking, mood swings and strenuous physical exercise—an "endorphin rush" has now become part of common parlance. What is by now firmly established, however, and of prime significance, is that they are, like morphine, both pain-killing and addictive (Richardson & Zaleski, 1986; Smith *et al.* 1982; Nathan, 1988). They are actually produced by pain or stress, and they relieve it by reducing neural excitability. Pleasure, so often referred to in the literature as "the reward factor", follows. It is perhaps noteworthy that ever since their discovery, endogenous opioids have been tested on the *vas deferens* dissected out of the mouse. The implication is that the relief of stress-produced nervous tension and the release of sexual tension in orgasm are parallel processes in both of which endogenous opioids participate. In fact, their active presence in both cases has now been amply demonstrated by experiment and assay (Wiesenfeld-Hallin & Sodersten, 1984; Meston & Frohlich, 2000). They are the mediators of pain relief by both acupuncture and TeNS (transcutaneous nerve stimulation) equipment which emits an adjustable electric pulse. There apparently exists a form of acupuncture known as sexual acupuncture. Princess Grace of Monaco is said to have undergone this during her connection with the Solar Temple, the cult which has since become notorious through mass ritualized suicides. Its orgasmic effects are associated with the release of these neuronal hormones.

Endogenous opioids and their receptors have been found in all species examined, both vertebrate and invertebrate. Neuroendocrine cells, secreting peptides, appeared at once in the evolution of the primitive nervous system and these neuropeptides have been conserved with very little change from species to species throughout evolution. They are thus both ancient and fundamental to the functioning of the organism. In mammals, they have been found at significant levels during pregnancy, in the placenta, the umbilical cord and the amniotic fluid, blood plasma levels of both mother and fetus peaking at the intensely stressful time of delivery (Petrucha *et al.* 1983). The craving to return to the womb, evinced every night, as Freud (1917*a*, *14*, p. 222) suggested, when we prepare for sleep, may thus be in part a craving for the primal undisturbed state of well-being mediated in the fetus by these endogenous opioids. For what it is worth (and that may be little or much indeed), a marked increase in (β-endorphin secretion has been reported as occurring shortly before death (Carr, 1981).

It is high time to retreat before the alarmingly pretentious scale of this discussion and return, finally, to a consideration of masochism, itself a highly complex phenomenon. Let us therefore leave aside the psychological and examine the physical aspect, confining ourselves, that is, to the masochistic perversion and, within that, only to the seeking of pain and stress, not the more complex aim of humiliation. The practising masochist is a person for whom 'normal' sexual release by means of the genitals is at best problematic. Often, the anus and buttocks are more erotogenic than the genitals. If one looks into the childhood of a masochist, one very frequently, if not invariably, finds an accident or illness involving intense, protracted, physical pain, or repeated corporal punishment, or a situation causing severe, prolonged stress. These events, usually only the beginning of a series, have not only psychological but also physiological consequences, one of these being the release of endogenous opioids which are, crucially, not only produced in response to pain or stress but also addictive. As painful event succeeds event, what happened at first by ill chance is later engineered. Puberty and adolescence bring added tension to a sexuality rendered incompetent through regression to discharge it. Sexual intercourse is often, as in T.E. Lawrence's case, eschewed altogether. But an alternative mode of relieving nervous tension has been adopted with pain as a trigger. There are three factors which may be brought together to link endogenous opioids with masochism: (a) they are produced in response to pain and stress, (b) they are addictive, (c) they produce what is often referred to in the literature as "the reward factor", a sensation of pleasure. To put it squarely, since the endogenous opioids are pain-released and addictive and since the adult masochist is addictively seeking pain, it seems not unreasonable to assume (particularly in view of all the evidence to support the assumption) that on the physiological, as distinct from the psychological, level the endogenous opioids must play a role in the etiology and practice of the masochistic perversion.

In this investigation, I encountered, as predicted, many cases of childhood injury and illness which inevitably involved prolonged pain, and many childhood situations which were severely and chronically stressful (Table 5.8). I therefore consider that my hypothesis of a physiological addiction involving these endogenous opioids, laid down in childhood and reinforced by later sadomasochistic practice, is supported by the facts revealed by many of my interviewees. They were addictively seeking pain and some of them even knew it and, like ES21, explicitly stated it.

LESCH-NYHAN SYNDROME

Several index subjects expressed a belief that their sadomasochism was inherited (Table 8.2). There is, of course, a remote genetical influence on all behavior—everything is ultimately 'genetical' in an attenuated sense since the instructions for our anatomical and physiological infrastructure are inherited—but the predisposition to sadomasochism is, surely, far more likely to be transmitted culturally by parental example or created fortuitously by adverse events after birth. There does exist, however, a tragic condition, Lesch-Nyhan syndrome (Lesch & Nyhan, 1964; Hoefnagel, 1965; Kelley & Wyngaarden, 1983; King & Stansfield, 1985; Wiedemann *et al.* 1992), featuring mental retardation, self-mutilation and sudden aggressive behavior, which is indeed an inherited defect of metabolism. This brief report is introduced at this point because some scepticism may have been aroused by the claim in the previous subsection that there can be a physiological addiction to pain—strictly speaking, not to pain but to the sensations which follow upon it and which are physiologically, as distinct from psychologically, mediated. Lesch-Nyhan syndrome, or HGPRT (hypoxanthine-guanine-phosphoribosyltransferase) deficiency, is the result of a mutation in a recessive structural gene which lies on the long arm of the X chromosome (Xq26). It is therefore transmitted by a carrier-mother to her son and has a prevalence of 1 in 10,000 males. It results in an abnormally high production of uric acid which, present at a raised level in the saliva, may be a direct irritant of the buccal mucosa, accounting to some extent for the biting of lips and lining of the mouth. The finger joints may also be irritated (as in gout) and similarly be bitten. However, no such direct explanation could apply to the following: (a) hitting the head against objects, (b) placing extremities in between the spokes of a wheelchair, (c) hitting out at others, spitting, using abusive language, whilst apologizing.

One explanation would be that these self-mutilating habits are akin to an addiction, i.e., the use of severe pain to obtain a release of endogenous opioids and thus obtain some relief from the unremitting discomfort of hyperuricemia. The outward aggression might be an attempt, as ill-directed violent gestures in general often are, to obtain some release of the nervous tension, constantly accumulating as a result of this same sustained discomfort.

The fact that sufferers beg to have their hands or arms left in restraint would seem, if anything, to confirm the hypothesis of addiction, in the same way that a heroin addict struggles to stay off the drug by seeking external restraint. Where this applies to one arm only, it suggests that a *formula* for satisfaction, or assuagement, has been established, using this particular arm. These suggestions are, of course, pure speculations, but the condition itself points to the fact that a physical, indeed physiological, basis for masochistic behavior must be considered alongside the psychological.

Way Stations on the Road to Sadomasochism

Gosselin & Wilson (1980) concluded from their large sample that the male fetishists stood as an intermediate group in terms of their sexual behavior, with male sadomasochists overlapping on one side and male transvestites on the other: "There are more transvestites and sadomasochists with a fetishistic interest on top of their own predilection than there are transvestites interested in sado-masochism" (p. 152). Many of my own subjects (e.g. ES8, ES40, ES63, ES71, ES76) described sexually colored incidents in their childhood involving rubber or plastic articles, and attributed their lifelong interest in rubber or shiny plastic as sexual stimuli to these incidents.

Fetishes may bear some resemblance to the 'transitional objects' postulated by Winnicott (1953). Bowlby preferred the term 'substitute objects', explaining that inanimate objects simply have 'certain components of attachment behavior' directed or redirected towards them because the attachment figure herself is unavailable. Like her, they are sought particularly when a child is tired or sick or upset (Bowlby, 1969, pp. 312–313). One might perhaps add also when a child is bored, and one might continue to speculate that at such a time, the physical properties of the substitute object itself might become salient. In a final step, they might become sexual stimuli through masturbation.

In pursuit of their fetish, several index subjects found themselves confronted with pornographic literature which led them into the SM 'scene'. In other words, what they at first encountered in sex shops as a contiguous interest gradually extended its fascination and became central to their deviance. As to the fetishistic paraphernalia on sale in sex shops, a telling observation is made by John Liggett (1974) in his wide-ranging book, *The Human Face*. Writing of the tribal medicine man or *feticheur* (the word 'fetish' comes from the Portuguese *feitiço*, meaning 'charm' or 'sorcery', and was used by explorers to describe some of the symbolic artefacts they encountered on voyages to the African coast during the 17th century), he observes: "The more frightening and mystifying he makes his mask, the more effective will be his treatment ... The distinctive mask which he wore served to enhance and confirm his importance; it concealed his miserably ordinary personal identity and created for him an entirely new and powerful personality. Like a uniform, it defined his role and confirmed his status" (Liggett, 1974, p. 166).

The Role of Comics and Science Fiction

A surprising number of index subjects (e.g., ES1, ES27, ES30, ES37, ES41, ES42, ES52, ES57, ES62, ES74), when asked to trace the development of their sadomasochistic interests, mentioned comics as a strong influence. They spent much time reading them in childhood, savouring the beatings received by the hapless characters figuring in them week by week. These reading habits frequently progressed to science fiction, where the visual images are quite plainly identical with the stereotypes of SM apparel. However, it is not only a question of these externals of science fiction magazines, films and television providing the raw materials for SM fantasies, a sort of visual framework. The mindless ruthlessness of most sci-fi is identical with the sadomasochistic compulsion to win at any price, with the philosophy of victory in defeat, with the preoccupation with power and, when ingested as a steady diet, can only help to create or reinforce such a mind-set.

The protest might be raised: "But this is monstrous! This is 'Reds under the bed'! Would you deny kids their comics and their computer games?" My response is that I am simply reporting a finding of this investigation. It might be set alongside the easily verifiable observation that for decades the subject matter of short cartoon films such as the *Tom and Jerry* series has been glaringly sadistic. The only further inference I am prepared to draw is that considerable cynicism must lie behind their creation.

CONCLUSIONS

(1) As found by earlier investigators (e.g., Spengler, 1977; Litman & Swearingen, 1972), sadomasochism is more prevalent in males than in females, at least as an overt sexual deviance.

(2) As observed by Theodor Reik (1939, 1941), sadomasochists are, characteristically, eager to reveal themselves personally and to discuss their sexuality in particular.
(3) Sadomasochism is a heterogeneous phenomenon with a variety of etiologies, almost all, however, likely to start at an early age (Figure 8.3).
(4) The childhood of the sadomasochists taking part in this study was frequently either harsh, lonely, stifling or smothering, leading to two main effects: (a) insecurity of emotional attachment, (b) underdevelopment of metacognitive capacity. Both these effects were likely to militate against successful human relationships on a psychological level and to be largely responsible for sadomasochistic preoccupation with the physical.
(5) Although some features were shared by sadomasochistic subjects and depressed controls, the latter possessed significantly more coherence and capacity to 'mentalize' (Tables 5.5–5.7; Figure 7.3).
(6) The index subjects showed clear evidence of a sadomasochistic mind-set (Tables 6.3, 6.6, 6.7). Since no similar bias in mental processing was discernable in the control group, this finding supports the postulate of mental rigidity attributed to sadomasochists before undertaking this empirical investigation (Chapter 4).
(7) Responses to the last item of the Beck Depression Inventory regarding loss of libido showed that the depressed index subjects were anomalous (Table 7.3). Their retained interest in sex tended to support the theory that sadomasochism acts as a defence against depression by the erotization of suffering (Panel, 1984).
(8) There were significantly more adopted subjects in the index group than would be expected by chance, and they had all received unfortunate adoptive parenting, creating, for the most part, a dismissing or devaluing internal model of attachment. The high incidence of adoptees in the sadomasochistic group suggests (a) the importance of a genetic relationship as a biological basis for good parenting, (b) that, since they differed greatly one from another as individuals, parenting probably plays a more important role than genetic inheritance in the development of sadomasochism (though this plausible assumption could only be confirmed or refuted by information about natural parents which was not available).
(9) The causes advanced by sadomasochistic subjects in explanation of their deviant sexuality were not notably perceptive, and some were bizarre (Table 8.2), again pointing to a low capacity for metacognition or low 'reflective-self function' (Fonagy *et al.* 1991*a*).

(10) In agreement with other studies (e.g., Gosselin & Wilson, 1980), more index subjects presented themselves as submissive than dominant (Table 8.1).

(11) The role of fantasy as a quintessential characteristic of sadomasochism (Reik, 1939) was amply confirmed (e.g., Table 8.3). The fantasies of self-styled masochists appeared to be predominantly sadistic (Table 8.5), underlining the observation made at the end of Chapter 3 that sadomasochism is one entity.

(12) As postulated (Chapter 4), self-deception, hypocrisy and, above all, lack of coherence emerged as characteristic of even the more intelligent, articulate and educated sadomasochists when considering their attititudes toward (a) cruelty and (b) love (Chapter 8, Table 8.6, Figure 8.4).

(13) The sadomasochistic relationships many of the index subjects formed could be related, through their own accounts, to a 'core complex' (Glasser, 1979, 1996) comprising a primitive longing for union conflicting with a terror of being taken over completely by another person, originally the mother. The transformation of aggression (the response to this fear) into sadism enabled some sort of link to be maintained.

(14) On the basis of their interviews, these sadomasochistic subjects' preoccupation with control could be ascribed in some cases to this anxiety about the loss of a fragile identity in any close contact with another human being, in other cases to the need to become master of situations which had once been suffered helplessly.

(15) As discussed in a previous publication under my maiden name (Turner, 1991, pp. 412–416), some sadomasochists, as a result of severe and prolonged pain or stress in childhood, acquired a physiological addiction, probably mediated by the body's endogenous opioids, to painful and stressful situations. This is, in fact, Freud's 'erotogenic masochism' (Freud, 1924*a*).

(16) One danger of addiction is its escalation. This can take the form of an intensification in the individual or an increased prevalence in the population.

Part III

THE PHILOSOPHY OF SADOMASOCHISM AND ITS EFFECTS

CHAPTER 10

THE QUESTION OF CONTROL

SUMMARY

The masochist's philosophy of 'victory through defeat' has a destructive effect on those nearest to him. That human beings can only relate to each other in terms of domination and submission is a needlessly limiting view of close relationship.

The main thrust of this study has been to determine the characteristics of masochism and to investigate its etiology. Both of these are heterogeneous and, because they are dependent upon definition, elusive. But for all that, masochism exists as a phenomenon. People know what is meant when an attitude or a behavior is dubbed 'masochistic'. Freud wrestled with the enigma of masochism thoughout his professional life and saw it "in the light of a great danger" (Freud, 1924*a*, p. 159). He was never in doubt as to its destructive nature: "Its danger lies in the fact that it originates from the death instinct" (p. 170). Whether this is taken literally or metaphorically, it implies an attitude to life, a *Weltanschauung*, a creed. It is generally appreciated that masochism is, almost by definition, self-destructive, but the self-destructive tendency has aggressive as well as self-punitive and erotic components (Menninger, 1938). A philosophy of life is likely to have wider repercussions than those affecting only the individual who holds it, and it is likely to be judged on those wider repercussions. What, then, is the philosophy of masochism—for this is not immediately obvious to all—and what are its effects? The justification for broadening the enquiry at this late stage, rather than concluding it, is twofold: (1) to grasp the nature of masochism, it is advisable to know its rationale; (2) to judge its morbidity, it is wise to be informed concerning its sequelae. These are likely to differ according to the manner in which it manifests and the degree of satisfaction it achieves.

CONTROL

> The only conception capable of explaining the movement of the locomotive is that of a force commensurate with the movement observed. The only conception capable of explaining the movement of peoples is that of some force commensurate with the whole movement of the peoples. (Leo Tolstoy, 1869)

Many of those practising sadomasochism will tell you that it is all about control. Their explanations are, however, seldom adequate to the impenetrability of the phenomenon they are addressing. Here is a verbatim extract from my third interview with a subject who had, from the start, emphasized his academic interest in my research. Roman type denotes ES19, italics denote the interviewer, myself, and an oblique stroke denotes an interruption.

> I have given it a good deal of thought. I think I might be about to slightly disappoint you because I can't say that I've been able to—I can't say that I've been able to think of too much, but I would—to me, basically, the philosophy has to be—as long as it's freely entered into—the basic philosophy has to be the pursuit of pleasure—em—both physical and emotional, I suppose. Beyond that there is, of course, the well-documented—as regards the submissive—there's the well-documented achievement of relinquishing control to the dominant person, *(Yes)* which for a lot of people is attractive and, of course, for the one playing the dominant role, there is the achievement of the dominant position, the acting out of it, the enjoying of it, which they may not be able to undergo in ordinary life. So there's obviously that—that side of it as well but, of course, they both, I suppose, come under the heading of the pursuit of pleasure. I know for a fact that, when you're in the dominant role, although an outsider, who is not familiar with these activities—an outsider would probably regard the dominant role as the—on the face of it, the more attractive one, the more inviting, maybe the easier one, but, having experienced these situations, I can assure anyone that it is not the easier one, because when you're in control, when you're the dominant, *you* are the driving force, effectively, for the entire proceedings. You've got to keep the whole thing going, you've got to instigate things, you've got to control things, you've got to order things, you've got to be in charge, and that is an awful lot easier—an awful lot more difficult than just, effectively, relinquishing all influence, all power, and taking what the dominant person is dishing out. That is fairly easy as long as you can cope with the

discomfort, of course. So really, on the point of philosophy, other than being an aspect of the pursuit of pleasure, I haven't really been able to tie things down as regards the philosophy of SM, much more than that.

* * * * *

If you're saying that the main thing you have come up with, having thought quite a bit about it, is the pursuit of pleasure/

/If it's entered into freely and with consent.

Yes. There is just one question that follows from that. I mean one can pursue pleasure in more obvious ways than, you know, being caned.

Oh yes. Some people wouldn't dream of likening the infliction of pain to the pursuit of pleasure, no. Other people's ideas of pleasure wouldn't necessarily be mine.

So what do you think is the other factor in this that makes it—that more or less determines that the pursuit of pleasure is by this particular means?

Well this is *one* means of pursuing pleasure. Because if pleasure isn't by this particular means alone, this is *a* method of pursuing pleasure, certainly not the only one/

/Why is it pleasurable?

Why is it pleasurable? *(Mm)* Well, as I mentioned earlier, if one is dominant, there is the thrill of power; if one is submissive, there is the satisfaction of abandoning control to another person; there is a degree of physical stimulation once the moment of pain has past; and there is for me the—perhaps exhibitionism or the flaunting of oneself in what might be regarded as somewhat of an exotic outfit, i.e., an outfit that is basically that that would be worn by [inaudible].

But in a way that puts it just one remove—in other words, as dominant it's the sense of power, but you can have a sense of power in various ways, you know.

You can have a sense of power in a lot of ways—the prime minister has a sense of power.

Well I mean, a pop singer perhaps.

Yes, they have power over their fans, don't they? The fans worship them whatever they do.

And you can also cast off—as the submissive—cast off responsibility—you can do that in other ways also—you can go on holiday, you know, and lounge about on the beach.

That's something I certainly don't do. I would regard lounging about on the beach as a complete waste of time. I just don't do that.

Yes, but I mean it is possible. (Oh yes) *So, again, why this particular means?*

Inexplicable, I would say. Inexplicable, probably even to myself, why we—why some of us find some things pleasurable and others not, and why other people cannot understand that certain people find things pleasurable that they don't. Inexplicable, to my mind.

You don't have any further sort of insight on that field?

I don't think so. Sorry to disappoint you!

It might be argued that ES19 is right, that any person might be at a loss to explain precisely how he obtains his sexual pleasure. However, the sadomasochist is often an educated man who is well aware that he is dealing in pain and humiliation. This underlines that there is, of course, a disincentive to any attempt to acquire a theory of mind in later years, assuming it were possible. The more aware one becomes of other people's thoughts and feelings, the more likely it becomes that their aspirations will interfere with one's own, that one will be gradually, like Prince Myshkin in Dostoevsky's *Idiot,* torn apart by their problems and their miseries. Not to put too fine a point on it, there is a cynical argument for pursuing one's own pleasure, oblivious of the mental state of the human object providing it. As the Marquis de Sade—and who could question *his* authority on the subject?—observed through the nobleman, Noirceuil (*Histoire de Juliette: Les Prospérités du Vice,* 1792): "There is no passion more egotistic than that of sensuality; not one that demands to be served more sternly. One must absolutely never think about anyone but oneself."

Control over Unpleasant Things One Could not Escape

As Freud pointed out (Freud, 1920*a*, *S.E. 18*, pp. 16–17; 1926, *S.E. 20*, p. 167), a child will repeat an unpleasant experience in its play in order to gain control of it. Play is the instinct to master. Sadism too, derives from this instinct for mastery in a pregenital stage of sexuality (Freud, 1905, *S.E. 7*, p. 193).

When considering the etiology of masochism in Chapter 9, it was mentioned that the depressed index subject, ES27, had his back teeth extracted at the age of four. These are his actual words and 'she' is, of course, his mother: "I never trusted her. She was the first person that ever betrayed my trust... suddenly there would be like all these smiling, well-meaning people sort of pushing me into a chair to be gassed and have my teeth taken out... I was like, you know, forcibly—had these things done to me on about three or four separate occasions as a kid kind of—and I'd always be 'conned' about it... She was the first person I kind of like—you know, I kind of like trusted and respected as a kid, I mean, as you do, who was then up to something very sinister behind my back." During our discussion after the more formal procedures of the interview, he said he would now probably indulge in the fear that was generated by such incidents in the past until he reached orgasm. Being forced to do something had become his favourite sadomasochistic fantasy and 'activity'. His mother had dressed him in girls' clothes as a young child, and he had triumphed by making cross-dressing a major source of sexual pleasure. However, the consequences of this mechanism for obtaining defiant pleasure are plain: a distortion of attitude which will not be comprehensible but alienating to many people, which may be damaging to the individual concerned in some circumstances and which leads to a confused perception of 'active' and 'passive'. The point is that it is attempting to go further than the replacement of helplessness by control—with characteristic overambition the masochist insists on pleasure. How successful it is as a psychological defense against helplessness is debatable. In relating the incidents, ES27 added: "I'm not generally these days a very trusting person."

Thus, the masochist, who has never grown up, *recreates* not once but many times, the situation he fears in order that he shall not, in retrospect, be the hapless victim of it but, indeed, its instigator. This is not likely to benefit those in his path! If he fears to live alone, he will systematically destroy one marriage, or intimate relationship, after another. If he fears to present an indelicate image to the world, he will not shave or wash for weeks. If he has invariably, clumsily, broken his toys, he will continue to break radios, chairs, even lavatories throughout his life because *he chooses* to be clumsy. It is not difficult to know when these 'mishaps' are 'deliberate', as distinct from truly inadvertent, because he will never apologize or express regret. (The single quotes refer to the fact that he is constantly operating on the level of what Freud termed the primary processes.)

Even the rubber fetish probably started in infancy, as in the case of the 77-year-old depressed subject, ES40, as intense discomfort in clammy rubber pants or lying, soaked, on a rubber cot-sheet (Appendix 3). Powerless then to escape the situation, the only means of controlling it in retrospect was to assert: "I adore the smelliness, stickiness, sweaty unpleasantness of rubber next to my skin!"

THE EFFECTS OF MASOCHISM IN EVERYDAY LIFE

In the course of this research, a letter arrived from a woman who seemed the disturbingly typical victim of what one might describe as 'the suburban masochist', the deviant who seeks, both overtly and covertly, to impose his sexuality on an unwilling partner. Her letter described her husband's behavior during their 30-year marriage: "He says I don't treat him right, I am not cruel enough and I don't enjoy the power that I could have over him. The trouble is he is right—I don't enjoy having a man as a slave, I cannot understand his behavior and I just don't know how to cope with him." This man was not only tormenting her day by day, but doing so in an attempt to deform her personality.

I would refer the reader back to the beginning of this Part III, where I adumbrate a justification for its inclusion though of a broader nature than the empirical study reported in Part II, indeed I would refer him back to its title: The philosophy of sadomasochism *and its effects*. (The use of the first person should alert the reader to the fact that, again, personal observations are to follow and that they are subject to the *caveat* placed at the beginning of Part I, namely, that, however accurately observed, they cannot be wholly objective and cannot claim general validity.) This woman's letter has led me to present a picture, a composite picture, of the likely effects of masochism in everyday life. I have personally witnessed all the details of this picture many times and with different protagonists. The 'man-in-the-street' masochist usually has a bad start in life. (Although, in coming forward, they are what might be termed the tip of the iceberg, whereas I am here depicting the iceberg hidden beneath, the index subjects I interviewed for empirical study supplied background material which might, in most cases and with their own concurrence, be regarded as a bad start in life; Appendix 3.) He develops an awkwardness and pursues incompetence for sexual pleasure (Freud, 1924*a*, pp. 169–170). He engineers situations in which he feels powerless, and he enjoys feeling powerless. (This is akin to the cryptic defiance of bondage: "I am deprived of any possibility of satisfaction yet, even so, I will have satisfaction"—in the same way as ES27 stated that he could now reach orgasm by 'indulging' in the fear created by traumatic situations.) He becomes obsessed with control, but control in a positive sense is precisely what he does not have by this time. 'Primary process' mentation may result in an intuitive grasp of some element in another person's unconscious, but it is not capable of a theory of mind, of accurately assessing another's reactions where they are conscious, logical and, one might have thought, obvious. Having thus probably arrived at an undistinguished and unsatisfying position in life, he seeks a partner, and with this unfortunate (or desperate) woman he engages in a day-to-day acrimonious tussle over trivia. This is a crazy ritual of pain and frustration, but it is all he has in lieu of being in genuine, positive control of a situation. Andreas Spengler (1977) in his empirical study of sadomasochism in 245 German males, reviewed in Part I, put it in moderate terms: "An especially difficult situation occurs in marriage: the deviant desires are frequently incompatible with the interests of the wife" (p. 444). The woman remains baffled, disbelieving, until she realizes that living with a masochist is like living with an enemy. It is not easy for her to perceive this for three reasons: (a) she may have entered the relationship in the expectation of an affectionate helpmate; (b) his behavior is highly ambivalent; (c) his hostility is partly hidden by the banal nature of his provocations. This latter point, already made in Chapter 4, lends a dismal quality to the unhappiness. Theodor Reik (1939), in explaining the masochistic characteristic he designated 'the suspense factor', used the analogy of the child reserving the portion of his meal which he likes best to the last and pointed to the danger "that the child finally renounces entirely that particular bit of food" (p. 40). Probably as a result of fixation, food has frequently remained from childhood onwards, an opportunity and a device for provoking. For instance, time and effort have gone into the preparation of a meal, but the adult masochist's approach to food, as I have noticed on many occasions, is to obtain the maximum unpleasure from it Typically, he will perhaps eat steadily through the vegetables on his plate without any meat or gravy—like a spoilt child he dislikes vegetables. After he has dawdled an hour, the gravy is, of course, cold and congealed. If he has a favourite dish in front of him, he promptly chokes.

Ultimately, then, after many tearful struggles to find a sane interpretation, the realization dawns on this woman that, though superficially, sporadically, he may be loving, there is an undercurrent which is relentlessly damaging, that this is treatment which would only be meted out to an enemy. As Hilde Lewinsky observed over fifty years ago, the masochist demands with no giving in return: "There is thus no other way of fulfilling this condition than by what may be called an unpleasant relationship" (Lewinsky, 1944, p. 154). She is not acquiescing to the role he wants to force on her—she is denying him the enactment of his fantasies. Unconsciously, and therefore unchangingly, he has perhaps perceived her as an enemy from the start. His first love objects may well have been experienced as enemies, they may even have been enemies—indeed 'other people' in general may thence be deemed, primarily, enemies. From this position, there can only be swings of the pendulum towards idealization, immature infatuation, sentimentality. But the pendulum will always swing back. As it swings forward, he sees people as awe-inspiring or threatening; as it swings back, he undervalues their capabilities and sees them as objects of contempt; he is either intimidated or irritated. (The fluctuation between overvaluation and undervaluation of the self, with which the corresponding fluctuation in the assessment of others is linked, was noticeable in several sadomasochistic subjects who came to be interviewed—it was most marked perhaps in the cases of ES35 and ES36—and was already discussed towards the end of Chapter 5 under the subheading 'Claims to superior ability'.)

The woman whose unenviable position we have been considering can *never win* against her masochistic partner. All values are reversed—in her efforts, she is aiming at success, but he is aiming at failure, he is entropy incarnate. He enjoys transgressing *and* being punished for transgression.

He can even enjoy the opprobrium attaching to his masochistic indulgences. It is useless to remonstrate with him—she cannot sting him into changing. However hurtful the accusation, it will not pain him, for his pain is his pleasure. It leaves him not contrite, not shattered, but cheerful, refreshed—and unchanged, always immovably unchanged. Even if, long-suffering and fully cognizant, she manages somehow to endure the ceaseless provocations with a minimum of reprisal, even if she contrives to ignore them, to anticipate and circumvent them, to deflect them, to rob them wherever possible of their destructiveness, refusing to be forced into the 'dominatrix' role, she will not be able to salvage a viable relationship for she is starving him of precisely that sexual gratification which is craved. There is no longer any spice in the relationship, she is no longer attractive to him, and he grows bored. (During one of several discussions of the topic with the 53-year-old masochist ES15, he pronounced his sexual interest in his wife to be 'zilch'.) Again, it requires to be underlined that in imposing his internal model of attachment, which is one of domination and submission, the masochist is destroying this woman, who had no part in the injuries he received in his childhood. He is prepared to warp her personality until it finally fits his model.

These observations may, of course, apply *mutatis mutandis* to female masochism. Undoubtedly there are women who deliberately goad their husbands or partners to violence. There are women, nowadays fewer, who elect the role of martyr at every opportunity. The women, mostly young women, who practise self-mutilation are not usually doing so for sexual gratification. Their behavior may be devastating to those closest to them, but it is differently motivated from that of the male masochist characterized above. The harm really is aimed primarily at the self, and it is primarily to relieve unbearable tension, replacing one pain by another. Those working clinically in this field, for example, Gloria Babiker and Lois Arnold, have become convinced that when these schoolgirls or young women cut their arms with glass or pencil-sharpener blades, it is as "a distracter from distress" (Babiker & Arnold, 1997, p. 5). They have "such self-hatred and despair as to wish to destroy and annihilate any real experience of self, in order to carry on functioning at some other level" (p. 6). True, they may be expressing anger and frustration, but their chief motive in injuring themselves is to regulate distress and soothe anxiety so as to carry on with life, not destroy it.

The Intergenerational Cycle

Many masochists do not marry or do not remain married. Latent homosexuality, an inhibited or fearful attitude to conventional sexual intercourse, instilled in childhood, or insecurity in forming relationships condemn them to a solitary life of fantasy and prostitutes. Those who enter and remain in lasting, if tortured, relationships rarely have any desire, themselves, for children. Their sexual behavior is rarely compatible with the biological function of procreation and, in fact, some deliberately sabotage their partners' chances of conceiving in order to torture them. The two adopted index subjects ES4 and ES50 had adopted children. Should a child arrive, usually through no intention of his, the laziness, the passivity, the preoccupation with self, the refusal to relinquish the child's role himself, make the masochist a neglectful and unproviding parent. He recreates the way *he* felt as a child—the insecurity, the betrayal, the destructiveness. He recreates this unwholesome state of affairs for the same prime reason that all behavior is repeated—because, since he is not open to fresh experience, it is the only situation he knows. As Bernhard Berliner (1940, 1947, 1958) puts it, this is the only love he knows. Revenge is really only a subsidiary motive. This is Freud's 'compulsion to repeat'. This is the 'intergenerational cycle' of attachment theory. Human mentation is not often able to create something truly new. When it happens, it is probably by the recognition of a propitious accident. The corollary of this observation is, of course, that if one wants to know how the masochist suffered as a child, the subtler elements of his suffering, it is only necessary to study closely and define the suffering he inflicts day by day on the family he lives with.

The Masochist's Rewards

The effects of the masochist's philosophy on others are likely to be negative, with the exception of those few professionals who are prepared to benefit from the money and domestic services of a 'slave'. It is also difficult to foresee many positive consequences for the masochist himself in pursuing his obsession with control and, at the same time, attempting to subvert the pleasure principle. At this point, however, it is advisable to define which aspect of the heterogeneous, amorphous phenomenon of masochism we have been looking at and which aspect we are now proposing to examine. We have just been looking at the masochist who may or may not admit to himself that he has a sexual deviance but who nevertheless seeks to impose it on others who do not acquiesce in it, and furthermore, this deviance has spread into his personality. We now turn, in the interests of fairness, to see whether those who are open about their unusual sexual interests, who act out their sadomasochism in an explicitly sexual context, have anything more positive to contribute. ES58 took money for her services of domination but also enjoyed bestowing them. She generously sent me some of her writing on SM themes, including some poems. The following excerpt is from a piece of prose, highly anatomical in content, headed 'Reflection': "Sometimes, she imagines scenarios, staged tableaux, in which his body is the living prop. He is usually static, in her mind she rarely sees him in motion, he is restrained or waiting to be restrained. Stretched over metalwork; hung by the neck; kneeling; crucified; it is the same. He is waiting to be done unto, to be undone. He is waiting for her." The 27-year-old 'gay' submissive to whom she administered wrote: "I was able to act out fantasies I had harboured for years—like a crucifixion 'thing' I'd had since I was 7 years old ... When the unpleasant—but at the same time pleasant—stimuli became unbearable and were replaced by total loving concern and care from the same person that five minutes previously had been beating the shit out of me—dichotomy again—the state I was left in was literally out of this world. It was how I imagine heaven is supposed to be—or the buddhists' nirvana."

There are several features of this duo which are worth noting: (a) the physical nature of the interaction; (b) its insulated, egocentric nature; (c) its dehumanizing effect—'his body is the living prop'—'beating the shit out of me'; (d) its compartmentalizing effect—'dichotomy again'. The mystical apotheosis is perhaps better left, without comment, for individual judgment.

Those who acknowledge their sadomasochism do, however, gain an advantage over those who do not in the effectiveness of their mental processing. There is a greater openness in the flow of information, both incoming and outgoing, which is noticeable even at the level of conversation. It seems likely that this difference turns around an internal model of the self which can accommodate what many would find unacceptable. In overt sadomasochists there is, therefore, less necessity for processes of defensive exclusion to come into operation (Bowlby, 1980, chapter 4) than in those who do not acknowledge their sadomasochism.

Hierarchical Situations

Several life situations, all involving control, power, a hierarchical system, lend themselves to sadomasochistic relations within the situation. The most obvious of these figure regularly in SM rituals—the school, the army, the justice system. Potential sadists gravitate to positions of power like bees to a honey pot.

Supposedly on his thirtieth birthday, T.E. Lawrence, whose diverse gifts made his self-destructiveness all the more poignant, conducted an exceptional piece of self-examination and self-revelation. He placed it towards the end of *Seven Pillars of Wisdom*, as Chapter 103, with the running head: 'Myself'. In his incisive style, he paints a portrait of asceticism, of grandiosity, of quintessential masochism: "There seemed a certainty in degradation, a final safety. Man could rise to any height, but there was an animal level beneath which he could not fall" (p. 581). He reviews the men with whom he had associated during the 1916–18 Arab Revolt in unmistakably masochistic terms: "It was a part of my failure never to have found a chief to use me. All of them, through incapacity or timidity or liking, allowed me too free a hand; as if they could not see that voluntary slavery was the deep pride of a morbid spirit, and vicarious pain its gladdest decoration" (p. 582).

Hierarchical systems are, by their structure, conducive to bullying. Having been forced at every stage to defer to the person immediately above and having resented yet coveted the privileges just out of reach, the 'upwardly mobile' individual is only too ready, on promotion, to demand deference from the person immediately beneath and to guard any privileges now acquired. It is true that other species, including primates, establish hierarchies, but it is characteristic of the human species to seek—whether with ultimate success remains to be seen—social values which are more humane than the indifference of the natural law. There is apparently a current trend towards democratization. Hardly reaching beyond the political and business spheres as yet, it still has a long way to go.

Take, for example, the recent adverse publicity surrounding training methods for classical ballet in England. The junior branch of the Royal Ballet School at White Lodge, Richmond, dispensed unnecessary bullying and suffering, it was alleged in *The Times* of Friday, 8 August 1997. It is not alone in attracting an above-average proportion of potentially masochistic, anorexic pupils. Ballet is a "theatre of the body" (McDougall, 1989), frequently involving pain, always demanding discipline.

In the so-called 'professions'—a snobbish designation if ever there was one—and even in the heartland of academia, a hierarchical structure can encourage intellectual bullying, the imposition of ideas. A self-perpetuating élite is created on criteria seldom subjected to review; abilities are categorized with little awareness of possible change; certain opinions are automatically deferred to, others disregarded.

Bureaucracy is frequently cruel. The Nazi atrocities could not have been perpetrated without the administration presided over by the bureaucratic mind, operating through a hierarchy of ever more mindless bureaucrats. The brilliance of Franz Kafka was to recognize and to portray the human predicament in terms of hierarchical situations where it was impossible to win against a succession of bureaucrats. The cruelty arises from psychical rigidity, from intolerance of anomaly, of troublesome individual difference. It manifests as an insensitivity to suffering. Like the masochist, the bureaucrat has little understanding of the mental states or emotions of others. Procedures must be strictly adhered to; rituals must be ordered as prescribed. Like the masochist, he has little insight into his own narrowly determined mental processes. He can never fathom how the bureaucratic muddles he creates could arise. Even if this is explained to him, he cannot accept it!

Nobody would suggest that all bureaucrats are sadomasochists, any more than that all sadomasochists are bureaucrats, but that, demonstrably, they have certain characteristics in common. Angus Calder (1971) alleges in *The People's War* (p. 223) that bureaucrats in some of the London Borough Councils displayed not only incompetence but callousness with respect to suffering caused by the 1940–41 blitz, that they were only concerned with their own prestige. (Prestige was an issue which surfaced in several interviews with sadomasochists conducted in my own empirical study, most notably perhaps in the case of ES41.) In his compelling and highly readable book *On the Psychology of Military Incompetence*, Norman Dixon (1976) writes of the "ritualistic observance of the dominance-submission relationships of the military hierarchy, extreme orderliness and a preoccupation with outward appearances" (p. 177). Like masochistic ritual, military 'bullshit' is, amongst other things, a defense against anxiety. Theodor Adorno *et al.* (1950), in their study of *The Authoritarian Personality*, list as some of its salient characteristics: a rigid adherence to conventional values, a submissive, uncritical attitude to authority, a tendency to condemn and punish those not conforming, an opposition to the imaginative and tender, a belief in magic, a habit of thinking in rigid categories, a preoccupation with the dominance-submission dimension, a 'puritanical' prurience with respect to sex. Their findings from the presentation of actual Nazi statements to over 2000 Americans are in many ways similar to those of Eysenck (1954, 1970) in England. They depict attitudes I encountered in my own research on sadomasochism reported in Part II.

The complex interactions of adults in hierarchical systems can thus present opportunities for cryptic sadomasochism, or at least the addictive control of one human being by another. More generally, however, the prototypic dominance/submission situation is still the home in early childhood. The infant is born and remains for some years, relatively helpless.

THE CASE OF ALFRED C. KINSEY

In a recent article in *The New Yorker* (25 August and 1 September 1997), "Annals of Sexology: Dr. Yes", the Kinsey biographer, James H. Jones, has revealed the principal author of the two famous Reports (Kinsey *et al.* 1948, 1953) as himself, not only bisexual, but "from childhood on, a masochist who, as he grew older, pursued an interest in extreme sexuality with increasing compulsiveness. His secret life was shared with a small circle of intimates, a few of whom became his sexual partners, sometimes in the name of 'research'" (p. 101). The excruciating torture he inflicted on his own genitals by sudden and brutal constriction of the scrotum is described in convincing detail. He had it filmed, in fact, in his attic.

At his Institute for Sex Research at Indiana University, Kinsey "was a strong-willed patriarch who created around himself a kind of utopian community in which sexual experimentation was encouraged" (p. 100). His appetite for control extended beyond his family to members of his staff and some trusted outsiders, amongst them high-profile sado-masochists. He "decreed that the men could have sex with each other, and that the wives, too, could be free to embrace whatever sexual partners they liked" (p. 110). He himself participated in these activities, and he pressured the other participants to agree to being filmed in them. He insisted, however, on controlling their sexual behavior. Any proposed extramarital affair had first to receive his assent.

Kinsey was born in 1894 of parents who were evangelical Protestants, whose Old Testament God "knew a person's every thought and deed and punished those who broke the Commandments" (p. 101). The eldest of three children, he suffered from rickets, rheumatic fever and typhoid fever. He was in pain and kept in bed over protracted periods until he was ten, when his health improved with the family's removal from the Hudson waterfront town of Hoboken, New Jersey, to South Orange where he could collect butterflies and observe birds in the hills and marshes. Although a campus leader at Bowdoin College, Maine, he was remembered by members of the fraternity he joined as 'a loner'. He studied under William Morton Wheeler, a world authority on the social behavior of insects, at the Bussey Institution, Harvard, and completed his dissertation in 1920 on the taxonomy of gall wasps. In August of that year, he took a post as assistant professor of zoology at Indiana University and within months had met and married a woman who had been a top chemistry undergraduate. "Lively and robust, Clara, who dressed in masculine clothes and enjoyed long nature hikes ... considered herself a freethinker, kept him waiting for two weeks before accepting ... Throughout their lives, they called each other by nicknames" (pp. 102–103). The union was only consummated when Clara had undergone minor corrective surgery, but then produced four children. The eldest, Donald, was diabetic and died when only three. The Kinseys' marriage was not as 'companionate', as egalitarian, as the progressive 1920s ideal—Clara gave up her chemistry for cooking—but on holiday in 1934 in the Great Smoky Mountains, the whole family bathed naked together in the stream beside their cabin, and over eighteen years Alfred continued to collect, from all corners of the continent, hundreds of thousands of gall wasps.

Kinsey's textbook *An Introduction to Biology* had been published only a year after the Tennessee science teacher, John Scopes, had championed Darwinian evolution at the 'monkey trial' in the summer of 1925. On field trips, Kinsey, the descriptive biologist, would question his students about their sex lives, often also volunteering information about his own, and thus he started to elaborate the protocol of his future interview which was not written but memorized to encourage openness. Any record would be unintelligible hieroglyphs on the form he devised. He studied the body language of those he subsequently interviewed, using staccato questions, avoiding euphemism and, above all, maintaining eye contact with them. From June 1939, he began to interview the gay communities of Chicago and other large cities, as time went on targeting other subcultures which had received little prior scientific attention. He would follow-up, sometimes he would even contact the parents of his subjects, until by December 1940, he had 1700 sexual histories and applied for funding from the Rockefeller Foundation. As the money flowed generously his way, he built his research institute, with library and archive, engaged his staff, interviewed far and wide until even he, the compulsive collector of large samples, concluded that the amount of data justified publication. He began to write *Sexual Behavior in the Human Male* and, almost directly, suffered a collapse which he blamed on physical tiredness. Ill health impeded him relentlessly, however, from 1945, through the publication of *Sexual Behavior in the Human Female* in 1953, until his death from an embolism in 1956.

James Jones points to the proselytizing tone underlying the two Reports: human sexual behavior was fluid with few individuals scoring at either extreme end of the famous 7-point scale as totally heterosexual or exclusively homosexual. With the orgasm as the basic unit of measurement, all methods of sexual release were equally acceptable, indeed valuable.

Kinsey was adept at controlling the media at the time of the first Report's publication. Journalists were presented with a detailed preview or promised access to the proofs provided their reviews were, in return, submitted to him for vetting, ostensibly for factual correctness. Mainstream reaction was thus manipulated with resounding success, but, to his irritation, criticism of statistical method came from Geoffrey Gorer in the New York *Herald Tribune* and Margaret Mead, speaking in March 1948 at a New York conference on the Report, accused Kinsey of reducing sex "to the category of a simple act of elimination". This criticism was taken further by Lionel Trilling (1948) in the April issue of *Partisan Review*: "We are led to see that their whole definition of a sexual experience is comprised by the physical act ... The Report never suggests that a sexual experience is anything but the discharge of specifically sexual tension ... But the Report, as we shall see, is most resistant to the possibility of making any connection between the sexual life and the psychic structure. This strongly formulated attitude of the Report is based on the assumption that the real reality of sex is anatomical and physiological" (pp. 467–468). "This awkwardness in the handling of ideas is characteristic of the Report. It is ill at ease with any idea that is in the least complex and it often tries to get rid of such an idea in favor of another that has the appearance of not going beyond the statement of physical fact ... The Report, we may say, has an extravagant fear of all ideas that do not seem to it to be, as it were, immediately dictated by simple physical fact" (p. 470). Trilling points to two important consequences: "removing the human subject from its human implications ... preventing the consideration of the consequences of certain forms of human conduct" (p. 476).

Trilling's criticism, by no means totally hostile, focuses on what was lacking in Kinsey's work and, one may reasonably infer, in Kinsey himself—a theory of mind. In its place there seems to have been a mind-set, a very frequent concomitant of masochism, I would contend. Looking at his life from the outside, the hallmarks of masochism are there: the restrictive, puritanical upbringing, the protracted painful illnesses in childhood, the nicknames, the 'demonstrative factor' (Reik, 1939) as evidenced by the nudity and unconstrained display of bodily functions, the homosexual vein, the downward spiral and compulsive risk-taking which set in with middle age. As to the inside, one might again use Trilling's words: "The act of understanding becomes an act of control" (p. 463). This observation is also the conclusion reached by Jones (1997): "Kinsey had always used sex research to gain control over others" (p. 113).

The Case of T.E. Lawrence

That Lawrence of Arabia was a potential masochist was probably known to James Elroy Flecker before the First World War; that he was a practising masochist was known to Professor Arnold Lawrence shortly after his brother's death in 1935, and known to the world at large after the 'revelations' of Colin Simpson and Phillip Knightley in the *Sunday Times* (1968).

Even if it had not been so well known that Lawrence was a practising masochist, at least during the last twelve years of his short life, little perspicacity would have been needed to guess this from his own words in *Seven Pillars of Wisdom* (1935). The mere history of the manuscript would have alerted one. Who but a masochist could possibly have lost almost the entire book, a year's concentrated work, almost a quarter of a million words, whilst changing trains at Reading station?! What academic, apart from Lawrence, an erstwhile archeologist employed by the British Museum, would have been perverse enough to destroy his wartime notes as each section of the book was constructed? And after it had been "built again with heavy repugnance", all but one page was burnt as soon as a third condensed text was ready for private printing by staff of the *Oxford Times* in eight copies! Whilst working a further four years, under almost imposssible circumstances, on the lavishly illustrated final version, he consistently denigrated the book and discouraged subscribers. It was completed at ruinous expense only in 1926. The abridged version *Revolt in the Desert* (1927), slashed out of the longer text with Indian ink and a brush (he had broken his right wrist shortly before), was withdrawn as soon as it had covered the debts incurred by the subscribers' edition, leaving Jonathan Cape with thousands of unsold copies but still very much richer. A similar perverse procedure was then instigated in connection with *The Mint* (1955)—with similar ultimate success, it must be noted. If Richard Aldington (1955) was right about one thing, it was that Lawrence's devious handling of his books amounted to genius. He was, as he wrote to Bernard Shaw's wife, Charlotte (14 April 1927), "a bag of tricks—too rich and full a bag for them to control" (British Museum MSS ADD.45903, 45904; Brown 1988). His manipulations generated a huge interest when the books were finally released, but this is, after all, to say little more than that Lawrence was daring and very clever—like many masochists.

In *Seven Pillars of Wisdom*, his exhortation of the Serahin culminates:

> To the clear-sighted, failure was the only goal. We must believe, through and through, that there was no victory, except to go down into death fighting and crying for failure itself, calling in excess of despair to Omnipotence to strike harder, that by His very striking He might temper our tortured selves into the weapon of His own ruin (p. 422).

In gauging the way into these fierce desert minds, could he have made a clearer statement of that cornerstone of the masochist's philosophy which may be summed up as 'victory through defeat'?

The much-cited incident at Deraa (*Seven Pillars of Wisdom*, pp. 451–454), thought by some of the less sympathetic biographers (James 1990, pp. 209–221) to have been a wishful fantasy, was rewritten, according to Lawrence in a letter to Charlotte Shaw (30 July 1925) about nine times. Captured and tortured by the Turks in November 1917, his account reaches this crescendo:

> At last when I was completely broken they seemed satisfied. Somehow I found myself off the bench, lying on my back on the dirty floor, where

> I snuggled down, dazed, panting for breath, but vaguely comfortable. I had strung myself to learn all pain until I died, and no longer actor, but spectator, thought not to care how my body jerked and squealed. Yet I knew or imagined what passed about me.
>
> I remembered the corporal kicking with his nailed boot to get me up; and this was true, for the next day my right side was dark and lacerated, and a damaged rib made each breath stab me sharply. I remembered smiling idly at him, for a delicious warmth, probably sexual, was swelling through me: and then that he flung up his arm and hacked with the full length of his whip into my groin. This doubled me half-over, screaming, or, rather, trying impotently to scream, only shuddering through my open mouth. One giggled with amusement. A voice cried, 'Shame, you've killed him.' Another slash followed. A roaring, and my eyes went black: while within me the core of life seemed to heave slowly up through the rending nerves, expelled from its body by this last indescribable pang (p. 454).

Though the trauma of Deraa was seen by Lawrence himself and many of his biographers as a turning point in his life, it did not happen in a void but was, in fact, the most dramatic link in a chain of events, all concerned with physical pain. The list of Lawrence's illnesses and injuries is startling. When he was about sixteen, he broke his right leg near the ankle in a scuffle with another boy at the Oxford City High School. He limped back to his classroom after the morning break and was wheeled home on a bicycle by his brothers at lunchtime. The family doctor set it in a splint, but the leg took a long time to mend and was blamed for stunting his growth to only 5 feet 5 inches. Even seven years later, during a journey on foot through Northern Mesopotamia, he noted in the diary he kept (26 July 1911):

> ... my right instep has again collapsed. I suppose it will never get over the smash after my leg was broken. It is painful now in the morning, and after every rest, however short (Garnett 1938, p. 116).

It had not, however, deterred his marathon cycling tours through France when, in 1908, he first contracted malaria, nor his 1909 Syrian trek for his B.A. thesis (*Crusader Castles*, 1936). He wrote to his mother from Aleppo on the 22nd of September that his feet were "all over cuts & chafes & blisters". He had also, according to his letter of the 24th of September to Sir John Rhys, the Principal of Jesus College, "had the delay of four attacks of malaria when I had only reckoned on two" and been "robbed & rather smashed up". During those 1911 explorations around the Euphrates, already mentioned, he suffered an abscess on a wisdom tooth, blisters on both feet, a sore on his hand, then contracted typhoid and was nursed by Hamoudi, the site-foreman at the Carchemish archaeological dig, in his own house.

On their forlorn mission (March–April 1916) to relieve Major-General Townshend's besieged force at Kut-el-Amara by offering a million pound bribe to the Turkish leader Khalil, Lawrence's companion, Aubrey Herbert, states: "Lawrence had hurt his knee and could not ride." In a report of the 16th April 1917 to Lieutenant-Colonel C.E. Wilson, the British Resident in Jidda, Lawrence explains:

> I had to stay in Abdulla's camp [at El Ain in Wadi Ais] from March 15th to March 25th. On the way up I developed boils, which made camel riding uncomfortable, and on top of them first a short attack of dysentery, and then somewhat heavy malaria for about ten days. This combination pulled me down rather, so that I was unable either to walk or ride.

By November 1917 we have this account of his approach to Deraa (*Seven Pillars of Wisdom*, p. 450):

> I was in Halim's wet things, with a torn Hurani jacket, and was yet limping from the broken foot [1922 Oxford text has "toe"] acquired when we blew up Jemal's train. The slippery track made walking difficult, unless we spread out our toes widely and took hold of the ground with them: and doing this for mile after mile was exquisitely painful to me. Because pain hurt me so, I would not lay weight always on my pains in our revolt: yet hardly one day in Arabia passed without a physical ache to increase the corroding sense of my accessory deceitfulness towards the Arabs, and the legitimate fatigue of responsible command.

Precisely five years after his flogging at Deraa, he wrote in a draft preface to Edward Garnett's proposed abridgement of the Oxford text:

> I do not wish to publish secret documents, nor to make long explanations: but must put on record my conviction that England is out of the Arab affair with clean hands. Some Arab advocates (the most vociferous joined our ranks after the Armistice) have rejected my judgment on this point. Like a tedious Pensioner I showed them my wounds (over sixty I have, each scar evidence of a pain incurred in Arab service as proof I had worked sincerely on their side.

No doubt a gross exaggeration, reminiscent of Falstaff, as Richard Aldington (1955, p. 376) points out, but hardly a total untruth.

He left the Paris Peace Conference in April 1919 to collect his papers and belongings from Cairo, flying in one of an ill-fated squadron of Handley-Page bombers. Just outside Rome his plane crashed, killing the pilot outright and the co-pilot. Lawrence suffered a fractured collar-bone, scapula and ribs (one rib dug into a lung) and mild concussion.

His training as an R.A.F. recruit at the Uxbridge Depot in the last months of 1922 was a chronicle of unremitting pain. On the 14th May 1923, he wrote to Lionel Curtis from the Tank Corps that he had a split thumb. His postscript to Charlotte Shaw on the 26th March 1924 informs her that his "mixture of flu and malaria is over: all but the weariness after" and his letter to her of the 10th June that he is "nursing a broken rib". By the 27th July, he was writing to his fellow train-wrecker, Colonel Alan Dawnay, who had helped him into the Tank Corps, of "having my face damaged and my lately-broken rib re-broken (I think) by four drunks after lights out in the hut".

On his readmission to the R.A.F., giving such a catalogue of broken bones to the medical orderly that the latter could barely list them, he kept in touch with Private "Posh" Palmer. He wrote from Cranwell Cadet College on the 10th December 1925:

> Crashed off the Brough last Monday: knee, ankle, elbow being repaired ... Hobble like a cripple now.

The following spring he had measles which left him "very tired and heavy-headed", then his right arm was broken, cranking a car for its elderly driver after an accident. Before 1926 was out, he crashed on his motorbike in Islington High Street, damaging his knee. In September 1930, he broke two ribs in his chest—"(those are worse than stomach-ribs)".

Even allowing for exaggeration and a degree of hypochondria, this catalogue of woes, by no means complete, surely establishes one fact, that Lawrence lived much of his life, from adolescence onwards, against a background of physical pain. On the sixth anniversary of Deraa, he found it necessary, almost incredibly, to supplement his miseries in the Tank Corps by paying the nineteen-year-old John Bruce to beat him (Knightley & Simpson 1969). Yet, with the ambivalence common to us all but glaring in the masochist, he was to write to Charlotte Shaw from his cottage the following summer (19 July 1924):

> Kreutzer Sonata being played by Bruce (a Scotsman, inarticulate, excessively uncomfortable). He comes up here often on Sundays, will enter only if I'm alone, glares and glowers at me till I put some Beethoven on the gramophone, and then sits solid, with a heroic aura of solidity about him: my room after four hours of Bruce feels like a block of granite, with myself a squashed door-mat of fossilised bones, between two layers. Good, perhaps, to feel like a pre-historic animal, extinct, and dead, and useless: but wounding also.

Whilst he suffered at Bovington Camp, Lawrence seemed to inhabit a sort of no-man's-land between insight and 'double-think'. In 1923 he wrote a series of letters of self-scrutiny (Garnett 1938, 410–421) to Lionel Curtis, editor of the *Round Table* and also a Fellow of All Souls:

> (14 May 1923) It's terrible to hold myself voluntarily here: and yet I want to stay here till it no longer hurts me: till the burnt child no longer feels the fire.

> Do you think there have been many lay monks of my persuasion? One used to think that such frames of mind would have perished with the age of religion: and yet here they rise up, purely secular. It's a lurid flash into the Nitrian desert: seems almost to strip the sainthood from Anthony. How about Teresa?

Professor Arnold Lawrence has explained gently that his brother sought to purge his sexual desires after the model of the saints, and, no doubt, this was indeed an element in the ritual beatings. It is characteristic of a masochist springing, as Lawrence did, from a puritanical background that he cannot admit to himself that his release is a gratification, and a sexual one, that his motivation is, albeit in the depths, sexual pleasure. Astonishingly enough, there is one exceptional instance: "... a delicious warmth, probably sexual, was swelling through me ..." he wrote of Deraa.

What of the other side of the coin—the sadistic obverse? Were the lurid passages in *Seven Pillars of Wisdom* a catharsis or a deliberate self-denigration? Much has been written of the massacre of Turkish prisoners at Tafas, but this was after his own experience at Deraa and after the discovery of the Turks' own atrocities in the village. I would cite first a more obscure incident mentioned in a letter written on Boxing Day 1913 to C.F. Bell (of the Ashmolean, Magdelen and the National Portrait Gallery) in flippant tone from Carchemish:

> I found the cat groaning about midnight and put it out of its misery. The misery was so great that it ended only at the eleventh bullet.

Of course, one has no idea of the immediate circumstances and Lawrence was undoubtedly a fantast. He was, however, also a crack shot. He practised assiduously throughout his teens, joined the Oxford High School Old Boys' Rifle Club (Marriot, private publication, p. 63) and the Oxford University Officers' Training Corps. The incident calls to mind the darker and more puzzling account in *Seven Pillars of Wisdom* (p. 187) of his execution of the murderer, Hamed, to prevent a blood feud between the Ageyl and the Moroccans:

> I stood in the entrance and gave him a few moments' delay which he spent crying on the ground. Then I made him rise and shot him through the chest. He fell down on the weeds shrieking, with the blood coming out in spurts over his clothes, and jerked about till he rolled nearly to where I was. I fired again, but was shaking so that I only broke his wrist. He went on calling out, less loudly, now lying on his back with his feet towards me, and I leant forward and shot him for the last time in the thick of his neck under the jaw. His body shivered a little, and I called the Ageyl; who buried him in the gully where he was.

Whether self-damaging fantasy or fact, the account is chilling.

In Freudian terms Lawrence's sexuality might be described as fixated at the anal-sadistic phase, with attendant reaction-formations, such as his struggles, under the most adverse conditions, to procure himself a daily bath. The digestive processes were as repugnant to him as the reproductive processes—witness his early vegetarianism, his reluctance to dine in Hall either at Jesus College or All Souls. "I eat breakfast only," he wrote to Lionel Curtis from Bovington (14 May 1923), and to Bernard Shaw from Miranshah (19 July 1928): "Up here I have begun to think with pleasure of the idea of eating ... once or twice." Yet he begins *The Mint* (1955) with a 'melting of the bowels' and entitles the brilliant chapter on refuse disposal: 'Shit-cart'. The notes made on his voyage to India on the troopship Derbyshire, *Leaves in the Wind*, possibly to be incorporated in *The Mint*, describe the unblocking of the wives' lavatory by the Orderly Officer:

> He pulled off his tunic and threw it at me to hold, and with a plumber's quick glance strode over to the far side, bent down, and ripped out a grating. Gazed for a moment, while the ordure rippled over his boots. Up his right sleeve, baring a forearm hairy as a mastiff's grey leg, knotted with veins, and a gnarled hand: thrust it deep in, groped, pulled out a moist white bundle. 'Open that port' and out it splashed into the night. 'You'd think they'd have had some other place for their sanitary towels. Bloody awful show, not having anything fixed up. ' He shook his sleeve down as it was over his slowly-drying arm, and huddled on his tunic, while the released liquid gurgled contentedly down its re-opened drain (Garnett 1938, 503).

I have introduced this discussion of anal-sadistic sexuality, which would otherwise be gratuitous, in order to point to two derivatives which importantly affected Lawrence's life. First, his extraordinary ambivalence towards money—the anal component. He was either disposing of millions of pounds (as at Kut-el-Amara) or counting pence (as in the opening chapter of *The Mint* and very many of his letters). Second, his extraordinary ambivalence towards mastery—the sadistic component. He was either a kingmaker or, at his own insistence, the lowest rank of the two services in which he spent over a quarter of his short life. In all branches of that life, he was a manipulator, even of the men who flogged him. John Bruce was 'in charge' of his punitive swims in the icy North Sea, but the 'Old Man' (Lawrence, or his pitiless 'superego') was pulling the strings. "The terror of being run away with, in the liberty of power, lies at the back of these many renunciations of my later life," he wrote to Charlotte Shaw (28 September 1925). John Mack quite rightly calls him 'Lawrence the Enabler', but, sadly, the pornographic magazines would have classified him 'submissive/dominant'.

In *The Economic Problem of Masochism*, Freud saw masochism arising from a defusion of the life instinct (Eros) and the death instinct: "Its danger lies in the fact that it originates from the death instinct" (Freud, 1924, p. 170). Lawrence wrote twice to E.M. Forster from Karachi (27 October and 21 December, 1927) about Forster's homosexual ghost story Dr. Woolacott. After detailed comments, he concluded (21 December 1927):

> I suppose you will not print it? Not that it anywhere says too much: but it shows far more than it says: and these things are mysteries. The Turks, as you probably know (or have guessed, through the reticences of the *Seven Pillars)* did it to me, by force: and since then I have gone about whimpering to myself Unclean, unclean. Now I don't know. Perhaps there is another side, your side, to the story. I couldn't ever do it, I believe: the impulse strong enough to make me touch another creature has not yet been born in me: but perhaps in surrender to such a figure as your Death there might be a greater realisation—and thereby a more final destruction—of the body than any loneliness can reach.

According to his boyhood friend, E. F. Hall, Lawrence was fascinated by a brass-rubbing of a man eaten by worms and for a time insisted on sleeping in a box resembling a coffin. A schoolboy's delight in the macabre, one might say, but evidence of a death instinct in ascendancy in Lawrence is not difficult to find from the date of his enlistment in the ranks onwards.

Three factors have generally been cited to account for Lawrence's decision, at the high-point of public recognition, to bury himself in the ranks, and to explain his self-denigration and nihilism. First, the Amfortas' wound of his illegitimacy, second, Deraa:

> ... how in Deraa that night the citadel of my integrity had been irrevocably lost (Lawrence, 1935, p. 456).

and third, his sense of duplicity in getting the Arabs to fight on the strength of promises which he knew would not be fulfilled:

> We are calling them to fight for us on a lie, and I can't stand it (British Museum MSS ADD.45915; Minorities, 1971, p. 33).

This brings us to an examination of that inevitable component of masochism—guilt. The guilt Lawrence felt at deceiving the Arabs was probably on the intellectual, rational level of consciousness and was apparently assuaged by his efforts before, during and after the 1919 Paris Peace Conference and the Middle East settlements he achieved with Winston Churchill through the 1921 Cairo Conference. Neither his illegitimacy nor his humiliation at Deraa were his fault—they were misfortunes which befell him, and one might well argue that any guilt should belong to others, the perpetrators, namely his parents and the Turks, especially Hacim Bey. However, masochistic guilt is not rational, is often not conscious, and is usually linked to sexuality. The two matters under consideration have sex and beating in common. His mother at the end of her long life would often repeat: "God hates the sin but loves the sinner." Her rigorous moral code and religious observance were part of her own struggle with guilt. After taking Thomas Robert Tighe Chapman from his wife and four daughters, she made him "a teetotaller, a domestic man, a careful spender of pence". She also frequently beat her headstrong son Ned (T.E.) on his bare buttocks, as part of her striving towards redemption and allegedly on one occasion after he had been apprehended with another boy at school engaged in mutual masturbation. Ned was brought up with four brothers, entered an all-boys school, an all-male college where his friend Vyvyan Richards formed an openly homosexual attachment to him, engaged in an all-male archeological dig at Carchemish, found love and intimacy with the handsome young Dahoum, shared experiences of appalling violence with alien men whose necessarily homosexual practices he witnessed—against this background, could his beating and homosexual rape at Deraa have been anything other than shattering and, from a soil of ambivalence thus prepared for such a culmination, could anything other than guilt have sprung? So that he would write to Charlotte Shaw (26 March 1924):

> The trial scene in *Joan*. Poor Joan, I was thinking of her as a person not as a moral lesson. The pain meant more to her than the example. You instance my night in Deraa. Well, I'm always afraid of being hurt: and to me, while I live, the force of that night will lie in the agony which broke me, and made me surrender. It's the individual view. You can't share it.
>
> About that night. I shouldn't tell you, because decent men don't talk about such things. I wanted to put it plain in the book, and wrestled for days with my self-respect ... which wouldn't, hasn't, let me. For fear of being hurt, or rather to earn five minutes respite from a pain which drove me mad, I gave away the only possession we are born into the world with—our bodily integrity. It's an unforgivable matter, an irrecoverable position: and it's that which has made me forswear decent living, and the exercise of my not-contemptible wits and talents.
>
> You may call this morbid: but think of the offence, and the intensity of my brooding over it for these years. It will hang about me while I live, and afterwards if our personality survives. Consider wandering among the decent ghosts hereafter, crying 'Unclean unclean!'

And therein lies the vicious circle of masochism: guilt requiring punishment, punishment with its yield of sexual pleasure creating more guilt, requiring in its turn more punishment, the concept of expiation being vital since without it the whole pathological process would be starkly and intolerably revealed. The floggings (already initiated) and the contrived physical ordeals at the hands of John Bruce and others would have had to be acknowledged not only as rituals of expiation and purgation but as means of sexual release and concomitant gratification, governed by that instinctual bedrock, the compulsion to repeat.

Finally it is perhaps not amiss to consider something extremely obvious, namely, the overwhelming effect of the war experiences on Lawrence. How could such devastating sights and acts have failed to damage a sensitive nature, nurtured on mediaeval chivalric ideals? "This killing and killing of Turks is horrible," he wrote on the 24th September 1917 to E. T. Leeds (D. G. Hogarth's successor at the Ashmolean). "When you charge in at the finish and find them all over the place in bits, and still alive many of them ..." At all events, psychological defense mechanisms seem to have come into operation after the war. The memories of killing and maiming were externalized in the *Seven Pillars*, and the guilt which might be expected to attach to them (and no doubt did, but was intolerable) became largely transposed to his surrender at Deraa. It is characteristic of the sadomasochist that he displays little remorse where remorse would most be justified, whilst clinging to his burden of guilt about things that were not his fault.

I believe that the 1916–18 Arab Revolt with its hardships, its dangers and its horrors tipped the balance in favour of pleasure through pain both psychologically and physiologically. It gave Lawrence of Arabia his place in history but at a tragic personal price. He was a born leader, farsighted, daring, but also a child and, for all his toughening preparations, very vulnerable. In *Memory Hold-the-Door*, John Buchan (1940) wrote:

> I am not a very tractable person or much of a hero-worshipper, but I could have followed Lawrence over the edge of the world. I loved him for himself, and also because there seemed to be reborn in him all the lost friends of my youth (p. 218).

George Bernard Shaw wrote in the front of his wife's copy of *Seven Pillars of Wisdom*: "His great abilities and interests were those of a highly gifted boy."

It bears testimony to those great abilities that he achieved so much in spite of the psychological impedimenta he was carrying. His achievements as archeologist, intelligence agent, guerrilla leader, diplomat, mechanic and writer (and translator: The Odyssey of Homer, 1986) are set out in the last section of Stephen Tabachnick and Christopher Matheson's excellent book *Images of Lawrence* (1988). A superabundance of biographical information exists (Caudwell 1938; Gorman 1940; Hyde 1977; Tabachnick 1978;

Winstone 1982; Yardley 1985; Brown & Cave 1988; Wilson 1989), but for a detailed examination of Lawrence's sexual problems I would recommend the sympathetic account given by John E. Mack in the penultimate chapter of his extremely painstaking biography *A Prince of Our Disorder: The Life of T.E. Lawrence* (1976). This chapter, 'Intimacy, Sexuality and Penance', sets out Lawrence's sufferings in a sensitive manner. It is not, like the present somewhat heartless portrait, a study of masochism, but a personal study of Lawrence, and there is little missing or to disagree with in Dr Mack's interpretations. I would only underline one of his concluding observations—that the remedy Lawrence chose for his sexual conflicts, the elaborate rituals he was driven to arrange during the last years of his life, probably entailed the expenditure of a great deal of psychic energy. My own view is that this is something of an understatement, in keeping with Dr Mack's compassionate review of what he calls 'a flagellation problem'. Apparently this problem peaked, as masochistic practices are wont to do (one might well assert, more generally, as established addictions are wont to do) with the lugubrious coarsening of middle age, in 1933, but the drain of psychic energy and the pervasive self-destructive drive of masochism are apparent from the war years onwards. In that remarkable feat of introspection 'Myself' (*Seven Pillars of Wisdom*), Lawrence states:

> I liked the things underneath me and took my pleasures and adventures downward. There seemed a certainty in degradation, a final safety. Man could rise to any height, but there was an animal level beneath which he could not fall. It was a satisfaction on which to rest (p. 581).

In this self-examination on his thirtieth birthday, overwrought or poignant depending on the reader, he speaks of 'mind-suicide', as in several of his later letters. In these he even contemplates an escape into madness. He threatened suicide, and, according to John Bruce, once actually attempted it. When he saw the boy-cyclists in his path on the 13th May 1935 he swerved and turned the injury against himself—in essence perhaps the only noble aspect of masochism, which must command admiration? It must have happened so quickly. It seems more likely the instant reaction of a man who was, amongst other things, noble.

King George V telephoned the hospital and Winston Churchill wept at his funeral, but John Bruce described this man of extraordinary talents, impossibly high ideals and extreme fastidiousness in 1923 as ragged, worn-out, dirty, broke and sleeping rough. Lawrence wrote to Charlotte Shaw (28 September 1925):

> Garnett said once that I was two people, in my book: one wanting to go on, the other wanting to go back. That is not right. Normally the very strong one, saying 'No', the Puritan, is in firm charge, and the other poor little

> vicious fellow, can't get a word in, for fear of him. My reason tells me all the while, dins into me day and night, a sense of how I've crashed my life and self and gone hopelessly wrong: and hopelessly it is, for I'm never coming back, and I want to.

VICTORY THROUGH DEFEAT

At the end of *Masochism in Modern Man*, Theodor Reik (1941) seeks the common denominator in the various manifestations of masochism—sexual deviance and personality disorder alike—and finds it in the formula 'victory through defeat'. This is indeed the kernel of masochism and there is no doubt that the highly specific victory is total. The man whose aim is to be defeated cannot be defeated—he has achieved a desperate invulnerability. The considerations raised by this philosophy of paradox are all simple ones. As Daniel C. Dennett remarked so pithily, "in crashing obviousness lies objectivity" (Dennett, 1991, p. 80). The first is the question—a victory through defeat for whom? Well, obviously, for the masochist alone; nobody associated with him stands to win, only to lose. The second is the nature of the victory. This can only be the satisfaction arising out of self-assertion and defiance: 'Come hell or high water, I will have my way!' The third is the price of defeat. If the masochist is a gifted individual, his disablement through his own agency is a tragic waste. If he has no talents, his self-damage is pointless for his perversity will not make him more interesting. The last consideration is the implication of it all turning out well in the end—the victory is a future one—but, as John Maynard Keynes pointed out with cheerful brutality, 'in the long run we're all dead!'

The masochist who operates primarily through deviant sexual practices, the 'supersensualist' (Sacher-Masoch, 1870), defiantly obtains gratification in spite of every obstacle, every delay, every embargo, but there is surely something deranged in the insistence on physical gratification, not only at the expense of self-respect, but dependent upon the loss of self-respect. The masochist who, in each situation life presents, systematically ruins his chances of happiness and success, who is locked within a vicious circle of guilt, requiring punishment, punishment affording masochistic satisfaction, thus begetting more guilt, requiring more punishment, presumably has an attitude of *après moi le déluge*, for it is difficult to see how a negative life aim can eventuate in a positive legacy.

The Prognosis

The downward spiral which sets in inevitably with aging is reinforced by masochism to a desperate, hopeless situation for the masochist in his 70s and 80s. All that is left is, in most cases, a monstrous obstinacy. Obstinacy, which might in earlier years have passed as fortitude, is in fact what has seen him through so many self-imposed ordeals, so many disasters brought down upon himself. At last it stands revealed for what it has always been—unproductive, childish obstinacy. The provocations of a child are offset by the charm of mischievous youthful fun. The provocations of an old man have no intrinsic charm. Old age is likely to be even lonelier for him than it is for most people. No effort is made to use intelligence to counter declining physical performance. On the contrary, getting up from an armchair, climbing out of the bath, become opportunities for displays of physical awkwardness. The body which has always been his medium of expression, which has sustained so many insults, is breaking down from year to year, finally from day to day. (In a conversation of the 6th December 1993 Mr Don Campbell, training analyst and Chairman of the Portman Clinic, Hampstead, London, for the treatment of sexual deviance, spoke to me in precisely these terms of the cheerless prospect likely to confront his masochistic patients as the aging process advances and "the body begins to break down"—out of years of experience, his very words.)

Sometimes the sorrows of old age are more dramatic. As already mentioned in Part I, Leopold von Sacher-Masoch himself is said to have spent the last ten years of his life in a mental institution in Mannheim where he died in 1905, his confinement there having been kept secret and his death having been announced in 1895 (Cleugh, 1951). More recently, Howard Hughes, the inventor and entrepreneur, and Lafayette Ron Hubbard, the founder of Scientology, after lives spent in the ruthless pursuit of money and power, always attempting to dominate and control others, both ended up as paranoid recluses with long hair, long fingernails and an obsessive fear of dust and germs. One is reminded of Freud's frequently expressed conviction that sadomasochism and obsessive compulsive neurosis stand in the relation of positive and negative to one another.

One might say that the masochist with all the predictability ensuing from his rigidity, is 'compulsion in action'—certainly he is obsessed by sex—reactionary, like Yukio Mishima with his samurai code, proceeding relentlessly towards self-destruction. The *minimalist* composer Philip Glass was an appropriate choice for the film *Mishima*. His insistent music has the inexorability to accompany a personality that is closed, a fate that is sealed.

Surely there must be an alternative path to Hegelian 'recognition' of self other than through 'lordship and bondage'. Surely there must be a way of relating to another human being, as a thinking, feeling, intentional being, other than only in terms of domination and submission. And if there *is* not, then surely there *ought to be*. In this vale of tears, where the only certainty for the individual is death, preceded or not, as the case may be, by old age and infirmity, where one species can only survive by feeding on another, the deliberate pursuit of suffering would seem gratuitous.

APPENDICES

APPENDIX 1

Criteria laid down in the Diagnostic and Statistical Manual of Mental Disorders (Third Edition Revised) of the American Psychiatric Association (DSM-III-R) for sexual masochism, sexual sadism, sadistic personality disorder and self-defeating personality disorder.

Diagnostic Criteria For Sexual Masochism (pp. 286–287)

A. Over a period of at least six months, recurrent intense sexual urges and sexually arousing fantasies involving the act (real, not simulated) of being humiliated, beaten, bound, or otherwise made to suffer.

B. The person has acted on these urges, or is markedly distressed by them.

Diagnostic Criteria for Sexual Sadism (pp. 287–288)

A. Over a period of at least six months, recurrent intense sexual urges and sexually arousing fantasies involving acts (real, not simulated) in which the psychological or physical suffering (including humiliation) of the victim is sexually exciting to the person.

B. The person has acted on these urges, or is markedly distressed by them.

Diagnostic Criteria for Sadistic Personality Disorder (pp. 369–371)

A. A pervasive pattern of cruel, demeaning, and aggressive behavior, beginning by early adulthood, as indicated by the repeated occurrence of at least four of the following:

(1) has used physical cruelty or violence for the purpose of establishing dominance in a relationship (not merely to achieve some noninterpersonal goal, such as striking someone in order to rob him or her)
(2) humiliates or demeans people in the presence of others
(3) has treated or disciplined someone under his or her control unusually harshly, e.g., a child, student, prisoner, or patient
(4) is amused by, or takes pleasure in, the psychological or physical suffering of others (including animals)
(5) has lied for the purpose of harming or inflicting pain on others (not merely to achieve some other goal)
(6) gets other people to do what he or she wants by frightening them (through intimidation or even terror)
(7) restricts the autonomy of people with whom he or she has a close relationship, e.g., will not let spouse leave the house unaccompanied or permit teen-age daughter to attend social functions
(8) is fascinated by violence, weapons, martial arts, injury, or torture

B. The behavior in A has not been directed toward only one person (e.g., spouse, one child) and has not been solely for the purpose of sexual arousal (as in Sexual Sadism).

Diagnostic Criteria for Self-Defeating Personality Disorder (pp. 371–374)

A. A pervasive pattern of self-defeating behavior, beginning by early adulthood and present in a variety of contexts. The person may often avoid or undermine pleasurable experiences, be drawn to situations or relationships in which he or she will suffer, and prevent others from helping him or her, as indicated by at least five of the following:

(1) chooses people and situations that lead to disappointment, failure, or mistreatment even when better options are clearly available
(2) rejects or renders ineffective the attempts of others to help him or her
(3) following positive personal events (e.g., new achievement), responds with depression, guilt, or a behavior that produces pain (e.g., an accident)
(4) incites angry or rejecting responses from others and then feels hurt, defeated, or humiliated (e.g., makes fun of spouse in public, provoking an angry retort, then feels devastated)

(5) rejects opportunities for pleasure, or is reluctant to acknowledge enjoying himself or herself (despite having adequate social skills and the capacity for pleasure)
(6) fails to accomplish tasks crucial to his or her personal objectives despite demonstrated ability to do so, e.g., helps fellow students write papers, but is unable to write his or her own
(7) is uninterested in or rejects people who consistently treat him or her well, e.g., is unattracted to caring sexual partners
(8) engages in excessive self-sacrifice that is unsolicited by the intended recipients of the sacrifice

B. The behaviors in A do not occur exclusively in response to, or in anticipation of, being physically, sexually, or psychologically abused.

C. The behaviors in A do not occur only when the person is depressed.

APPENDIX 2

Classification system of the Adult Attachment Interview (Main & Goldwyn, 1985–1994): Summary of criteria governing main classifications and their subclassifications

Source: Main, Mary, and Goldwyn, Ruth (1994). Adult Attachment Classification and Scoring System. Unpublished manuscript, University of California at Berkeley.

This appendix provides a very brief overview of the criteria governing the main classifications and subclassifications of the Adult Attachment Interview, and could in no way serve as a guide to classification or coding in itself. For a further and more elaborated description of the protocol and scoring system, see Hesse, E. (1999) The Adult Attachment Interview: Historical and Current Perspectives, in J. Cassidy and P. Shaver, *Handbook of Attachment: Theory, Research, and Clinical Applications*, pp. 395–433, New York: The Guilford Press.

Persons seeking training in the system should contact Dr Hesse or Dr Main at the Social Development Project, Department of Psychology, University of California at Berkeley, California 94720 (Fax: 510 642 5293).

GENERAL PRINCIPLES

The subject's final classification is arrived at in two ways: (a) as a global assessment of the whole interview transcript, (b) on the basis of scores awarded on 17 carefully defined 9-point scales. The scales fall into 3 main groups: those assessing probable past experiences with parents (the period of time being rated is from earliest memories to 14 years old), those evaluating patterned or organized states of mind (internal models), and those representing unresolved/disorganized states of mind (resulting from loss or trauma). The overall attachment classification is always based on the subject's current state of mind with respect to attachment.

9-POINT SCALES

Scales for inferred past experience with parents (Mother and father judged separately)

Loving (Loving vs unloving parenting in childhood, based on memories of physical love, comfort, forgiveness, support)

Rejecting (Aversion to child's expression of attachment, either inferred or directly described)

Involving/role-reversing (Attempts to elicit child's attention and involvement, to be parented by the child)

Pressure to achieve (Child expected to excel or to tackle adult tasks)

Neglecting (Parent inaccessible, preoccupied, even when physically available)

NOTE: Whereas the preceding 5 scales assess a parent's inferred behaviour in the past, the following scales are devised to assess the subject's current state of mind with respect to attachment. Out of many possible scales for the mental representation of attachment, these scales were selected for their power to distinguish individuals whose current state may be classified as Secure/autonomous (F), Dismissing of attachment (Ds), Preoccupied/entangled with respect to attachment experiences (E), or Unresolved/disorganized with respect to traumatic events (U).

Scales for states of mind with respect to parents (Mother and father considered separately)

Idealizing (Discrepancies between positive generalized descriptors of parent and descriptions of actual behaviour)

NOTE: High scores (5 or over) for idealization and insistence on lack of recall lead to a Ds1, or if there is some limited admission of parent's faults, to a Ds3 classification.

Involving anger (Current preoccupying anger towards a parent)

NOTE: A high score (6 or over) for involving anger leads to an E2 classification. A score of 5 leaves the judge free to decide, after reviewing the interview as a whole, whether it better fits the Preoccupied (E) or the Secure-autonomous (F) category (probably F5).

Derogation (Active derogating dismissal of parents or of attachment-related experiences such as loss)

NOTE: A high score (6 or over) for derogation leads to a Ds2 classification. A score of 5 leaves this classification dependent on the overall features of the interview.

<u>Scales for overall states of mind</u> (Patterned or organized mental representations of attachment)

Derogation (As summarized above, this scale assesses subject's attitude to attachment-related issues, not only relationship with parents)

Inability to recall (Insistence upon lack of memory, especially when used to block further discourse)

NOTE: a high score for inability to recall, coupled with a high score for idealization (5 or over), pointing to a self-deceptive defense mechanism, leads to a Ds1 classification or, where less marked, to a Ds3 classification. Where complete absence of memory for a frightening event points to traumatic memory loss, this is noted, and E3b classification is likely. Claims to very early memories, well before the age of 5, are often asociated with F4, F5 and E classifications.

Metacognitive monitoring (Ability to report on processes of thinking and recall taking place while the interview is in progress)

NOTE: A high score for metacognitive monitoring points to an Autonomous (F) classification, although one or two sentences suggestive of metacognitive monitoring may appear in Ds or E transcripts.

Passivity of thought processes (Inability to focus on a topic, to find words or complete sentences)

NOTE: A high score (5 or over) for passivity leads to an El classification, provided the overall criteria for the Preoccupied state of mind are met and the subject seems to have a 'hallowed' sense of the past yet a feeling that he has failed to please his parents.

Fear of loss (The subject's current fear of the death of an existing or imagined child)

NOTE: A high score (6 or over) for fear of loss leads to a Ds4 classification. A score of 5 means that the transcript should be seen to fit the general descriptors of the Dismissive category before the classification is made.

Coherence of transcript (Ability to present and assess the past in a reaonable, understandable manner, without contradictions)

NOTE: A high score (5 or over) for coherence of transcript is likely to lead to an F classification. A score of 7 or more is likely to lead to F3. High scores on the scales for idealization and insistence on lack of recall imply a lowered score for overall coherence. Preoccupying anger and some lapses of dialogue associated with unresolved mourning will also lower coherence.

Coherence of mind (The judge not only considers the rating already assigned to coherence of transcript but also the nature of the subject's apparent beliefs)

NOTE: A score of 7 or more for coherence of mind is likely to lead to an F3 classification, but scores ranging between 4 and 8 may have been given to subjects assigned to other F subcategories. Coherence of mind is expected to predict, better than any other single scale, a subject's overall functioning insofar as it is related to attachment. Fear of loss, where unrelated to source, or irrational beliefs arising as indices of unresolved trauma may result in a lower score for coherence of mind than for coherence of transcript.

<u>Scales for Unresolved/disorganized states of mind</u> (Unresolved experiences of loss through death or unresolved abusive experiences)

Unresolved loss through death (Disorientation in reasoning, discourse or behaviour)

NOTE: A score of 6 or more leads to an Unresolved (U) classification. A rating of 5 indicates that Unresolved status is uncertain. An alternative, best-fitting Ds, E or F classification is always awarded in addition.

Unresolved trauma (Includes unresolved/disorganized responses to abuse)

NOTE: A score of 6 or more leads to a U classification, while 5 indicates some uncertainty. An alternative, best-fitting Ds, E or F classification is also made. This scale has features running parallel to the scale for unresolved loss. The detailed criteria of both scales are, in fact, considered before a decision regarding U classification is reached.

FINAL CLASSIFICATION CATEGORIES

Category Ds: Dismissing of Attachment

Dismissing, devaluing or cut off from intimate relationships and experiences

Subjects' state of mind indicates a current attempt to limit the influence of attachment in thought, feeling or everyday life. They preserve an organization of thought which permits the attachment mechanism to remain relatively de-activated. This can be achieved either by imagining that parents would be ideally responsive whenever needed, or by devaluing parents so that they would be unworthy of approaching in any event. Except for subcategory Ds4 (cut off from fear of loss), there is an implicit claim to strength and normalcy.

Ds1: Absence of memory for childhood is presented as normal and to be expected. Idealization of one or both parents is strong. This is not supported by episodic memories, often making the interview shorter than usual.

Ds2: Cool, active derogation of one or both parents, or of attachment in general. Reliance on one's own personal strength which is frequently vaunted.

Ds3: Attachment issues are not entirely dismissed but their current influence is denied. The tone is upbeat and 'normalizing'. Feeling is restricted.

Ds4: Fear of the death of a healthy child, without any consciousness of the source of that fear. It might emanate from a loss in childhood which parents have tried to keep secret but somehow partly betrayed by their own fearful behaviour.

Category F: Secure, Therefore Autonomous, with Respect to Attachment

Freely valuing, forgiving, yet objective

Subjects are at home with attachment which remains an open subject for them. They are relatively coherent, reflective and thoughtful. Their responses are relevant and show balance and freshness.

F1: Some setting aside of attachment but this is conscious.

(a) These adults have achieved a redirection and re-evaluation of their personal lives after a harsh childhood. They have escaped to alternative friends or parent figures.
(b) There has always been a somewhat limited involvement with attachment, perhaps due to poverty or the incessant hard work required of the family. This has left little time for expressions of affection.

F2: These adults seem partially dismissing of attachment but this is belied by the affection, compassion or humour which soon breaks through. At first they may be defensive but ultimately show themselves to be caring or forgiving.

F3: This is the group representing a secure model of attachment. Individuals are varied but they all display strong coherence, lack of idealization and good memory for childhood. Because they are aware of their own shortcomings, they are willing to forgive.

(a) These adults had largely supportive families and childhood experiences. Their responses are clear and objective, often also simple.
(b) Difficult experiences during childhood have made these interviewees exceptionally thoughtful. They seem highly developed with a strong sense of self. Vivid memories are recounted with balance or humour.

F4: Relationships are strongly valued, but there is some preoccupation with attachment figures, with separations or past trauma, resulting in a slight tendency to 'psychologize'.

(a) A largely supportive childhood nevertheless held some difficulty in the character of one or other parent, or in early experiences. The speaker may sound young or sentimental, and the tone may be a little exaggerative.
(b) Difficult childhoods that may include trauma or early loss of a parent, even sexual or physical abuse. Any preoccupation or confusion is, however, limited to these events, and the interview as a whole is rational and contained within consciousness.

F5: These adults are still somewhat preoccupied and angry about childhood, but they remain coherent. They recognize and accept a continuing involvement. They are capable of a rational, often humorous, overview.

Category E: Preoccupied with Early Attachments or Trauma

Confused and mentally entangled with the past

Subjects are unable to move beyond their childhood experiences. Their sense of personal identity is weak. They cannot see any role apart from the family, they cannot focus, and they oscillate in their evaluations.

E1: Passivity of thought processes means that speech wanders, becomes irrelevant, vague, and often childlike. There is a somewhat 'hallowed' view of childhood, a tendency to extol the past, yet an almost silent sense of having failed to please.

E2: Continual involvement, interference, criticism, in some cases role-reversal, on the part of a parent have resulted in the child reaching adulthood in an angry conflicted state. Usually at great length, parental behaviour, past and present, is angrily related, dubious psychological interpretations of it are offered, and the agreement of the interviewer is sought. There is an inability to see the other's point of view and a *penchant* for jargon.

E3: Fearfully preoccupied by traumatic events of the past. These may include physical or sexual abuse, traumatic loss, psychosis in a parent, or the terrifying events likely to take place during war. The classification is thus fairly rare in normal samples.

(a) Confused, fearful and overwhelmed, the interviewee repeatedly describes these traumatic experiences even when questioned on other topics. They thus may be said to invade discourse and become a dominant theme.
(b) Distressing loss of memory with respect to events which were almost certainly traumatic. The subject not only lacks memories but is distressed by this memory loss, which thus constitutes an unconscious preoccupation with the events.

Category U: Unresolved (Disorganized/Disoriented) Attachment Status

This classification may be indicated in cases of either loss or abuse. It rests upon lapses in the monitoring of reasoning or discourse, or reports of extreme behavioural reactions to such trauma. There may, for instance, be a displaced reaction with respect to bereavement. Every effort must be made to assign the best-fitting alternative Ds, E or F classification, following U, although assignment to subcategories may be more difficult.

Category CC: Cannot Classify

This indicates that the individual cannot be assigned (as a primary classification) any of the 'organized' categories (Ds, F, E) either because no overriding organization is apparent or because he displays characteristics of mental states which are irreconcilable, which are pulling in opposing directions. It is occasionally indicated where he appears to undergo a complete shift in his state of mind in the middle of the interview or a completely different state of mind with respect to different people. Finally, alternative Ds, E, or F classifications are reviewed and listed after CC as 'forced' categories in order of descending fit.

APPENDIX 3

A summary, for all index subjects (14 depressed, 34 nondepressed), of early life circumstances which may have contributed to the development of sadomasochism

Depressed ($n = 14$)

ES7

1 year old: alimentary canal blockage. 10 years old: broken arm 11 years old: 'irritable bowel' syndrome. Jealous of younger sister. Parents gave no information about sex.

ES10

Confined to playpen, harnessed when taken out. Mother made him wait for sweets. Prolonged pain from tooth abscess. Bullied at school.

ES18

2 years old: mother gave enemas, then housekeeper. Smacked for every transgression by mother and housekeeper. Sister would provoke this. Bullied at school. 6 years old: finger broken by bully. Early puberty.

ES19

Adopted. 7 years old: shocked when informed of this by mother. Jealous of younger sister (also adopted). Sex was never discussed at home.

ES20

Precocious sexual development. Bullied at school. Tormented younger brother.

ES24

5–13 years old: excruciating earache, tonsillitis, adenoids, sinus operations. 14 years old: sexually abused by neighbouring couple.

ES27

Mother wanted a girl, dressed him in girls' clothes, stopped him from crying. 4 years old: back teeth extracted under gas, tonsils removed. 10 years old: broke arm. 11 years old: broke leg. Rheumatism. Influenced by comics. Probable latent homosexual.

ES28

Mother was 16 and already pregnant, father 18, when they married. Father walked out when subject was under 1 year old. 2–3 years old: mother beat him in front of a family friend. 3 years old: given girl's knickers for bathing trunks. 8 years old: felt pushed aside by birth of half-sister. First met father when 9 years old. Asthma: physiotherapy at hospital 3 mornings a week. 12 years old: beaten by father in front of sister. Beaten by schoolmistress.

ES29

Mother wanted a girl. 6 years old: mother had nervous breakdown. 7 years old: mother had 2nd nervous breakdown. She talked religion with him. Subject fostered with 2 brothers on a farm where they were treated sadistically. 12 years old: mother beat him in front of 5 of his friends.

ES40

Mother wanted a girl. Rubber sheet in cot, rubber pants round nappy, mother wore rubber apron when bathing him. ?Reality or fantasy: 4 years old: pretty nursemaid dressed him in sister's rubber mac, teased him, laughed at him.

ES52

Twin sister died at birth, probably malformed after *in utero* competition, but she is regarded as a person by his elder sister who bullied him until he was 7 years old. Influenced by comics. 7 years old: mother divorced father who was also a masochist. 8–18 years old: boarding school.

ES61

Mother belonged to Plymouth Brethren, used to beat him once a week with father's slipper. Father also submissive. 3 sisters got him into trouble, never played with him. Mutual masturbation with other boys at school. Caning at school an extension of master's interest.

ES71

Church 3 times a day on Sunday. Parents gave no information about sex. 9 years old: rubberized sheet for picnics pinned round him, naked, as a cape. Father's fetish: shiny macintoshes. 12 years old: put on mother's shiny mac which was hanging on the wall.

ES80

An old father who was violent and an alcoholic, an old mother who was role-reversing and 3 much older siblings. Strongly attached to brother who was 15–16 years older. Sucked his thumb whilst he stroked his face with brother's tie, dangled over his cot. 5 years old: threw tie on the fire. Sex only discussed with parents once, aged 13, when porn magazines confiscated from under his bed then returned.

NONDEPRESSED ($n = 34$)

ES1

Less than 10 years old: mother hospitalized for a year. Influenced by comics. 12–13 years old: boarding school.

ES2

8–9 years old: excited by taking physical risks, probably in emulation of father who had a dangerous occupation. 11 years old: threw himself deliberately down the stairs. 11–12 years old: boarding school, returning home for weekends. 12 years old: tied up by other boys whilst staying with father's colleagues. Father, whom he regarded as a nonfather, more like an uncle, moved out of his life altogether when he was 14. Lived with a devouring mother until 53 years old. Homosexual but no sex life with a partner.

ES4

Adopted. No love shown by either parent, though adoptive father might have been blood father. Rigid Victorian values. Chilblains each year so painful he had to wear slippers to school. Frequent caning at school and, at least once a month, at home. Influenced by reading.

ES8

8 years old onwards: affected by ladies' rubber garments, macintoshes, hot-water bottles. Mother "a very proper person", forever sacrificing

herself. Father had a harelip, a cleft palate, was incompetent. Subject followed in his 2 elder brothers' footsteps, only left home when he married at 32. Asthmatic.

ES11

3 years old: sent away to stay with a maternal aunt for 6 months. ? Reality or fantasy: 5 years old: mother ordered him to take his clothes off, to pick one of the straps from a collection laid out on the bed, and then, for several minutes, she chased him round the house with it. Subject used food as weapon against mother. Idolized father, who drank, but was disillusioned by father's unexpected slap across the face when subject, without looking, crossed the road to him. They used to threaten him with a Dr Barnardo's Home at the end of the street.

ES13

3–12 years old: bronchitis each year. 3–4 years old: watched mother, who had a Victorian figure, in old-fashioned corsets. Claustrophobic upbringing—mother tried to prevent relationships with girls.

ES15

Mother, of a theatrical temperament, wanted a girl. Nursery-school mistress wore riding mac and boots. 8–18 years old: boarding school, often Cadet camps in the vacations. Beaten by prep school headmaster first with a slipper, then with a cane.

ES17

From 3 months old: eczema covering whole body, bleeding, giving constant pain. Taken to hospital once or twice a week, treated with corticosteroids. Asthma, bronchitis, possibly polio, bad whooping cough, measles twice, German measles. 6 years old: tonsils removed. Tormented and beaten up at school even though his father taught there, tormented also by maternal grandfather, who locked him under the stairs in the dark.

ES21

Father, whom subject idealized, beat him with a bamboo cane and a belt, almost suffocated him under bedclothes, drove him to a children's home to scare him. 10 or 12 years old: sexual relationship with female cousin. 11–16 years old: recurrent tonsillitis, stabbing back pain for which he wore a support corset. 14 years old: father kicked him in the back. Jealous of younger brother.

ES22

'Borderline' personality. Alleged both his parents were masochistic. 4–6 years old: ritualized spanking by nanny who would threaten him and his sister (2 years younger) with a huge strap. 6–7 years old: miserable at school where games master, whom he was anxious to please, caned him. 7 years old: parents split up after a stormy relationship. Many injuries but asserted he was never bothered by physical pain.

ES23

Father beat him 4 or 5 times a month with a strap. Also caned at primary school 2 or 3 times a week but idolized the teacher who caned him. This man was a family friend. Jealous of sister (15 months younger). 16 years old: went into the army.

ES26

2–3 years old: walking reins (interest in bondage attributed to this by subject). Resented sister (5 years younger). Influenced by comics. Identified with mother. 12 years old: masturbated wearing mother's underclothes and high-heeled shoes. Father envious of his education. 14 years old: parents' marriage started to break up, leading to divorce.

ES30

2–3 years old: would get up in the morning, throw himself on the ground, beat the floor and scream with frustration for 20 minutes. Influenced by comics and science fiction on television. 14 years old: masturbated wearing mother's underclothes.

ES34

5 years old: remembers erection. Influenced by comics. Jealous of girl cousin (18 months younger). Excited by girls being caned at school—would masturbate that night.

ES35

Father made him feel an academic failure. Parents quarrelled constantly and ultimately separated. Mother had a collection of voices.

ES36

Mother wanted a girl. 15 years: masturbated in mother's clothes. Resented brother (4 years younger). Homosexual relations about once every 5 years.

ES37

Mother and 2 older sisters would gather round in a semicircle whilst father spanked him. 8 years old: mother threatened to take his trousers down and spank him out in the street. Paternal grandmother a strict disciplinarian. Would provoke the sister (13 years older) with whom he had rivalry. Influenced by comics. Bullied at school. 11 years old: pressured by father over entrance examination whilst he had glandular fever.

ES39

Born with umbilical cord wrapped around his neck—probably caused deafness in one ear. Claustrophic upbringing, both metaphorically and literally. 4–8 years old: bedroom above the shop had no window, only room for the bed. Father bullied his mother, a large woman, and his two sisters (8 and 10) years older. Mostly in the company of older people.

ES41

Jealous of her brother (4 years younger). 8–12 years old: reading of comics led to bondage fantasies (images of heroism, fighting against the odds).

ES42

Mother died before she was 2 years old. 4 years old: father remarried. Hated her controlling stepmother. Not trusted with her half-sister (5 years younger) who taunted her, nor with her half-brother (6 years younger), she developed a behaviour pattern of 'defy and lose'. Semi-incestuous closeness with father. Influenced by science fiction on television and in films. 10 years old: thought as a boy, developed male attitudes to sex.

ES50

Most probably adopted. Sex was taboo with his mother since her mother died in childbirth. 4–6 years old: felt his mother 'enveloped' him, was 'going to swallow' him. 6 years old: dressed in mother's clothes. Father scolded him. 8–9 years old: aware of sexual feelings towards schoolteacher.

ES51

Adopted. 8 months old: gastro-enteritis, nearly fatal. Mother frequently slapped him on the legs, threatened to make him put on girls' clothes which she was sewing. Sexually abused by an older male friend of his mother's. 7–13 years old: father took his trousers down and hit him with a belt. 12 years old: bullied at school—friend who protected him also dominated him. 15 years old: girlfriend provided clothes for cross-dressing. Father, also sadomasochistic, felt trapped in an unhappy marriage.

ES57

Frequently bored as a child. Influenced by comics. 9–10 years old: undressing game with 2 boy neighbours, putting on girls' clothes. 10 years old: mother decamped with lover who drank and became violent. Bullied by brother (10 years older).

ES58

Convinced she was hungry as an infant. 3 years old: attacked brother (2 years younger). 10 years old: menarche, no explanation from mother. 9–10 years old: sexually abused by brother (9 years older).

ES62

Lesbian. Congenital eye disease. 1 year old: broke her arm in a fall. 4 years old: fell from a tree and broke a rib. 8–9 years old: knocked down by a trolley-bus, serious and painful head injuries. Influenced by comics. Bullied at school but liked wrestling with boys.

ES63

1–2 years old: hospitalized for 3 months after being badly scalded. Brother (5 years older) teased him. Jealous of sister (1–2 years younger).

8 years old: mother dressed him in girl's jeans, with a fringe. 12–13 years old: parents separated, then divorced. 14 years old: put on mother's corset and stockings.

ES65

Recurrent painful earache. Prudish mother. 7–8 years old: spanked by father. 8 years old: spanked brother (4 years younger). 10 years old: premature puberty. Put on mother's underwear and asked brother to spank him. 11 years old: father's spanking led to an erection. 14 years old: excited by sadistic headmaster who caned both boys and girls.

ES66

Both parents, regular churchgoers, imparted prudishness about sex. 4 years old: fell into the fire and was badly burnt. Caned severely at school. Latent homosexuality.

ES69

Adopted, aged 2, after being abandoned as a baby. Extremely hostile to adoptive sister (14 months older). 4–14 years old: boarding schools. Frequently beaten by both adoptive parents but claimed to love mother. Beatings by mother and teacher became substitute-affection. 'Homophobic', self-styled, but probably some latent homosexuality.

ES74

Asthma. Slept in parents' bedroom until 7 years old. Enjoyed being 'caged' in his cot. Influenced by comics. Precocious sexual development. Eye problems—did not cry until 40 years old. Bisexual.

ES75

3 years old: mother hit her with wooden spoon. Jealous of brother (6 years younger). Teased at school for being overweight. 9 years old: mother hit her with belt.

ES76

Subject and his brother (4 years older) allowed to cut up mother's old plastic mac. Elder brother used to tease him. Jealous of younger brother (2 years younger). 9 years old: younger brother given plastic mac with sou'wester.

ES77

Born with umbilical cord wrapped around his neck, almost choked (interest in bondage attributed to this). Asthma. Bullied at school. Father, 9 years younger than mother, died an alcoholic. 12 years old: sexual contact with 8-year-old girl.

ES81

From 5 years old parents would go away, leaving him for a fortnight with a couple he did not care for. 7 years old: mother hit him with a coat hanger. 8–12 years: boarding school where he was bullied. Precocious sexual development.

APPENDIX 4

'Emotional' Stroop task: Mean response times (rounded to the nearest millisecond) of each subject for three categories of words (depressed-content, sadomasochistic-content, neutral-content) and overall mean response times.

Index and control groups subdivided into depressed (a) and nondepressed (b).

Index Subjects

	Word category			
	Dep	SM	Neut	All
(a)				
ES7	863	828	805	832
ES10	602	626	624	617
ES18	657	688	689	678
ES19	656	664	664	661
ES20	637	675	637	650
ES24	759	778	845	794
ES27	546	601	588	579
ES28	836	859	788	828
ES29	870	797	895	854
ES40	1168	1217	1224	1203
ES52	707	731	690	710
ES61	986	1007	975	989
ES71	1550	1624	1334	1503
ES80	528	533	525	529
(b)				
ES1	601	623	626	617
ES2	865	856	930	884
ES4	774	802	798	791
ES8	949	1027	974	984
ES11	542	544	563	550
ES13	849	920	869	880
ES15	693	681	704	692
ES17	1024	1064	1041	1043
ES21	632	678	631	647
ES22	939	990	945	958
ES23	636	673	665	658
ES26	867	900	884	884
ES30	637	669	670	659
ES34	737	777	742	752
ES35	870	908	905	894
ES36	607	599	604	603
ES37	968	1043	997	1002
ES39	1175	1047	964	1062
ES41	658	684	664	669

Index Subjects (*Continued*)

	Word category			
	Dep	SM	Neut	All
ES42	712	822	761	765
ES50	795	852	849	832
ES51	704	767	749	740
ES57	751	805	771	776
ES58	635	659	648	647
ES62	900	924	845	890
ES63	1082	1312	1003	1132
ES65	1020	1086	1082	1063
ES66	1158	1186	1056	1134
ES69	857	920	857	878
ES74	1024	1171	1029	1075
ES75	620	622	633	625
ES76	802	883	836	840
ES77	598	581	587	589
ES81	827	790	789	802

Control Subjects

	Word category			
	Dep	SM	Neut	All
(a)				
CS121	676	638	703	672
CS125	783	835	804	808
CS132	590	574	614	592
CS136	702	698	711	704
CS138	623	641	644	636
CS149	611	600	611	607
CS157	751	758	737	749
CS173	919	922	840	894
CS175	893	963	891	916
CS180	588	598	600	595
CS187	683	654	654	663
CS190	744	814	724	761
CS196	799	799	765	788
CS206	659	680	676	672
CS226	604	602	639	615
CS258	713	779	745	746
CS259	718	726	710	718
CS260	729	717	680	708
CS283	722	715	713	717
CS284	701	691	757	716

Control Subjects (*Continued*)

	Word category			
	Dep	SM	Neut	All
CS284	701	691	757	716
(b)				
NS101	722	725	710	719
NS103	910	917	935	920
NS104	873	924	844	880
NS108	655	620	649	641
NS111	967	920	894	927
NS122	736	736	742	738
NS146	761	780	793	778
NS172	723	710	758	730
NS176	764	788	769	773
NS217	555	561	578	565
NS222	776	731	766	758
NS229	713	727	723	721
NS269	1028	1033	1010	1024
NS278	1113	1033	955	1033
NS285	752	784	772	769

APPENDIX 5

Wording of the 4 questionnaires presented to the index group to obtain information concerning chronicity, practice and motivation of sadomasochism.

QUESTIONNAIRE 1: completed by all index subjects ($n = 48$)

Please underline the correct answer in the righthand column:

(1) Does your sex life in general involve SM activities	(a) Only sometimes? (b) Fairly often? (c) Nearly always?
(2) In your SM activities do you prefer to be	(a) Mostly or totally dominant? (b) Mostly or totally submissive?
(3) Can you switch dominant/ submissive roles	(a) Very easily? (b) Fairly easily? (c) With difficulty or not at all?
(4) Is your sexual orientation	(a) Totally or largely heterosexual?

	(b) Totally or largely bisexual?
	(c) Totally or largely homosexual?
(5) How long have you been in the SM 'scene'	(a) Less than three years?
	(b) Three to six years?
	(c) More than six years?
(6) Do you take on your SM role	(a) Mostly for your own enjoyment?
	(b) Equally for you and your partner's enjoyment?
	(c) Mostly for your partner's enjoyment?
(7) What type of enjoyment do you get out of SM?	(a) A sexual turn-on
	(b) A mental 'high'
	(c) A sense of power
	(d) A thrill from your partner's enjoyment
(8) Overall, how do you rate your sex life?	(a) Very satisfactory
	(b) Moderately satisfactory
	(c) Not satisfactory

Why do think you developed SM interests?

QUESTIONNAIRE 2: FANTASY QUESTIONNAIRE completed by all index subjects ($n = 48$)

Please indicate how often you fantasize about the following themes and how often you have actualized them in reality:

0 = Never, 1 = Rarely, 2 = Sometimes, 3 = Often

	Fantasy	Have done in reality
(1) Being forced to do something	______	______
(2) Forcing someone to do something	______	______
(3) Being whipped or spanked	______	______
(4) Whipping or spanking someone	______	______
(5) Being hurt by a partner	______	______
(6) Hurting a partner	______	______
(7) Being tied up	______	______
(8) Tying someone up	______	______

Please give the number of the single theme from the above list you find most exciting: (a) In fantasy _______ (b) In reality _______

Do you have a favourite fantasy that has been omitted? (Describe briefly)

QUESTIONNAIRE 3: INFORMAL QUESTIONS answered by all index subjects ($n = 48$)

(For the most part these were put verbally and responses were written on the form by the interviewer)

(Do you mind if I make notes?)

(1) When did you first notice you had SM interests?
(2) What happened on that occasion?
(3) How did you feel about it?
(4) Which activities do you prefer?
(5) How often?
(6) When was the last time?
(7) What do you get out of them?
(8) Can you describe your physical sensations?

QUESTIONNAIRE 4: REQUESTING YOUR OPINION—completed by 15 index subjects and returned by post

(1) Do you feel differently towards your SM partner than towards other people? If so, how is she/he different for you?
(2) How much is your sexuality focussed in the genitals?
(3) What are your thoughts on the subject of cruelty?
(4) Would you say that there might be an element of revenge in SM practice? If so, revenge for what?
(5) To what extent (not at all, somewhat, largely, completely) do you associate LOVE with

    TENDERNESS TEASING PAIN BETRAYAL

(6) Did you ever witness sexual intercourse as a child and take it to be an aggressive act?
(7) James Rusbridger's 'operational description of a generalised masochism':

"Masochistic pleasure occurs when the masochist voluntarily *suppresses* a reaction to a situation that they would tend to react strongly to, if that situation also contains exposure to a sexual stimulus" (my italics).

Would you agree with this? Could you please explain it to me?

REFERENCES

Abraham, K. (1911) Notes on the psychoanalytic investigation and treatment of manic-depressive insanity and allied conditions. In *Selected papers on psychoanalysis*, pp. 137–156. New York: Basic Books (1960).

Abraham, K. (1916) The first pregenital stage of the libido. In *Selected papers on psychoanalysis*, pp. 248–279. New York: Basic Books (1960).

Abraham, K. (1924) A short study of the development of the libido. In *Selected papers on psychoanalysis*, pp. 418–501. New York: Basic Books (1960).

Adorno, T. W., Frenkel-Brunswik, E., Levinson, D. J. & Sanford, R. N. (1950) *The authoritarian personality*. New York: Harper.

Ainsworth, M. D. S., Blehar, M. C., Waters, E. & Wall, S. (1978) *Patterns of attachment: A psychological study of the Strange Situation*. Hillsdale, N.J.: Erlbaum.

Aldington, R. (1955) *Lawrence of Arabia: A biographical enquiry*. London: Collins.

Alloy, L. B. & Abramson, L. Y. (1988) Depressive realism: four theoretical perspectives. In *Cognitive processes in depression* (Ed. L. B. Alloy). New York: Guilford.

Babiker, G. & Arnold, L. (1997) *The language of injury: Comprehending self-mutilation*. Leicester: The British Psychological Society.

Bak, R. (1946) Masochism in paranoia. *Psychoanal. Q. 15*, 285–301.

Bargh, J. A. (1982) Attention and automaticity in the processing of self-relevant information. *J. Personality Soc. Psychol. 43*, 425–436.

Bargh, J. A. & Pietromonaco, P. (1982) Automatic information processing and social perception: The influence of trait information presented outside of conscious awareness on impression formation. *J. Personality Soc. Psychol. 43*, 437–449.

Bargh, J. A. & Pratto, F. (1986) Individual construct accessibility and perceptual selection. *J. Exp. Soc. Psychol. 22*, 293–311.

Bateson, W. (1908) *The methods and scope of genetics*. An inaugural lecture delivered 23 October 1908. Cambridge: Cambridge University Press.

Beck, A. T. (1967) *Depression: Clinical, experimental, and theoretical aspects*. New York: Harper & Row.

Beck, A. T. & Lester, D. (1973) Components of depression in attempted suicides. *J. Psychol. 85*, 257–260.

Beck, A. T., Steer, R. A. & Garbin, M. G. (1988) Psychometric properties of the Beck Depression Inventory: twenty-five years of evaluation. *Clin. Psychol. Rev. 8*, 77–100.

Benoit, D., Zeanah, C. H. & Barton, M. L. (1989) Maternal attachment disturbances in failure to thrive. *Infant Ment. Health J. 10*, 185–202.

Berglas, S. (1989) Self-handicapping behavior and the self-defeating personality disorder: Toward a refined clinical perspective. In R. C. Curtis (Ed.), *Self-defeating behaviors: Experimental research, clinical impressions, and practical implications.* New York and London: Plenum Press.

Berliner, B. (1940) Libido and reality in masochism. *Psychoanal. Q. 9*, 322–333.

Berliner, B. (1947) On some psychodynamics of masochism. *Psychoanal. Q. 16*, 459–471.

Berliner, B. (1958) The role of object relations in moral masochism. *Psychoanal. Q. 27*, 38–56.

Bernstein, I. (1957) The role of narcissism in moral masochism. *Psychoanal. Q. 26*, 358–377.

Blumstein, A. (1959) Masochism and fantasies of preparing to be incorporated. *J. Am. Psychoanal. Assoc. 7*, 292–298.

Bonaparte, M. (1951) Some biopsychical aspects of sado-masochism. (Paper read before the Seventeenth International Psycho-Analytical Congress in Amsterdam, 1951, which appeared in a translation by John Rodker in the *International Journal of Psycho-Analysis*, vol.XXXIII, 1952.) In *The First Freudians* (Ed. H. M. Ruitenbeek), pp. 164–192. New York: Jason Aronson (1973).

Bowlby, J. (1969) *Attachment and loss*, Vol. 1. *Attachment*. London: Hogarth Press. New York: Basic Books.

Bowlby, J. (1973) *Attachment and loss*, Vol. 2. *Separation: Anxiety and anger*. London: Hogarth Press. New York: Basic Books.

Bowlby, J. (1980) *Attachment and loss*, Vol. 3. *Loss: Sadness and depression*. London: Hogarth Press. New York: Basic Books.

Bowlby, J. (1987) Attachment. In *The Oxford companion to the mind* (Ed. R. L. Gregory), pp. 57–58. Oxford: Oxford University Press.

Bowlby, J. (1988) *A secure base: Clinical applications of attachment theory*. London: Routledge.

Brenman, M. (1952) On teasing and being teased: and the problem of "moral masochism". *Psychoanal. Study Child 7*, 264–285.

Brenner, C. (1959) The masochistic character: genesis and treatment. *J. Am. Psychoanal. Assoc. 7*, 197–226.

Breslow, N., Evans, L. & Langey, J. (1985) On the prevalence and roles of females in the sadomasochistic subculture: report of an empirical study. *Arch. Sex. Behav. 14*, 303–317.

British Medical Bulletin (1983) *Opioid peptides* (Scientific Editor: J. Hughes; Introduction by J. Hughes and H. W. Kosterlitz; published for the British Council by Churchill Livingstone) *39*, 1–100.

Bromberg, N. (1955) Maternal influences in the development of moral masochism. *Am. J. Orthopsychiatry 25*, 802–809.

Brown, J. S. (1965) Theoretical note: a behavioural analysis of masochism. *J. Exp. Res. Personality 1*, 65–70.
Brown, J. S., Martin, R. C. & Morrow, M. W. (1964) Self-punitive behaviour in the rat: facilitative effects of punishment on resistance to extinction. *J. Comp. Physiol. Psychol. 57*, 127–133.
Brown, M., Ed. (1988) *The letters of T.E. Lawrence.* London: J.M. Dent & Sons.
Brown, M. & Cave, J. (1988). *A touch of genius: The life of T. E. Lawrence.* London: J. M. Dent & Sons.
Buchan, J. (1940) *Memory hold-the-door.* London: Hodder and Stoughton.
Buhrich, N. (1983) The association of erotic piercing with homosexuality, sadomasochism, bondage, fetishism, and tattoos. *Arch. Sex. Behav. 12*, 167–171.
Burt, M. R. (1980) Cultural myths and supports for rape. *J. Personality Soc. Psychol. 38*, 217–230.
Calder, A. (1971) *The people's war.* London: Panther.
Carr, D. B. (1981) Endorphins at the approach of death. *Lancet 1*, 390.
Cattell, J. M. (1886) The time it takes to see and name objects. *Mind 11*, 63–65.
Caudwell, C. (1938) *Studies in a dying culture.* II. T. E. Lawrence: A study in heroism, pp. 20–43. London: John Lane The Bodley Head.
Chodorwo, N. (1978) *The reproduction of mothering.* Berkeley: University of California Press.
Cixous, H. (1976) The laugh of the Medusa. In *New French feminisms* (Ed., E. Marks and I. de Courtivon). Sussex: Harvester Press (1981).
Cleugh, J. (1951) *The marquis and the chevalier.* London: Andrew Melrose.
Cohen, J. (1960) A coefficient of agreement for nominal scales. *Educ. Psychol. Meas. 20*, 37–46.
Crepault, C., Abraham, G., Porto R. & Couture, M. (1977) Erotic imagery in women. In *Progress in sexology* (Eds. R. Gemme and C. C. Wheeler), pp. 267–283. New York: Plenum Press.
Crepault, C. & Couture, M. (1980) Men's erotic fantasies. *Arch. Sex. Behav. 9*, 565–581.
Crowell, J. A. & Feldman, S. S. (1988) Mothers' internal models of relationships and children's behavioral and developmental status: A study of mother-child interaction. *Child Dev. 59*, 1273–1285.
Dannecker, M. & Reiche, R. (1974) *Der gewöhnliche Homosexuelle.* Frankfurt: Fischer.
Dennett, D. C. (1991) *Consciousness explained.* Harmondsworth: Penguin Books.
Deutsch, H. (1925) The psychology of women in relation to the functions of reproduction. *Int. J. Psychoanal. 6*, 405–418. In *The psychoanalytic reader* (Ed. R. Fliess), vol. I, pp. 192–206. New York: International Universities Press (1948).
Deutsch, H. (1930) The significance of masochism in the mental life of women. *Int.J. Psychoanal. 11*, 48–60. In *The psychoanalytic reader* (Ed. R. Fliess), vol. I, pp. 223–236. New York: International Universities Press (1948).
Deutsch, H. (1937) Absence of grief. *Psychoanal. Q. 6*, 12–22.
Dinnerstein, D. (1977) *The mermaid and the minotaur.* New York: Harper & Row.
Dixon, N. (1976) *On the psychology of military incompetence.* London: Jonathan Cape.

Donnerstein, E. (1980) Pornography and violence against women. *Ann. N.Y. Acad. Sci. 347*, 277–288.

Dsm-III-R. (1987) *American Psychiatric Association: Diagnostic and statistical manual of mental disorders*, Third Ed., Revised. Washington, DC: American Psychiatric Association.

Duman, R. S., Heninger, G. R. & Nestler, E. J. (1997) A molecular and cellular theory of depression. *Arch. Gen. Psychiatry 54*, 597–606.

Dyer, F. N. (1973) The Stroop phenomenon and its use in the study of perceptual, cognitive, and response processes. *Memory and Cognition 1*, 106–120.

Eidelberg, L. (1934) A contribution to the study of masochism. In *Studies in psychoanalysis*, pp. 31–40. New York: International Universities Press (1952).

Eidelberg, L. (1959) Humiliation in masochism. *J. Am. Psychoanal. Assoc. 7*, 274–283.

Eisler, R. (1951) *Man into wolf: An anthropological interpretation of sadism, masochism, and lycanthropy.* London: Routledge and Kegan Paul.

Eysenck, H. J. (1954) *The psychology of politics.* London: Routledge.

Eysenck, H. J. (1970) *The structure of human personality.* London: Methuen.

Fechner, G. T. (1873) *Einige Ideen zur Schöpfungs- und Entwicklungsgeschichte der Organismen* (Part XI, Supplement, 94). Leipzig.

Fein, M. L. (1999) *The limits of idealism: When good intentions go bad.* New York: Kluwer Academic/Plenum Publishers.

Fenichel, O. (1945) *The psychoanalytic theory of neurosis.* New York: W. W. Norton.

Ferenczi, S. (1925) (Trans. 1926) Psycho-analysis of sexual habits. In *Further contributions to the theory and technique of psycho-analysis*, Chap. XXXII.

Ferenczi, A. (1926) (Trans. 1926) The problem of acceptance of unpleasant ideas. In *Further contributions to the theory and technique of psycho-analysis*, Chap. LXXIII.

Fisk, A. D. & Schneider, W. (1984) Memory as a function of attention, level of processing, and automatization. *J. Exp. Psychol.: Learning, Memory, and Cognition 10*, 181–197.

Flavell, J. H., Flavell, E. R. & Green, F. L. (1983) Development of the appearance-reality disctinction. *Cognitive Psychol. 15*, 95–120.

Fleiss, J. L., Cohen, J. & Everitt, B. S. (1969) Large sample standard errors of kappa and weighted kappa. *Psychol. Bull. 72*, 323–327.

Fonagy, P., Leigh, T., Steele, M., Steele, H., Kennedy, R., Mattoon, G., Target, M. & GERBER, A. (1996) The relation of attachment status, psychiatric classification, and response to psychotherapy. *J. Consulting Clin. Psychol. 64*, 22–31.

Fonagy, P., Steele, H., Moran, G., Steele, M. & Higgett, A. (1991*a*) The capacity for understanding mental states: the reflective self in parent and child and its significance for security of attachment. *Infant Ment. Health J. 13*, 200–217.

Fonagy, P., Steele, H., & Steele, M. (1991*b*) Maternal representations of attachment during pregnancy predict the organization of infant-mother attachment at one year of age. *Child Dev. 62*, 891–905.

Fraiberg, S. (1982) Pathological defenses in infancy. *Psychoanal. Q. 51*, 612–635.

Freud, S. (1891) *Zur Auffassung der Aphasien.* Vienna: Deuticke. *On Aphasia.* Translated by E. Stengel, 1953. New York: International Universities Press.

Freud, S. (1893) Charcot. *Standard Edition 3*, 11–23.
Freud, S. (1895*a*) Project for a scientific psychology. *Standard Edition 1*, 295–387.
Freud, S. (1895*b*) Studies on hysteria. Case 5: Elisabeth von R. *Standard Edition 2*, 135–181.
Freud, S. (1896) Letter to Wilhelm Fliess dated 6 December, no. 52. *Standard Edition 1*, 233–239.
Freud, S. (1900) The interpretation of dreams. *Standard Edition 4–5*, 1–621.
Freud, S. (1905) Three essays on the theory of sexuality. *Standard Edition 7*, 135–243.
Freud, S. (1910) The psycho-analytic view of psychogenic disturbance of vision. *Standard Edition 11*, 20–218.
Freud, S. (1911) Formulations on the two principles of mental functioning. *Standard Edition 12*, 218–226.
Freud, S. (1913) The disposition to obsessional neurosis: A contribution to the problem of choice of neurosis. *Standard Edition 12*, 317–326.
Freud, S. (1914) On the history of the psycho-analytic movement. *Standard Edition 14*, 7–66.
Freud, S. (1915*a*) Instincts and their vicissitudes. *Standard Edition 14*, 117–140.
Freud, S. (1915*b*) The unconscious. *Standard Edition 14*, 166–204.
Freud, S. (1916–1917) Introductory lectures on psycho-analysis. *Standard Edition 15–16*, 15–463.
Freud, S. (1917*a*) A metapsychological supplement to the theory of dreams. *Standard Edition 14*, 222–235.
Freud, S. (1917*b*) Mourning and melancholia. *Standard Edition 14*, 243–258.
Freud, S. (1918) From the history of an infantile neurosis. *Standard Edition 17*, 7–122.
Freud, S. (1919) 'A child is being beaten': A contribution to the study of the origin of sexual perversions. *Standard Edition 17*, 17–204.
Freud, S. (1920*a*) Beyond the pleasure principle. *Standard Edition 18*, 7–64.
Freud, S. (1920*b*) The psychogenesis of a case of homosexuality in a woman. *Standard Edition 18*, 147–172.
Freud, S. (1921) Group psychology and the analysis of the ego. *Standard Edition 18*, 6–143.
Freud, S. (1923*a*) Two encyclopaedia articles. (B) The libido theory. *Standard Edition 18*, 255–259.
Freud, S. (1923*b*) The ego and the id. *Standard Edition 19*, 12–59.
Freud, S. (1924*a*) The economic problem of masochism. *Standard Edition 19*, 159–170.
Freud, S. (1924*b*) Letter to Le Disque Vert. *Standard Edition 19*, 290.
Freud, S. (1925) Some psychical consequences of the anatomical distinction between the sexes. *Standard Edition 19*, 248–258.
Freud, S. (1926) Inhibitions, symptoms and anxiety. *Standard Edition 20*, 87–172.
Freud, S. (1927) Fetishism. *Standard Edition 21*, 152–157.
Freud, S. (1928) Dostoevsky and parricide. *Standard Edition 21*, 177–194.
Freud, S. (1930) Civilization and its discontents. *Standard Edition 21*, 64–145.
Freud, S. (1931) Female sexuality. *Standard Edition 21*, 225–243.

Freud, S. (1933) New introductory lectures on psycho-analysis. *Standard Edition 22*, 7–182.

Freud, S. (1937) Analysis terminable and interminable. *Standard Edition 23*, 216–253.

Freud, S. (1940*a*) An outline of psycho-analysis. *Standard Edition 23*, 144–206.

Freud, S. (1940*b*) Splitting of the ego in the process of defense. *Standard Edition 23*, 275–278.

Fromm, E. (1973) *The anatomy of human destructiveness.* New York: Holt, Rinehart & Winston.

Frosh, S. (1987) *The politics of psychoanalysis: An introduction to Freudian and post-Freudian theory.* London: Macmillan.

Frosh, S. (1994) *Sexual difference: Masculinity and psychoanalysis.* London, New York: Routledge.

Gallop, J. (1982) *The daughter's seduction: Feminism and psychoanalysis.* London: Macmillan.

Garnett, D., ed. (1938) *The Letters of T.E. Lawrence.* London, Toronto: Jonathan Cape.

Glasser, M. (1979) Some aspects of the role of aggression in the perversions. In *Sexual deviation*, 2nd Ed. (ed. I. Rosen), pp. 278–305. Oxford: Oxford University Press.

Glasser, M. (1996) Aggression and sadism in the perversions. In *Sexual deviation*, 3rd ed. (Ed. I. Rosen), pp. 279–299. Oxford: Oxford University Press.

Glenn, J. (1984*a*) A note on loss, pain and masochism in children. *J. Am. Psychoanal. Assoc. 32*, 63–73.

Glenn, J. (1984*b*) Psychic trauma and masochism. *J. Am. Psychoanal. Assoc. 32*, 357–386.

Golin, S., Terrell, T. & Johnson, B. (1977) Depression and the illusion of control. *J. Abnormal Psychol. 86*, 440–442.

Golin, S., Terrell, T., Weitz, J. & Drost, P.L. (1979) The illusion of control among depressed patients. *J. Abnormal Psychol. 88*, 454–457.

Gorman, J. T. (1940) *With Lawrence to Damascus* (Great Exploit Series). London, New York, Toronto: Oxford University Press.

Gosselin, C. & Wilson, G. (1980) *Sexual variations: Fetishism, sadomasochism and transvestism.* London: Faber and Faber. New York: Simon and Schuster.

Gosselin, C. C., Wilson, G. D. & Barrett, P. T. (1991) The personality and sexual preferences of sadomasochistic women. *Personality and Individual Differences 12*, 11–15.

Gotlib, I. H. & Cane, D. B. (1987) Construct accessibility and clinical depression: a longitudinal investigation. *J. Abnormal Psychol. 96*, 199–204.

Gotlib, I. H. & McCann, C. D. (1984) Construct accessibility and depression: an examination of cognitive and affective factors. *J. Personality Soc. Psychol. 47*, 427–439.

Gray, C. & Hesetline, P. (1971) *Carlo Gesualdo, Prince of Venosa, musician and murderer.* Westport, Connecticut: Greenwood Press. (Originally published in 1926 by Kegan Paul, Trench, Trubner & Co., Ltd., London.)

Green, R. (1975) Sexual identity: Research strategies. *Arch. Sex. Behav. 4*, 337–352.

Greenberg, M. S. & Alloy, L. B. (1989) Depression versus anxiety: Processing of self- and other-referent information. *Cognition and Emotion 3*, 207–223.

Grice, H. P. (1975) Logic and conversation. In *Syntax and semantics III. Speech acts* (Eds. P. Cole & J. L. Moran), pp. 41–58. New York: Academic Press.

Grinker, R,. Miller, J., Sabshin, M., Nunn, R. & Nunnally, J. (1961) *The phenomena of depressions.* New York: Hoeber.

Grossman, W. I. (1986) Notes on masochism: a discussion of the history and development of a psychoanalytic concept. *Psychoanal. Q. 55*, 37–413.

Guthrie, E. R. (1935) *The Psychology of learning.* New York: Harper.

Hamilton, G. V. (1929) *A research in marriage.* New York: Boni.

Hartmann, H. (1950) Psychoanalysis and developmental psychology. *Psychoanal. Study Child 5*, 7–17.

Hayflick, L. (1965) The limited in vitro lifetime of human diploid cell strains. *Exp. Cell Res.* 37, 614–636.

Hegel, G. W. F. (1807) *Phänomenologie des Geistes* (Ed. J. Hoffmeister), IV, A, pp. 141–150: Herrschaft und Knechtschaft. Hamburg: Felix Meiner Verlag, 1952. Trans. J. B. Baillie: *The phenomenology of mind,* pp. 229–240: Lordship and bondage. London: George Allen & Unwin, revised ed., 1931.

Helman, C. G. (1985) Psyche, soma and society: The social construction of psychosomatic disorders. *Cult. Med. Psychiatry 9*, 1–26.

Helman, C. G. (1990) *Culture, health and illness: An introduction for health professionals,* 2nd ed. Oxford: Butterworth-Heinemann.

Helweg-Larsen, R., Hoffmeyer, H., Kieler, J., Thaysen, E. H., Thaysen, J. H. & Thygesen, P. (1952) Famine disease in German concentration camps. *Acta Med. Scand.* Suppl. 274, 235–250.

Hermans, H. J. M., Kempen, H. J. G. & Van Loon, R. J. P. (1992) The dialogical self: Beyond individualism and rationalism. *Am. Psychol.* 47, 23–33.

Hesse, E. (1996) Discourse, memory, and the Adult Attachment Interview: A note with emphasis on the emerging Cannot Classify category. *Infant Ment. Health J. 17*, 4–11.

Hilgard, E. R. (1973) A neodissociation interpretation of pain reduction in hypnosis. *Psychol. Rev. 80*, 396–411.

Hilgard, E. R. (1974) Toward a neodissociation theory: multiple cognitive controls in human functioning. *Perspect. Biol. Med. 17*, 301–316.

Hill, A. B. & Knowles, T. H. (1991) Depression and the 'emotional' Stroop effect. *Personality and Individual Differences 12*, 481–485.

Hirschfeld, M. (1930) *Geschlechtskunde auf Grund dreissigjähriger Forschung und Erfahrung bearbeitet,* Vol. 3, *Einblicke und Ausblicke.* Stuttgart: Julius Puttmann.

Hoefnagel, D. (1965) The syndrome of athetoid cerebral palsy, mental deficiency, self-mutilation and hyperuricemia. *J. Ment. Deficiency Res.* 9, 6–74.

Hoffman, R. R., Cochran, E. L. & Nead, J. M. (1990) Cognitive metaphors in experimental psychology. In *Metaphors in the history of psychology* (Ed. D. E. Leary), pp. 173–229. Cambridge: Cambridge University Press.

Hollingworth, H. L. (1915) Articulation and association. *J. Educ. Psychol. 6*, 99–105.

Horney, K. (1935) The problem of feminine masochism. *Psychoanal. Rev. 22*, 241–257.

Hotelling, H. (1931) The generalization of Student's ratio. *Ann. Math. Stat. 2*, 360–378.

Howell, D. C. (1987) *Statistical methods for psychology*, 2nd ed. Boston: PWS-Kent.

Hughes, J., Smith, T. W., Kosterlitz, H. W., Fothergill, L. A., Morgan, B. A. & Morris, H. R. (1975) Identification of two related pentapeptides from the brain with potent opiate agonist activity. *Nature 258*, 577–579.

Hunt, M. (1974) *Sexual behaviour in the 1970s*. Chicago: Playboy Press.

Hyde, H. Montgomery. (1977) *Solitary in the ranks: Lawrence of Arabia as airman and private soldier.* London: Constable.

Iles, T. C. (1993) Crossed and hierarchical analysis of variance. In *Biological data analysis: A practical approach* (Ed. J. C. Fry), pp. 41–80. Oxford: IRL Press at Oxford University Press.

Isakower, O. (1938) A contribution to the pathopsychology of phenomena associated with falling asleep. *Int. J. Psychoanal. 19*, 331–345.

Isserlin, M. (1922) Ueber Agrammatismus. *Zeitschrift für die gesamte Neurologie und Psychiatrie 75*, 332–416. Translated and edited by D. Howard, H. Droller & R. Campbell, *Cognitive Neuropsychology* 2, 303–345 (1985).

Jacques, T. (1993) *On the safe edge: A manual for SM play.* Toronto: WholeSM Publishing.

James, L. (1990). *The golden warrior: The life and legend of Lawrence of Arabia.* London: Weidenfeld and Nicolson.

Jensen, A. R. & Rohwer, W. D, Jr. (1966) The Stroop color-word test: A review. *Acta Psychologica 25*, 36–93.

Jones, J. H. (1997) Annals of sexology: Dr. Yes. *The New Yorker*, August 25 & September 1, pp. 98–113.

Kelley, W. & Wyngaarden, J. B. (1983) Clinical syndromes associated with hypoxanthine-guanine-phosphoribosyltransferase deficiency. In *The metabolic basis of inherited disease*, 5th ed. (Ed. J. B. Stanbury), chap. *51*, pp. 1115–1117. Maidenhead: McGraw-Hill.

Kelly, G. A. (1955) *The psychology of personal constructs*. New York: W. W. Norton.

Kernberg, O. F. (1988) Clinical dimensions of masochism. *J. Am. Psychoanal. Assoc. 36*, 1005–1029.

King, R. C. & Stansfield, W. D. (1985) *A dictionary of genetics*, 3rd edition. Oxford: Oxford University Press.

Kinsey, A. C., Pomeroy, W. B. & Martin, C. E. (1948) *Sexual behaviour in the human male*. Philadelphia, London: W.B. Saunders.

Kinsey, A. C., Pomeroy, W. B., Martin, C. E. & Gebhard. P .H. (1953) *Sexual behaviour in the human female.* Philadelphia, London: W.B. Saunders.

Klein, G. S. (1964) Semantic power measured through the interference of words with colour-naming. *Am. J. Psychol. 77*, 576–588.

Klein, M. (1934) A contribution to the psychogenesis of manic-depressive states. In *Contributions to psycho-analysis 1921–1945*, pp. 282–310. London: Hogarth Press (1948).

Knightley, P. & Simpson, C. (1969) *The secret lives of Lawrence of Arabia*. London: Nelson.
Kobak, R. & Sceery, A. (1988) Attachment in late adolescence: working models, affect regulation and representations of self and others. *Child Dev. 59*, 135–146.
Kohut, H. (1971) *The analysis of the self: A systematic approach to the psychoanalytic treatment of narcissistic personality disorders*. (The Psychoanalytic Study of the Child Monograph no. 4.) Madison, Connecticut: International Universities Press.
Kohut, H. (1977) *The restoration of the self*. New York: International Universities Press.
Krafft-Ebing, R. von (1886) *Psychopathia sexualis* (8th ed. 1893; 11th ed. 1901). Stuttgart: Ferdinand Enke.
Krainess, S. H. (1965) Manic-depressive syndrome: A diencephalic disease. Paper presented at the *Annual Meeting of the American Psychiatric Association*, New York, May 6, 1965.
Kral, V. A. (1951) Psychiatric observations under severe stress. *Am. J. Psychiatry 108*, 185–192.
Kral, V. A., Pazder, L. H. & Wigdor, B .P. (1967) Long-term effects of a prolonged stress experience. *Can. Psychiat. Assoc. J. 12*, 175–181.
Kucera, H. & Francis, W. N. (1967) *Computational analysis of present-day American English*. Providence, Rhode Island: Brown University Press.
Kucera, O. (1959) On teething. *J. Am. Psychoanal. Assoc. 7*, 284–291.
Lacan, J. (1958) The meaning of the phallus. In *Feminine sexuality* (Eds. J. Mitchell and J. Rose). London: Macmillan (1982).
Laforgue, R. (1930) On the eroticization of anxiety. *Int. J. Psycho-anal.* 11, 312–321.
Lagache, D. (1961) Situation de l'agressivité. *Bull. Psychol. 14*, 99–112.
Laing, R. D. (1976). *The facts of life*. Harmondsworth, UK: Penguin Books.
Lampl-De Groot, J. (1937) Masochismus und Narzissmus. *Int. Z. Psychoanal. 23*, 479–489.
Lawrence, T. E. (1926) *Seven pillars of wisdom: A triumph*. Harmondsworth, Middlesex: Penguin Books in association with Jonathan Cape (1986).
Lawrence, T. E. (1927) *Revolt in the desert*. London: Jonathan Cape.
Lawrence, T. E. (1936) *Crusader castles*. London: The Golden Cockerel Press. Michael Haag, 1986.
Lawrence, T. E. (1955) *The mint*. London: Jonathan Cape. Penguin Books, 1978.
Lawrence, T. E. (1971) *Minorities* (private anthology given to Charlotte Shaw in 1927), (Ed. J. M. Wilson.) London: Jonathan Cape.
Lawrence, T. E. (1986) Translation: *The Odyssey of Homer*. Gloucester: Alan Sutton. (A limited edition published on completion in 1932 in U.S.A. by Oxford University Press)
Lax, R. F. (1992) A variation on Freud's theme in "A Child is Being Beaten" — mother's role: some implications for superego development. *J. Am. Psychoanal. Assoc. 40*, 455–473.
Lenzer, G. (1975) On masochism: A contribution to the history of a phantasy and its theory. *Signs 1*, 277–324.
Lesch, M. & Nyhan, W. L. (1964) A familial disorder of uric acid metabolism and central nervous system function. *Am. J. Med.* 36, 561–570.

Lewin, B. D. (1950) *The psychoanalysis of elation.* New York: W. W. Norton (1951, London: Hogarth Press).

Lewinsky, H. (1944) On some aspects of masochism. *Int. J. Psychoanal. 25,* 150–155.

Lewinsohn, P. M., Mischel, W., Chaplain, W. & Barton, R. (1980) Social competence and depression: the role of illusory self-perceptions? *J. Abnormal Psychol. 89,* 203–212.

Liggett, J. (1974) *The human face.* London: Constable.

Light, P. (1979) *Development of a child's sensitivity to people.* London: Cambridge University Press.

Lindsley, O. R. (1956) Operant conditioning methods applied to research in chronic schizophrenia. *Psychiat. Res. Rep. 5,* 118–139.

Litman, R.E. & Swearingen, C. (1972) Bondage and suicide. *Arch. Gen. Psychiatry 27,* 80–85.

Loewenstein, R. M. (1957) A contribution to the psychoanalytic theory of masochism. *J. Am. Psychoanal. Assoc. 5,* 197–234.

Lunde, I., Rasmussen, O. V., Wagner, G. & Lindholm, J. (1981) Sexual and pituitary-testicular function in torture victims. *Arch. Sex. Behav. 10,* 25–32.

Mack, J. E. (1976) *A prince of our disorder: The life of T.E. Lawrence.* London: Weidenfeld and Nicolson.

Macleod, C. (1991) Half a century of research on the Stroop effect: An integrative review. *Psychol. Bull. 109,* 163–203.

Main, M. (1991) Metacognitive knowledge, metacognitive monitoring, and singular (coherent) vs. multiple (incoherent) models of attachment: Findings and directions for future research. In *Attachment across the lifecycle* (Eds. P. Harris, J. Stevenson-Hinde & C. Parkes), chap. *8,* pp. 127–159. New York: Routledge.

Main, M. & Goldwyn, R. (1984) Predicting rejection of her infant from mother's representation of her own experience: implications for the abused-abusing intergenerational cycle. *Child Abuse and Neglect 8,* 203–217.

Main, M. & Goldwyn, R. (1985–1994) *Adult attachment scoring and classification system.* Unpublished scoring manual. Department of Psychology, University of California, Berkeley.

Main, M., Kaplan, N. & Cassidy, J. (1985) Security in infancy, childhood, and adulthood: a move to the level of representation. In *Growing points of attachment theory and research* (Eds. I. Bretherton & E. Waters). *Monogr. Soc. Res. Child Dev. 50,* 66–104.

Malamuth, N. M. (1981) Rape fantasies as a function of exposure to violent sexual stimuli. *Arch. Sex. Behav.* 10, 33–47.

Malamuth, N. M. & Spinner, B. (1980) A longitudinal content analysis of sexual violence in the best-selling erotic magazines. *J. Sex Res. 17,* 226–237.

Maleson, F. G. (1984) The multiple meanings of masochism in psychoanalytic discourse. *J. Am. Psychoanal. Assoc. 32,* 325–356.

Marks, I. M., Rachman, S. & Gelder, M. G. (1965) Methods for assessment of averson treatment in fetishism with masochism. *Behav. Res. Ther. 3,* 253–258.

Marriot, P. J. *The young Lawrence of Arabia 1888–1910* (private publication).

Masserman, J. H. (1946) *Principles of dynamic psychiatry.* Philadelphia: W. B. Saunders.

Masson, J. M. (1984) *The assault on truth: Freud's suppression of the seduction theory.* Toronto: Collins.

Mathews, A. & Macleod, C. (1985) Selective processing of threat cues in anxiety states. *Behav. Res. Ther. 23,* 563–569.

Maxwell, S. E. & Delaney, H. D (1993) Bivariate median splits and spurious statistical significance. *Psychol. Bull. 113,* 181–190.

McDougall, J. (1985) *Theatres of the mind: Illusion and truth on the psychoanalytic stage.* (Translated from the French by the author.) London: Free Association Books.

McDougall, J. (1989) *Theatres of the body: A psychoanalytical approach to psychosomatic illness.* London: Free Association Books.

McGuire, R. J. & Vallance, M. (1964) Aversion therapy by electric shock: a simple technique. *Br. Med. J. 1,* 151–152.

Melvin, K. B & Brown, J. S. (1965) Neutralization of an aversive light simulus as a function of number of paired presentations with food. *J. Comp. Physiol. Psychiatry 58,* 350–353.

Melzack, R. & Wall, P. D. (1982) *The challenge of pain.* Revised edition 1988. Harmondsworth: Penguin Books.

Menaker, E. (1953) Masochism — a defense reaction of the ego. *Psychoanal. Q. 22,* 205–220.

Meninger, K. A. (1938) *Man against himself.* London: George G. Harrap.

Mental Measurements Yearbook, Vol. 11. (1992) (Eds. J. J. Kramer & J. C. Conoley.) Beck Depression Inventory (Revised ed.), pp. 72–81. Lincoln, Nebraska: University of Nebraska Press.

Meston, C. M. & Frohlich, P. F. (2000) The neurobiology of sexual function. *Arch. Gen. Psychiatry 57,* 1012–1030.

Miller, N. E. (1960) Learning resistance to pain and fear: Effects of overlearning, exposure, rewarded exposure in context. *J. Exp. Psychol. 60,* 137–145.

Mitchell, J. (1974) *Psychoanalysis and feminism.* Harmondsworth: Penguin.

Mitchell, J. & Rose, J., eds. (1982) *Feminine sexuality.* London: Macmillan.

Monchy, R. de (1950) Masochism as a pathological and as a normal phenomenon in the human mind. *Int. J. Psychoanal. 31,* 95–97.

Moser, C. & Levitt, E. E. (1987) An exploratory-descriptive study of a sadomasochistically oriented sample. *J. Sex Res. 23,* 322–337.

Mowrer, O. H. (1950) *Learning theory and personality dynamics.* New York: Ronald Press.

Myers, J. (1980) Adjectives rated as self-descriptive by depressed and manic psychiatric patients. Unpublished manuscript, University of Calgary, Calgary, Alberta, Canada.

Myers, W. A. (1980/81) The psychodynamics of a beating fantasy. *Int. J. Psychoanal. Psychother. 8,* 623–660.

Nacht, S. (1938) *Le masochisme.* Paris: Le François (1948).

Nathan, P. (1988) *The nervous system.* 3rd ed. Oxford, New York: Oxford University Press.

Novick, J. & Novick, K. K. (1972) Beating fantasies in children. *Int. J. Psychoanal. 53*, 237–242.
Novick, K. K. & Novick, J. (1987) The essence of masochism. *Psychoanal. Study Child 42*, 353–384.
O'Donnell, T. J. (1977) The confessions of T. E. Lawrence: The sadomasochistic hero. *Am. Imago 34*, 115–132.
Office of Population Censuses and Surveys. (1974) The Registrar General's Statistical Review of England and Wales for the Year 1972. Part II: Tables, Population, pp. 14, 92. London: Her Majesty's Stationery Office.
Olson, G. A., Olson, R. D., Kastin, A. J. & Coy, D. H. (1980–1987) Annual reviews: Endogenous opiates. *Peptides, 1*, 365–379; *2*, 34–369; *3*, 103–1072; *4*, 563–576; *5*, 975–992; *6*, 76–791; 7, 907–933; *8*, 1135–1164.
Osgood, C. E., Suci, G.J. & Tannenbaum, P. H. (1957) *The measurement of meaning.* Illinois: University of Illinois Press.
Panel (1956) The problem of masochism in the theory and technique of psychoanalysis. M.H. Stein, reporter. *J. Am. Psychoanal. Assoc. 4*, 526–538.
Panel (1981) Masochism: current concepts. N. Fischer, reporter. *J. Am. Psychoanal. Assoc. 29*, 673–688.
Panel (1984) The relation between masochism and depression. J. Caston, reporter. *J. Am. Psychoanal. Assoc. 32*, 603–614.
Pavlov, I. P. (1927) *Conditioned reflexes.* Oxford, London: Oxford University Press.
Pearce, J. & Morley, S. (1989) An experimental investigation of the construct validity of the McGill Pain Questionnaire. *Pain 39*, 115–121.
Peterson, J., Lanier, L. H. & Walker, H. M. (1925) Comparisons of white and negro children in certain ingenuity and speed tests. *J. Comp. Psychol.* 5, 271–283.
Petrucha, R. A., Goebelsmann, U., Hung, T. T., Haase, H. R. & Lobo, R. A. (1983). Amniotic fluid (-endorphin and (-lipotropin concentrations during the second and third trimesters. *Am. J. Obstet. Gynecol. 146*, 644–651.
Rado, S. (1928) The problem of melancholia. *Int. J. Psychoanal. 9*, 420–438.
Rado, S. (1933) Fear of castration in women. *Psychoanal. Quart.* 2, 425–475.
Raff, M. C. (1992) Social controls on cell survival and cell death. *Nature 356*, 397–400.
Rathbone, J. A. (1999). Anatomy of masochism. PhD thesis. University of London.
Reich, W. (1932) The masochistic character. In *Character analysis*, 3rd Ed., pp.208–247. New York: Orgone Institute Press (1949).
Reik, T. (1939) The characteristics of masochism. *Am. Imago 1*, 26–59.
Reik, T. (1941) *Masochism in modern man.* New York: Farrar and Rinehart.
Richardson, J. S. & Zaleski, W. A. (1986). Endogenous opiates and self-mutilation. *Am. J. Psychiatry 143*, 938–939.
Sacher-Masoch, L. von (?1870) *Venus im Pelz.* Privately printed.
Sacher-Masoch, W. von (1906) *Confessions de ma vie.* Paris: Tchou (1967).
Sade, D. A. F., Marquis de. (1792) *Histoire de Juliette: Les prospérités du vice.*
Sadger, I. (1926) A contribution to the understanding of sado-masochism. *Int. J. Psychoanal. 7*, 484–491.
Schatzman, M. (1992) Freud: Who seduced whom? *New Scientist* 133 (no.1813, 21 March), 34–37.

Schrenck-Notzing, A. von (1899) Literaturzusammenstellung über die Psychologie und Psychopathologie der Vita sexualis. *Z. Hypnot. 9*, 98.

Scott, E. M. & Delaney, H. D. (1993) Bivariate median splits and spurious statistical significance. *Psychol. Bull. 113*, 181–190.

Scott, J. E. & Cuvelier, S. J. (1987) Violence in Playboy magazine: A longitudinal analysis. *Arch. Sex. Behav. 16*, 279–288.

Seligman, M. E. P. (1974) Depression and learned helplessness. In *The psychology of depression: Contemporary theory and research* (eds. R. J. Friedman and M. M. Katz). Washington, DC: Winston-Wiley.

Seligman, M. E. P. & Beagley, G. (1975) Learned helplessness in the rat. *J. Comp. Physiol. Psychol. 88*, 534–541.

Shepherd, G. M. (1988) *Neurobiology* (2nd ed.). New York, Oxford: Oxford University Press.

Shore, M. F., Clifton, A., Zelin, M. & Myerson, P. G. (1971) Patterns of masochism: an empirical study. *Br. J. Med. Psychol. 44*, 5–66.

Simpson, C. & Knightley, P. (1968) The Secret Life of Lawrence of Arabia. *Sunday Times Weekly Review* 9, 16, 23, 30 June.

Siuciak, J. A., Lewis, D. R., Wiegand, S. J. & Lindsay, R. M. (1997) Antidepressant-like effect of brain-derived neurotrophic factor (BDNF). *Pharmacol. Biochem. Behav.* 56, 131–137.

Skinner, B. F., Solomon, H. & Lindsey, O. R. (1954) A new method for the experimental analysis of psychotic patients. *J. Nerv. Ment. Disease 120*, 404–406.

Smirnoff, V. N. (1969) The masochistic contract. *Int. J. Psychoanal. 50*, 665–671.

Smith, B. R., Brown, Z. W. & Amit, Z. (1982). Intraventricular self-administration of leucine-enkephalin by laboratory rats. *Life Sci. 31*, 1527–1530.

Snyder, C. R. (1990). Self-handicapping processes and sequelae: On the taking of a psychological dive. In R.L. Higgins, C.R. Snyder & S. Berglas (Eds.), *Self-handicapping: The paradox that isn't.* New York and London: Plenum Press.

Spengler, A. (1977) Manifest sadomasochism of males: results of an empirical study. *Arch. Sex. Behav.* 6, 441–456.

Spitz, R. A. (1945) Hospitalism: an inquiry into the genesis of psychiatric conditions in early childhood. *Psychoanal. Study Child 1*, 53–74.

Spitz, R. A. (1961) Some early prototypes of ego defenses. *J. Am. Psychoanal. Assoc. 9*, 625–651.

Spitz, R. A. & Cobliner, W. G. (1965) *The first year of life: A psychoanalytic study of normal and deviant development of object relations.* New York: International Universities Press.

Srouff, L. A. (1985) Attachment classification from the perspective of infant-caregiver relationships and infant temperament. *Child Dev.* 56, 1–14.

Steiger, J. H. (1980) Tests for comparing elements of a correlation matrix. *Psychol. Bull.* 87, 245–251.

Stein, M. (1975) *Lovers, friends, and slaves.* New York: Berkeley.

Stekel, W. (1929) *Sadism and masochism: The psychology of hatred and cruelty.* New York: Liveright. (Trans. 1968) New York: Washington Square.

Stoller, R. (1970) Pornography and perversion. *Arch. Gen. Psychiatry 22*, 490–499.

Stroim, A. (1968) *Norwegian concentration camp survivors.* Oslo: Oslo University Press.

Stroop, J. R. (1935) Studies of interference in serial verbal reactions. *J. Exp. Psychol. 18*, 643–662.

Sue, D. (1979) Erotic fantasies of college students during coitus. *J. Sex Res. 15*, 299–305.

Suttie, I. D. (1935). *The origins of love and hate.* London: Kegan Paul, Trench, Trubner.

Szasz, T. S. (1957) *Pain and pleasure: A study of bodily feelings* (2nd expanded ed. 1975). New York: Basic Books.

Tabachnick, S. E. (1978) *T. E. Lawrence.* Boston: G.K. Hall.

Tabachnick, S. E. & Matheson, C. (1988) *Images of Lawrence.* London: Jonathan Cape.

Tellenbach, H. (1961) *Melancholie.* Berlin: Springer-Verlag.

Thorndike, E. L. & Lorge, I. (1944) *The teacher's word book of 30,000 words.* New York: Bureau of Publications.

Thygesen, P., Hermann, K & Willanger, R. (1970) Concentration camp survivors in Denmark. *Dan. Med. Bull. 17*, 65–108.

Tolstoy, L. (1869) *War and peace,* Epilogue, Part 2, Chap. 3, p. 1409. (Translated by Rosemary Edmonds.) London: Penguin Classics.

Trilling, L. (1948) Sex and science: The Kinsey report. *Partisan Rev.* 15, 460–476.

Turner, J. (1986–7) Musorgsky. *Music Rev.* 47, 153–175.

Turner, J. (1991) T. E. Lawrence. *Am. Imago* 48, 395–416.

Van Ijzendoorn, M. H. & Balermans-Kranenburg, M. J. (1996) Attachment representations in mothers, fathers, adolescents, and clinical groups: a meta-analytic search for normative data. *J. Consulting Clin. Psychol. 64*, 8–21.

Ward, M. J., Carlson, E. A., Altman, S., Levine, L., Greenberg, R. H. & Kessler, D. B. (1990) Predicting infant-mother attachment from adolescents' prenatal working models of relationships. *Seventh International Conference on Infant Studies,* Montreal, April.

Ward, M., Botyanski, N., Plunket, S. & Carlson, E. (1991) The predictive and concurrent validity of the Adult Attachment Interview for adolescent mothers. Paper presented at the *Meeting of the Society for Research in Child Development,* Seattle.

Watkins, G. (1991) *Gesualdo: The man and his music.* 2nd ed. (1st ed. 1973). Oxford: Clarendon Press.

Watts, F. N., McKenna, F. P., Sharrock, R. & Trezise, L. (1986) Colour naming of phobia-related words. *Br. J. Psychol. 77*, 97–108.

Weinberg, M. & Williams, C. (1975) *Male homosexuals.* New York: Penguin Books.

Weisman, A. D. (1967) Self-destruction and sexual perversion. In *Essays in self-destruction* (Ed. E. S. Schneidman), pp. 265–299. New York: Science House.

Welldon, E. V. (1988) *Mother, madonna, whore: The idealization and denigration of motherhood.* New York, London: The Guilford Press.

Whitam, F. L. (1977) Childhood indicators of male homosexuality. *Arch. Sex. Behav. 6*, 89–96.

Wiedemann, H. -R., Kunze, J. & Dibbern, H. (1992) *An atlas of clinical syndromes: A visual aid to diagnosis for clinicians and practising physicians*, 2nd ed., pp. 522–523. London: Wolfe Publishing Ltd.

Wiesenfeld-Hallin, Z. & Sodersten, P. (1984) Spinal opiates affect sexual behaviour in rats. *Nature 309*, 257–258.

Wilkie, D. (1992) Early recollections of fungal genetics and the cytoplasmic inheritance controversy. In *The early days of yeast genetics and molecular biology* (Ed. M. A. Hall), pp. 111–119. New York: Cold Spring Harbor Laboratory Press.

Wilks, S. S. (1962) *Mathematical statistics*. New York: John Wiley & Sons.

Williams, E. J. (1959) The comparison of regression variables. *J. Roy. Stat. Soc., B, 21*, 396–399.

Wilson, A. N. (1990) *C.S. Lewis: A biography*. London: Collins.

Wilson, G. W. (1988) Measurement of sex fantasy. *Sexual Marital Ther. 3*, 45–55.

Wilson, J. (1989). *Lawrence of Arabia: The Authorised Biography of T. E. Lawrence*. London: Heinemann.

Winnicott, D. W. (1953) Transitional objects and transitional phenomena. *Int. J. Psycho-Anal. 34*, 1–9.

Winstone, H. V. F. (1982) *Leachman: 'O.C. desert': The life of Lieutenant-Colonel Gerard Leachman D.S.O.* London: Quartet Books.

Yardley, M. (1985) *Backing into the limelight: A biography of T. E. Lawrence*. London: Harrap.

Young-Bruehl, E. (1990) *Freud on women: A reader*. London: Hogarth Press.

Yourcenar, M. (1986) *Mishima: A vision of the void*. (Translated from the French by A. Manguel.) Salcombe, Devon: Aidan Ellis.

INDEX